NEW PERSPECTIVES IN MONITORING LUNG INFLAMMATION

Analysis of Exhaled Breath Condensate

NEW PERSPECTIVES IN MONITORING LUNG INFLAMMATION

Analysis of Exhaled Breath Condensate

EDITED BY

Paolo Montuschi, M.D.

Catholic University of the Sacred Heart
Rome, Italy

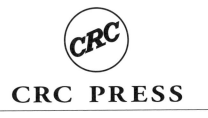

CRC PRESS

Boca Raton   London   New York   Washington, D.C.

Library of Congress Cataloging-in-Publication Data

New perspectives in monitoring lung inflammation : analysis of exhaled breath condensate
/ edited by Paolo Montuschi.
   p. ; cm.
  Includes bibliographical references and index.
  ISBN 0-415-32465-3 (alk. paper)
  1. Pneumonia—Diagnosis. 2. Breath tests. 3. Biochemical markers—Diagnostic use. I.
Montuschi, Paolo, 1964-
  [DNLM: 1. Lung—pathology. 2. Breath Tests—methods. 3. Diagnostic Techniques,
Respiratory System. 4. Inflammation—pathology. WF 600 N5317 2004]
RC771.N49 2004
616.2'41075–dc22   2004050319

Visit the CRC Press Web site at www.crcpress.com

© 2005 by CRC Press LLC

No claim to original U.S. Government works
International Standard Book Number 0-415-32465-3
Library of Congress Card Number 2004050319
Printed in the United States of America 1 2 3 4 5 6 7 8 9 0
Printed on acid-free paper

Dedication

To my father, Ferdinando, and my mother, Laura,
with everlasting gratitude.

Preface

There is increasing interest in exhaled breath condensate, a noninvasive method to study airway inflammation. Exhaled breath consists of a gaseous phase containing volatile substances (e.g., nitric oxide and carbon monoxide) and a liquid phase, termed exhaled breath condensate, that contains aerosol particles in which nonvolatile substances (e.g., inflammatory mediators) have been identified. Analysis of exhaled breath condensate is potentially useful for monitoring airway inflammation and pharmacological therapy. Identification of selective profiles of inflammatory markers in exhaled breath condensate in different lung diseases might be relevant to differential diagnosis. Given its noninvasiveness, this method might be suitable for longitudinal studies in patients with lung disease, including children.

This book provides an introduction to the analysis of exhaled breath condensate. To provide an overview of lung inflammation, basic and clinical pharmacology of leukotrienes, prostanoids, cytokines, chemokines, and tachykinins in the respiratory system is presented.

Current knowledge on the physicochemical properties of exhaled breath condensate and its formation in the airways is presented, and the methods for collection of exhaled breath condensate are described. Particular emphasis is put on the methodological issues because they are essential for future development of this technique. The number of molecules identified in exhaled breath condensate is rapidly increasing. Information on biomarkers and/or classes of biomarkers of airway inflammation that have been measured in this biological fluid are presented in single chapters. One chapter takes into consideration the potential applications of analysis of exhaled breath condensate in children. At present, the quantification of lung inflammation is mainly based on invasive or semi-invasive methods or on measurement of inflammatory biomarkers in biological fluids that are likely to reflect systemic rather than lung inflammation. Assessment of lung inflammation is relevant for diagnosis and management of inflammatory lung diseases because the inflammatory process often precedes the onset of symptoms and decrease in lung function. The availability of sensitive noninvasive biomarkers of lung inflammation might indicate the need for beginning anti-inflammatory therapy at an earlier stage and have a significant impact on the management of lung diseases including asthma and chronic obstructive pulmonary disease. Measurement of inflammatory biomarkers in exhaled breath condensate might provide more sensitive end points for clinical trials in respiratory medicine — a uniquely valuable approach to establish the effectiveness of dose regimens of current drugs and a rational basis for assessing new pharmacological therapies. The potential implications of analysis of exhaled breath condensate for diagnosis and therapy of respiratory diseases are thoroughly discussed in this book, and indications for future research in this area are provided.

Standardization and validation of analysis of exhaled breath condensate currently are the main priority in this research area. At present, the lack of a standardized technique makes it difficult to compare the results from different laboratories. Robust analytical methodology usually precedes the application of a new technique. In the case of exhaled breath condensate, the initial enthusiasm, the search for new molecules in this biological fluid, and the availability of immunoassays for several inflammatory mediators led researchers to overlook a rigorous analytical approach, leaving open the question of the specificity and reliability of measurements. Because several methodological issues still need to be addressed, whether and when the analysis of exhaled breath condensate will be applicable to the clinical setting is difficult to predict. However, considering the importance of inflammation in the pathophysiology of lung disease, the relative lack of noninvasive methods for monitoring airway inflammation and therapy, and the relevance of its potential applications, further research on exhaled breath condensate analysis is warranted. Identification of breath "fingerprints" might open a new era in respiratory medicine. These are the promises. Future research will attest whether they are a reality.

Editor

Paolo Montuschi was born in Rome in 1964 and is Associate Professor of Pharmacology in the Faculty of Medicine of the Catholic University of the Sacred Heart in Rome, Italy. He is also Senior Registrar in the Clinical Pharmacology Unit of the University Hospital Agostino Gemelli in Rome. He graduated in Medicine in 1989. He was Fellow in Pharmacology from 1990 to 1994 when he became Assistant Professor of Pharmacology. In 1996, he was Visiting Scientist at the Centers for Disease Control (CDC), in Morgantown, West Virginia. From 1997 to 2000, he was Visiting Clinical Research Fellow at Imperial College, School of Medicine, at the National Heart and Lung Institute, Department of Thoracic Medicine, in London, United Kingdom.

He was awarded two NATO-Italian Research Council Fellowships in 1996 and 1998, and two Italian Research Council Fellowships in 1997 and 1999. He served as a Temporary Adviser of the World Health Organization/International Programme on Chemical Safety, in Geneva, Switzerland.

His scientific activity is focused on basic and clinical pharmacology of the respiratory system.

He is author or coauthor of more than 130 publications, 40 of them as full papers in peer-reviewed journals. He serves as a reviewer of the *American Journal of Respiratory and Critical Care Medicine*, *Thorax*, and *European Respiratory Journal.*

Contributors

Peter J. Barnes
National Heart and Lung Institute
Imperial College School of Medicine
London, England

Christopher A. Bates
National Jewish Medical and Research
  Center
Denver, Colorado

Julie Biller
Department of Medicine
Medical College of Wisconsin
Milwaukee, Wisconsin

P.N. Richard Dekhuijzen
Department of Pulmonary Diseases
University Medical Centre
Nijmegen, The Netherlands

Katelijne O. De Swert
Department of Respiratory Diseases
Ghent University Hospital
Ghent, Belgium

Louise E. Donnelly
National Heart and Lung Institute
Imperial College School of Medicine
London, England

Marshall Dunning
Department of Medicine
Medical College of Wisconsin
Milwaukee, Wisconsin

Ryszard Dworski
Center for Lung Research
Vanderbilt University Medical Center
Nashville, Tennessee

Richard M. Effros
Department of Medicine
Harbor-UCLA Medical Center
Torrance, California

Jon L. Freels
Respiratory Science Center
The University of Arizona Medical
  Center
Tucson, Arizona
and
Carl T. Hayden VA Medical Center
Phoenix, Arizona

Benjamin Gaston
Pediatric Respiratory Medicine
University of Virginia School of
  Medicine
Charlottesville, Virginia

Umur Hatipoğlu
Department of Medicine
University of Illinois at Chicago
Chicago, Illinois

John F. Hunt
Department of Pediatric Respiratory
  Medicine
University of Virginia School of
  Medicine
Charlottesville, Virginia

Quirijn Jöbsis
Department of Pediatrics
University Hospital Maastricht
Maastricht, The Netherlands

Guy F. Joos
Department of Respiratory Diseases
Ghent University Hospital
Ghent, Belgium

Sergei A. Kharitonov
Department of Thoracic Medicine
National Heart and Lung Institute
Imperial College of Medicine
London, England

Paolo Montuschi
Department of Pharmacology
Faculty of Medicine
Catholic University of the Sacred Heart
Rome, Italy

Romain A. Pauwels
Department of Respiratory Diseases
Ghent University Hospital
Ghent, Belgium

R. Stokes Peebles, Jr.
Center for Lung Research
Vanderbilt University Medical Center
Nashville, Tennessee

Richard A. Robbins
Respiratory Science Center
The University of Arizona Medical
  Center
Tucson, Arizona
and
Carl T. Hayden VA Medical Center
Phoenix, Arizona

Philippe P.R. Rosias
Department of Pediatrics
University Hospital Maastricht
Maastricht, The Netherlands

Israel Rubinstein
Departments of Medicine and
  Biopharmaceutical Sciences
Colleges of Medicine and Pharmacy
University of Illinois
and VA Chicago Health Care Sytem
Chicago, Illinois

Reza Shaker
Department of Medicine
Medical College of Wisconsin
Milwaukee, Wisconsin

James R. Sheller
Center for Lung Research
Vanderbilt University Medical Center
Nashville, Tennessee

Philip E. Silkoff
224 Spruce Tree Road
Radnor, Pennsylvania

Suzanne L. Traves
Department of Thoracic Medicine
National Heart and Lung Institute
Imperial College
London, England

Wendy J.C. van Beurden
Department of Pulmonary Diseases
Catharina Hospital Eindhoven
Eindhoven, The Netherlands

Contents

1 Exhaled Breath Condensate: A New Approach to Monitoring Lung Inflammation

Peter J. Barnes

CONTENTS

I. INTRODUCTION

Inflammation plays a critical role in the pathophysiology of many pulmonary diseases, but traditionally it has been difficult to measure this in airway and peripheral lung disease because invasive methods, such as bronchial biopsy, lung biopsy, or bronchoalveolar lavage, have been necessary. This has been a particular problem in patients with severe disease and with children. The invasiveness of these measurements also means that repeated measurements are not possible, so it is difficult to follow disease progression or the response to therapy.

A. NONINVASIVE MARKERS

Traditionally, asthma control has been monitored by symptoms and lung function measurements, particularly peak expiratory flow. Airway inflammation underlies asthma symptoms but, as discussed above, is difficult to measure directly because this involves invasive procedures. More recently, the less invasive procedure of sputum induction has been introduced.[1] Although this is more acceptable to patients, some patients find it unacceptable and it is not possible to obtain adequate samples from other patients. It also is particularly difficult to apply in young children. The procedure of sputum induction with hypertonic saline itself induces airway inflammation, so it cannot be repeated frequently.[2,3]

This has led to a search for less invasive ways to measure airway and lung inflammation to aid diagnosis, to assess response to anti-inflammatory treatments, to predict loss of disease control, and to assess the response to novel treatments. There is increasing evidence that measurement of biomarkers in the breath may reflect pulmonary disease. Direct sampling from the lung has major advantages compared with sampling from the blood or urine, when dilution and metabolism of inflammatory markers arising in the lungs make interpretation very difficult. Many biomarkers in exhaled breath have now been explored.[4] This is a rapidly advancing field with the potential for enormous clinical impact. It provides new opportunities to explore the underlying inflammatory process in asthma, chronic obstructive pulmonary disease (COPD), interstitial lung disease, as well as providing a potential means of monitoring systemic disease.

B. VOLATILE GASES

Most progress has been made with volatile gases that are detected in the gaseous phase, including nitric oxide (NO), carbon monoxide (CO), and hydrocarbons, such as ethane. Exhaled NO has been particularly intensively investigated and appears to be a useful marker of asthmatic inflammation, so that it is useful for monitoring response to corticosteroid therapy and ensuring adequate control of the underlying inflammatory disease.[5] Measurements of exhaled NO are still a research tool but are increasingly being used in the clinic. As less expensive analyzers are developed, it is likely that this measurement will become much more widely used; with advances in technology, it may even be possible for patients to measure NO at home.

II. EXHALED BREATH CONDENSATE

Exhaled breath condensate (EBC) contains many biomarkers of inflammation and oxidative stress[6,7] (Table 1.1). The principle of sampling the airways by EBC is that mediators from airways are released from the airway lining fluid, carried up by exhaled breath, and subsequently collected by condensation of the exhalate by

---

TABLE 1.1
Inflammatory Markers in Exhaled Breath Condensate

Markers of Oxidative and Nitrative Stress
Hydrogen peroxide
8-Isoprostane
Thiobarbituric acid
Nitrite/nitrate
3-Nitrotyrosine
S-Nitrosothiols

Inflammatory Mediators
Leukotriene B_4
Cysteinyl-leukotrienes
Prostaglandins
Histamine
Adenosine
Interleukin-4
Interleukin-6
Interleukin-8
Interferon-γ
Hydrogen ions (pH)

---

breathing into a cooled tube. EBC collection appears to be a simple and non-invasive method to sample the lower respiratory tract, which can be performed in young children and severely ill patients and can be repeated several times with no adverse effects. There are now numerous publications on EBC, but published studies have been characterized by a variation in mediator levels and methods used for collection of EBC, much of which are likely to be related to the nature of EBC formation. This has led to the setting up of a task force by the European Respiratory Society and the American Thoracic Society to make recommendations about how measurements of EBC should be standardized and to facilitate research into the methodological issues surrounding EBC collection. This has been very important in facilitating research and clinical development in exhaled NO.[8]

The first studies identifying surface-active properties, including pulmonary surfactant, of exhaled condensate were published in Russian in the 1980s,[9,10] and since then an increasing number of inflammatory mediators, oxidants, and ions have been identified in EBCs.

A. ORIGIN

Potentially, EBC is derived from the mouth (oral cavity and oropharynx), respiratory tract, and alveoli, but the origin of individual biomarkers in EBC has not yet been determined. It is assumed that airway surface liquid becomes aerosolized during turbulent airflow, so that the content of the condensate reflects the composition of airway surface liquid, although large molecules may not aerosolize as well as small soluble molecules. It is possible that some lipid mediators may be volatile at body temperature and dissolve in the condensate during collection. Much more research is needed to establish the origin of biomarkers in EBC and to compare its composition with airway lining fluid.

B. FACTORS AFFECTING MEASUREMENTS

Several methods of condensate collection have been described. The most common approach is to ask the subject to breathe tidally via a mouthpiece through a non-rebreathing valve in which inspiratory and expiratory air is separated. During expiration, the exhaled air flows through a condenser, which is cooled to 0°C by melting ice or to –20°C by a refrigerated circuit, and breath condensate is then collected into a cooled collection vessel. A low temperature may be important for preserving labile markers such as lipid mediators during the collection period, which usually takes between 10 and 15 min to obtain 1 to 3 ml of condensate. Exhaled condensate may be stored at –70°C and is subsequently analyzed by gas chromatography and/or extraction spectrophotometry, or by immunoassays (enzyme-linked immunosorbent assay [ELISA]).

Salivary contamination may influence the levels of several markers detectable in EBC. Thus, high concentrations of some eicosanoids (thromboxane B_2, leukotriene [LTB_4], prostaglandin [$PGF_{2\alpha}$]), but low levels of prostaglandin E_2 (PGE_2) and prostacyclin have been found in saliva, so it is important to minimize and monitor salivary contamination. Subjects should rinse their mouth before collection and keep the mouth dry by periodically swallowing their saliva. Salivary contamination, measured by amylase concentration of condensate, should be monitored routinely. In most of the studies reported, amylase has been measured in condensate and no salivary contamination has been detected.[11,12] The quantity of exhaled condensate is dependent on the ventilation volume per unit time (minute volume), but this does not affect the concentration of mediators.[13,14]

The major component of EBC is condensed water vapor and this may lead to variable dilution of EBC constituents. This is likely to be less of a problem with volatile mediators, but a greater problem with soluble mediators, such as hydrogen peroxide and proteins that are present in airway lining fluid. This is one of the factors contributing to the variability in measurements and a dilution marker is needed to correct for this variable dilution. Cation concentrations, urea, and conductivity (after removal of ammonium ions) have been suggested as a way of correcting for this variable water vapor dilution,[15] but more studies are needed to test the validity of this approach.

C. MARKERS OF OXIDATIVE STRESS

Exhaled hydrogen peroxide (H_2O_2) levels are increased in adults and children with asthma, particularly those with severe disease,[16–19] and are correlated with airway hyperresponsiveness.[20] The concentrations of H_2O_2 in exhaled condensate are reduced in asthmatic patients after treatment with inhaled corticosteroids.[21] The concentration of H_2O_2 is also increased in patients with COPD[22] and bronchiectasis.[11] However, this marker is relatively unstable and there is a large diurnal variability.[23]

8-Isoprostane is a more stable marker of oxidative stress that is formed nonenzymatically by oxidation of arachidonic acid. Levels of 8-isoprostane are increased in exhaled condensate of asthmatic patients and are correlated with disease severity.[24] 8-Isoprostane is also increased in patients with COPD and cystic fibrosis.[13,25] 8-Isoprostane may be well suited to assessment of oxidative stress in asthma and could be used to assess the effects of antioxidant therapies.

D. MARKERS OF NITRATIVE STRESS

Elevated levels of nitrite and nitrate are detectable in exhaled breath of patients with asthma and COPD and in normal smokers.[26–28] Nitrosothiols, formed from an interaction of NO with low-molecular-weight thiols such as glutathione or with thiol groups on cysteine residues of proteins, are also elevated in asthma.[28] S-Nitrosothiols have bronchodilator effects, and deficiency of S-nitrosothiol concentrations in the airways have been linked causally to asthmatic respiratory failure in children.[29] The interaction of NO with superoxide anions formed from oxidative stress results in the formation of peroxynitrite, which is unstable but interacts with tyrosine residues in proteins to form stable 3-nitrotryosine. 3-Nitrityrosine levels are increased in exhaled breath of patients with asthma and cystic fibrosis.[30,31] It is likely that increased 3-nitrotyrosine levels in the breath might occur during exacerbations of asthma when oxidative stress increases.

E. INFLAMMATORY MEDIATORS

Several mediators of inflammation have been detected in the breath of patients with inflammatory airway diseases. There is an increase in the levels of LTB_4 and cysteinyl-leukotrienes (cys-LTs) in asthmatic patients.[31–34] LTB_4 concentrations in EBC appear to be relatively reproducible and are measurable even in normal subjects, making changes with disease easier to interpret.[35] In COPD patients there is a greater increase of exhaled LTB_4 than seen in asthma, but no increase in cys-LTs (as in asthma) and an increase in exhaled PGE_2.[36] There is an additional increase in exhaled LTB_4 concentrations during exacerbations.[37] Several other mediators, including ATP and adenosine, also might be detectable in the breath.[6] Even cytokines might be detectable in EBC, and in children with asthma there is an increase in the concentrations of interleukin (IL)-4 and a decrease in interferon-γ compared with normal children[38] and an increase in IL-6 concentrations in smokers.[39] There is also an increase in the peptide endothelin-1 and vitronectin in patients with interstitial lung disease.[40] However, the variability of cytokine measurements is high, presumably because these proteins are carried in the droplets. Many cytokines, including IL-8, IL-13, and tumor necrosis factor α, are not detectable in EBC, although they are readily detectable in sputum. Acidification of EBC (low pH) also might indicate acute inflammation in patients with asthma[41] and COPD.[42]

III. FUTURE DEVELOPMENTS

A. USE IN CLINICAL PRACTICE

Exhaled breath condensate is a simple, entirely noninvasive procedure that can be used in patients with severe disease and in children older than 4 years. The apparatus is relatively simple to use and operate and is inexpensive, making it possible to conduct studies in a general practice setting that might be particularly appropriate for common lung diseases, such as asthma and COPD. In a recent study, we measured EBC of COPD patients during and following an exacerbation, demonstrating an increase in exhaled 8-isoprostane and LTB_4, presumably reflecting the increase in oxidative stress and neutrophilic inflammation.[37] Interestingly, we demonstrated a very slow recovery to baseline values, indicating that the increase in inflammation associated with an acute exacerbation is very prolonged in COPD. Measurements can be used repeatedly so that the kinetics of drugs can be investigated. The measurement of specific mediators and biomarkers means that it might be used to explore the effects of specific inhibitors, as well as anti-inflammatory effects. For example, measurement of LTB_4 or cys-LTs can be used to study the efficacy of a 5-lipoxygenase inhibitor, or exhaled 8-isoprostane can be used to study the effect of an antioxidant.

B. GUIDELINES

It is clear that EBC contains many potential biomarkers. It is important to optimize their measurement and study the clinical value of monitoring biomarkers in the breath in a variety of lung diseases and to establish the reproducibility of these measurements. This is a complex task — each biomarker needs to be considered differently because of differing solubility, stability, volatility, and amount.

C. INCREASED SENSITIVITY OF ASSAYS

One of the current limitations of EBC measurements is the low concentration of many biomarkers so that their measurement is limited by the sensitivity of assays. It is likely that more sensitive assays will be developed as more potent antibodies are developed and new molecular detection techniques are introduced. Metabonomics is a recent technique that might be particularly applicable to EBC analysis. Metabonomics involves the detection of hundreds of thousands of metabolites in a biological fluid, usually using high-resolution nuclear magnetic resonance (NMR) spectrometry or liquid chromatography/mass spectrometry. Powerful pattern recognition computer programs recognize patterns of metabolites that are sensitive to disease, effects of treatment, and disease severity. Metabonomics of EBC (a breathogram) might therefore prove to be useful in screening lung diseases, following disease progression, predicting responses to treatment, and monitoring response to therapy.[43,44]

D. ON-LINE MEASUREMENTS

A relative disadvantage of EBC measurements is that they require a subsequent analysis; it is likely that there will be important advances in on-line detection of particular biomarkers using sensitive biosensors. For example, it is possible to detect H_2O_2 on-line (in real time) using a silver electrode or by coating a platinum electrode or polymer with horseradish peroxidase.[45,46] Similar enzyme detector systems also might be developed for real-time monitoring of various lipid mediators, including 8-isoprostane, prostaglandins, and leukotrienes. It is relatively easy to monitor the pH of EBC; this is readily amenable to real-time detection. Several molecular biosensors are in development and have the potential to detect very low concentrations of various relevant biomarkers.[47] Ultimately, it might be desirable to collect EBC to monitor patients in clinical practice using disposable detector sticks.

E. PROTEOMICS

Proteomics, which applies high-resolution gel electrophoresis or mass spectrometry to detect multiple proteins in biological samples, might also be a useful approach to analyze the proteins in EBC. This might reveal disease-specific patterns and lead to the identification of novel proteins for detection of disease and identification of new therapeutic targets.[48] However, several technical problems have to be overcome before this becomes a useful approach.

IV. CONCLUSIONS

EBC is an exciting new approach to monitoring inflammatory lung diseases. The technique might have great potential in the future. Far more information is needed about the technical aspects of measurement, and we need to understand better the factors that affect the measurements so that reliable and reproducible measurements can be made. Because the technique is relatively inexpensive, it might be useful in large clinical studies and in clinical practice. This could require the development of on-line measurements. In the future, it might be possible to detect multiple biomarkers in EBC to aid diagnosis, to predict the most effective therapies, and to monitor the response to treatment in a variety of pulmonary diseases.

FURTHER READING

1. Parameswaran, K. et al., Clinical judgement of airway inflammation versus sputum cell counts in patients with asthma, *Eur. Respir. J.*, 15, 486, 2000.
2. Magnussen, H. and Holz, O., Monitoring airway inflammation in asthma by induced sputum, *Eur. Respir. J.*, 13, 5, 1999.
3. Nightingale, J.A., Rogers, D.F., and Barnes, P.J., Effect of repeated sputum induction on cell counts in normal volunteers, *Thorax*, 53, 87, 1998.
4. Kharitonov, S.A. and Barnes, P.J., Exhaled markers of pulmonary disease, *Am. J. Respir. Crit. Care Med.*, 163, 1693, 2001.
5. Kharitonov, S.A. and Barnes, P.J., Clinical aspects of exhaled nitric oxide, *Eur. Respir. J.*, 16, 781, 2000.
6. Montuschi, P. and Barnes, P.J., Analysis of exhaled breath condensate for monitoring airway inflammation, *Trends Pharmacol. Sci.*, 23, 232, 2002.
7. Mutlu, G.M. et al., Collection and analysis of exhaled breath condensate in humans, *Am. J. Respir. Crit. Care Med.*, 164, 731, 2001.

8. Kharitonov, S.A., Alving, K., and Barnes, P.J., Exhaled and nasal nitric oxide measurement: recommendations, *Eur. Respir. J.*, 10, 1683, 1997.
9. Kurik, M.V. et al., Physical properties of a condensate of exhaled air in chronic bronchitis patients, *Vrach. Delo*, 37, 1987.
10. Sidorenko, G.I., Zborovskii, E.I., and Levina, D.I., Surface-active properties of the exhaled air condensate (a new method of studying lung function), *Ter. Arkh.*, 52, 65, 1980.
11. Loukides, S. et al., Elevated levels of expired breath hydrogen peroxide in bronchiectasis, *Am. J. Respir. Crit. Care Med.*, 158, 991, 1998.
12. Scheideler, L. et al., Detection of nonvolatile macromolecules in breath, *Am. Rev. Respir. Dis.*, 148, 774, 1993.
13. Montuschi, P. et al., Exhaled 8-isoprostane as a new non-invasive biomarker of oxidative stress in cystic fibrosis, *Thorax*, 55, 205, 2000.
14. Reinhold, P. et al., Breath condensate — a medium obtained by a noninvasive method for the detection of inflammation mediators of the lung, *Berl Munch. Tierarztl. Wochenschr.*, 112, 254, 1999.
15. Effros, R.M. et al., A simple method for estimating respiratory solute dilution in exhaled breath condensates, *Am. J. Respir. Crit. Care Med.*, 2003 (in press).
16. Antczak, A. et al., Increased hydrogen peroxide and thiobarbituric acid-reactive products in expired breath condensate of asthmatic patients, *Eur. Respir. J.*, 10, 1235, 1997.
17. Dohlman, A.W., Black, H.R., and Royall, J.A., Expired breath hydrogen peroxide is a marker of acute airway inflammation in pediatric patients with asthma, *Am. Rev. Respir. Dis.*, 148, 955, 1993.
18. Horváth, I. et al., Combined use of exhaled hydrogen peroxide and nitric oxide in monitoring asthma, *Am. J. Respir. Crit. Care Med.*, 158, 1042, 1998.
19. Jöbsis, Q. et al., Hydrogen peroxide in exhaled air is increased in stable asthmatic children, *Eur. Respir. J.*, 10, 519, 1997.
20. Emelyanov, A. et al., Elevated concentrations of exhaled hydrogen peroxide in asthmatic patients, *Chest*, 120, 1136, 2001.
21. Antczak, A. et al., Inhaled glucocorticosteroids decrease hydrogen peroxide level in expired air condensate in asthmatic patients, *Respir. Med.*, 94, 416, 2001.
22. Dekhuijzen, P.N.R. et al., Increased exhalation of hydrogen peroxide in patients with stable and unstable chronic obstructive pulmonary disease, *Am. J. Respir. Crit. Care Med.*, 154, 813, 1996.
23. van Beurden, W.J.C. et al., Variability of exhaled hydrogen peroxide in stable COPD patients and matched healthy controls, *Respiration*, 69, 211, 2002.
24. Montuschi, P. et al., Increased 8-isoprostane, a marker of oxidative stress, in exhaled condensate of asthma patients, *Am. J. Respir. Crit. Care Med.*, 160, 216, 1999.
25. Montuschi, P. et al., Exhaled 8-isoprostane as an *in vivo* biomarker of lung oxidative stress in patients with COPD and healthy smokers, *Am. J. Respir. Crit. Care Med.*, 162, 1175, 2000.
26. Balint, B. et al., Increased nitric oxide metabolites in exhaled breath condensate after exposure to tobacco smoke, *Thorax*, 56, 456, 2001.
27. Ganas, K. et al., Total nitrites/nitrate in expired breath condensate of patients with asthma, *Respir. Med.*, 95, 649, 2001.
28. Corradi, M. et al., Increased nitrosothiols in exhaled breath condensate in inflammatory airway diseases, *Am. J. Respir. Crit. Care Med.*, 163, 854, 2001.
29. Gaston, B. et al. Bronchodilator *S*-nitrosothiol deficiency in asthmatic respiratory failure, *Lancet*, 351, 1317, 1998.

30. Balint, B. et al., Increased nitrotyrosine in exhaled breath condensate in cystic fibrosis, *Eur. Respir. J.*, 17, 1201, 2001.
31. Hanazawa, T., Kharitonov, S.A., and Barnes, P.J., Increased nitrotyrosine in exhaled breath condensate of patients with asthma, *Am. J. Respir. Crit. Care Med.*, 162, 1273, 2000.
32. Antczak, A. et al., Increased exhaled cysteinyl-leukotrienes and 8-isoprostane in aspirin-induced asthma, *Am. J. Respir. Crit. Care Med.*, 166, 301, 2002.
33. Csoma, Z. et al., Increased leukotrienes in exhaled breath condensate in childhood asthma, *Am. J. Respir. Crit. Care Med.*, 166, 1345, 2002.
34. Montuschi, P. and Barnes, P.J., Exhaled leukotrienes and prostaglandins in asthma, *J. Allergy Clin. Immunol.*, 109, 615, 2002.
35. Montuschi, P. et al., Validation of leukotriene B_4 measurements in exhaled breath condensate, *Inflamm. Res.*, 52, 69, 2003.
36. Montuschi, P. et al., Exhaled leukotrienes and prostaglandins in COPD. *Thorax*, 58, 585, 2003.
37. Biernacki, W.A., Kharitonov, S.A., and Barnes, P.J., Increased leukotriene B_4 and 8-isoprostane in exhaled breath condensate of patients with exacerbations of COPD, *Thorax*, 58, 294, 2003.
38. Shahid, S.K. et al., Increased interleukin-4 and decreased interferon- in exhaled breath condensate of children with asthma, *Am. J. Respir. Crit. Care Med.*, 165, 1290, 2002.
39. Carpagnano, G.E. et al., Increased inflammatory markers in the exhaled breath condensate of cigarette smokers, *Chest*, 124, 1386, 2003.
40. Carpagnano, G.E. et al., Increased vitronectin and endothelin-1 in the breath condensate of patients with fibrosing lung disease, *Respiration*, 70, 154, 2003.
41. Hunt, J.F. et al., Endogenous airway acidification. Implications for asthma pathophysiology, *Am. J. Respir. Crit. Care Med.*, 161, 694, 2000.
42. Kostikas, K. et al., pH in expired breath condensate of patients with inflammatory airway diseases, *Am. J. Respir. Crit. Care Med.*, 165, 1364, 2002.
43. Brindle, J.T. et al., Rapid and noninvasive diagnosis of the presence and severity of coronary heart disease using 1H-NMR-based metabonomics, *Nat. Med*, 8, 1439, 2002.
44. Nicholson, J.K. et al., Metabonomics: a platform for studying drug toxicity and gene function, *Nat. Rev. Drug Discov.*, 1, 153, 2002.
45. Razola, S.S. et al., Hydrogen peroxide sensitive amperometric biosensor based on horseradish peroxidase entrapped in a polypyrrole electrode, *Biosens. Bioelectron.*, 17, 921, 2002.
46. Thanachasai, S. et al., Novel hydrogen peroxide sensors based on peroxidase-carrying poly[pyrrole-co-[4-(3-pyrrolyl)butanesulfonate]] copolymer films, *Anal. Sci.*, 18, 773, 2002.
47. Nakamura, H. and Karube, I., Current research activity in biosensors, *Anal. Bioanal. Chem.* 377, 446, 2003.
48. Zhu, H., Bilgin, M., and Snyder, M., Proteomics, *Annu. Rev. Biochem.*, 72, 783, 2003.

2 Analysis of Exhaled Breath Condensate: Methodological Issues

Paolo Montuschi

CONTENTS

I. INTRODUCTION

There has been growing interest in the identification of biomarkers for inflammatory airway diseases. Ideally, these biomarkers should (1) identify those patients who are more susceptible to the disease; (2) reflect the degree of pulmonary inflammation and the disease severity; (3) be reproducible in stable clinical conditions; (4) be noninvasive (i.e., easy to obtain for repeated measurements in the longitudinal follow-up of the patients); (5) be elevated during exacerbations; (6) be useful for monitoring pharmacological therapy; and (7) be of prognostic value.[1] Inflammation has an important pathophysiological role in lung diseases such as asthma and chronic obstructive pulmonary disease (COPD).[2–5] The assessment of lung inflammation is relevant to the management of respiratory diseases because it may indicate that pharmacological intervention is required in an early stage in the disease process. Moreover, monitoring airway inflammation might be useful in the follow-up of patients with lung disease, and for guiding drug treatment. At present, quantification of inflammation in the lungs is based on invasive methods such as the analysis of bronchoalveolar lavage (BAL) fluid and bronchial biopsies,[6] semi-invasive methods such as sputum induction,[7] and the measurement of inflammatory markers in plasma and urine, which are likely to reflect systemic rather than lung inflammation. Exhaled breath consists of a gaseous phase that contains volatile substances (e.g., nitric oxide, carbon monoxide, and hydrocarbons) and a liquid phase, termed exhaled breath condensate (EBC), that contains aerosol particles in which nonvolatile substances have been identified.[8] Since its discovery in the exhaled air of humans in the early 1990s, measurement of exhaled nitric oxide (NO) has become a widely used method for monitoring airway inflammation in patients with asthma who are not being treated with corticosteroids.[9]

Recently, attention has focused on analyzing EBC as a noninvasive method for studying the composition of the fluid that lines the respiratory tract.[10,11] Using urea (a freely diffusible molecule) as a marker, it has been shown that a measurable fraction (1 in 24 parts) of the EBC in healthy subjects is derived from aerosolized airway lining fluid.[12] EBC analysis of inflammatory markers is a noninvasive method that has the potential to be useful for monitoring lung inflammation in patients with respiratory diseases, including children.[10,11] Given that it is completely noninvasive, EBC also is suitable for longitudinal studies and for monitoring the efficacy of pharmacological therapy. Moreover, different biomarkers might reflect different aspects of lung inflammation or oxidative stress, which is an important component of inflammation. Identification of selective profiles of biomarkers in different inflammatory airway diseases might be relevant to differential diagnosis in respiratory medicine. However, several methodological issues, such as standardization of sample collection and validation of analytical methods, need to be addressed before this approach can be applicable to the clinical setting. This chapter describes the experimental setup for EBC sample collection, discusses methodological issues, presents advantages and limitations of EBC analysis, and proposes future directions of this promising method.

II. EXPERIMENTAL SETUP

The collection of EBC samples is easy to perform. In most studies, the equipment is homemade and generally consists of a mouthpiece with a one-way valve connected to a collecting system that is placed in either ice or liquid nitrogen to cool the breath.[8] The collecting system is a condensing chamber with a double wall of glass, the inner wall of which is cooled by ice (Figure 2.1)[13]; alternatively, jacketed cooling pipes or tubes in buckets of ice have been used.[8] Generally, subjects wear a noseclip and are asked to breathe tidally for 15 min through a mouthpiece connected to the condenser. Exhaled air enters and leaves the chamber through one-way valves at the inlet and outlet while the chamber is kept closed. If the condenser consists of two

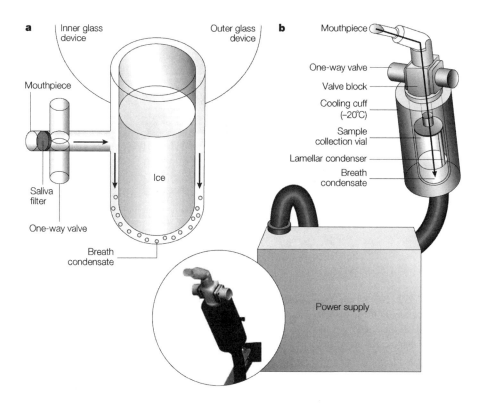

FIGURE 2.1 Schematic representation of EBC collecting systems. (A) Homemade EBC collecting system, which consists of a glass condensing chamber that contains a double wall of glass for which the inner side of the glass is cooled by ice. EBC is collected between the two glass surfaces and drops to the bottom of the outer glass container in a liquid form. (A) Schematic representation of a commercially available condenser (EcoScreen). Frozen EBC is collected in the collecting vial, as indicated by the arrow. (Modified from Montuschi, P., *Nature Reviews Drug Discovery, Vol. 1, Indirect Monitoring of Lung Inflammation,* Macmillan Magazines, 2002, pp. 238–242. With permission.)

glass containers, EBC is collected between the two glass surfaces and drops at the bottom of the outer glass container in a liquid form.[13] Usually, 1.0 to 2.5 ml of EBC is collected depending on respiratory parameters (minute ventilation, respiratory rate, tidal volume), condenser material and temperature, and turbulence of airflow.

Commercially manufactured condensing chambers are also available.[14,15] The EcoScreen® (Jaeger Toennies, Hoechberg, Germany) is an electric refrigerated system consisting of a mouthpiece with a one-way valve and a collecting system connected to a power supply by an extendable arm (Figure 2.1). Subjects sitting upright on a chair breathe through the mouthpiece that is connected to a valve block in which inspiratory and expiratory air are separated. The valve block, in turn, is connected to the collecting system (lamellar condenser and sample collection vial) that is inserted into a cooling cuff maintained at a cold temperature by a refrigerator. According to the information provided by the manufacturers, the temperature inside

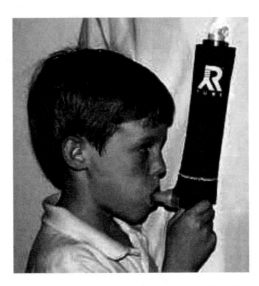

FIGURE 2.2 The RTube is a portable device that consists of a disposable polypropylene condensation chamber with an exhalation valve that also serves as a syringe-style plunger to pull fluid off the condenser walls. Cooling is achieved by placing an aluminum cooling sleeve over the disposable polypropylene tube.

the cooling cuff is maintained at $-10°C$. During expiration, the air flows through the lamellar condenser, condenses on the inner wall of the lamellar condenser, and drops into the vial. Currently, there is no evidence of advantages of this condenser over homemade devices, except for the possible immediate freezing of the samples, which can be important for chemically unstable compounds, such as leukotriene (LT) E_4. However, because the temperature inside the cooling cuff is probably higher than $-10°C$, is not maintained at $-10°C$ throughout the test, and/or other possible technical problems, samples usually are collected in a liquid or in a mixed liquid/frozen form. Inconsistencies in collection of samples (liquid, frozen, or liquid/frozen) may affect the concentrations of labile compounds in EBC and explain part of the variability in their concentrations reported by different studies. In any case, even if the sample is collected frozen, when measuring more than one marker, the sample must be thawed at the time of collection to make sufficient aliquots. The high cost of this commercial condenser also should be taken into account when considering a large-scale application of this technique.

The RTube® (Respiratory Research, Inc., Charlottesville, VA), another commercially available condenser, is a portable device that consists of a disposable polypropylene condensation chamber with an exhalation valve that also serves as a syringe-style plunger to pull fluid off the condenser walls (Figure 2.2).[16] Cooling is achieved by placing an aluminum cooling sleeve over the disposable polypropylene tube (Figure 2.2). The temperature of the cooling sleeve can be chosen by the investigator. The device inherently prevents salivary contamination, and no detectable concentrations of amylase in EBC have been reported.[16] An attachable microbial filter (0.3 μm) is provided to prevent transmission of infectious particles. The RTube is particularly suitable for pH measurement in EBC samples, which requires deaeration for removal of carbon dioxide.[16] A separate device, the pHTube® (Respiratory Research, Inc.), can be used for this purpose.[16] The RTube has three advantages: (1) it is portable, allowing for collection of EBC samples at home, which is particularly suitable for longitudinal studies or when collection of several samples a day is required; (2) the EBC sample contained in the polypropylene tube can be stored in the freezer at home; and (3) a sample of EBC for pH measurement can be collected in as little as 1 min.[16] However, EBC samples need to be brought to the laboratory for biochemical assays, and storage conditions in freezers at home should be as similar as possible to those in the laboratory, particularly when chemically unstable mediators are to be measured.

Careful sterilization of the EBC equipment is essential for avoiding cross-contamination. However, collection of EBC from patients with severe infections (e.g., methicillin-resistant *Staphylococcus aureus* and *Burkholderia cepacia*) should be avoided. Although standardized procedures for sterilization of condensers are not available, it is reasonable to leave the EBC collecting system in an antibacterial solution (e.g., 1% aqueous solution of sodium hypochlorite) for at least 1 h. This procedure limits the number of samples that can be collected, unless several devices are available. This is particularly relevant when very expensive parts of the condenser need to be sterilized, such as the valve block in the EcoScreen condenser. A possible approach to overcome this problem is the use of completely disposable material such as with the RTube or some homemade condensers. After sterilization, the EBC collecting system needs to be washed thoroughly with water to remove completely the antiseptic solution and dried accurately to avoid dilution of EBC. Some investigators use Teflon® (E.I. du Pont de Nemours & Company, Inc., Wilmington, DE) tubes or Teflon-coated lamellar condensers as in the EcoScreen to avoid adhesion of biomolecules to the EBC collecting system walls and, therefore, an artifactual decrease in their concentrations in the EBC samples. A condenser with borosilicate glass coating may be superior to silicone, aluminium, polypropylene, and Teflon for detection of albumin in EBC.[17] Moreover, the physicochemical effects of the sterilization procedures on the EBC collecting system materials are not currently known and studies to clarify this important issue are required. It needs to be clarified whether the sterilizing solutions interact and damage the coating material of the collecting devices. Technical improvements in the design of new condensers would allow measurement of flow rate, total exhaled volume, tidal volume, respiratory rate, and minute ventilation. A device that can be applied to the condenser for measuring respiratory parameters during the collection of EBC has recently been manufactured by Jaeger Toennies. Alternatively, the EcoScreen can be connected to a pneumotachograph and a computer for online recording of respiratory parameters. Condensers should also be designed to collect simultaneously several frozen aliquots that will allow different markers to be measured without thawing the whole sample. The possibility of using selective sensors to make on-line measurements of hydrogen peroxide[18] and possibly other specific inflammatory mediators in the breath is currently under investigation, but, because of the expected high cost, it is unlikely that this method will be used routinely.

III. WHAT IS MEASURED

Several biomolecules, including markers of inflammation, have been measured in the EBC of healthy subjects, and of patients with different inflammatory lung diseases (Table 2.1 and Figure 2.3). In most studies, exhaled markers were measured by immunoassays that still need to be validated with more specific analytical methods, such as gas chromatography/mass spectrometry (GC/MS), liquid chromatography/mass spectrometry (LC/MS), or high-performance liquid chromatography (HPLC). These methods also will provide a more accurate analytical determination of the concentrations of the different biomarkers in EBC. The presence of 8-isoprostane and prostaglandin E_2 (PGE$_2$) in EBC has been confirmed by GC/MS.[19] Malondialdehyde and other aldehydes in EBC have been measured by LC/MS,[20] whereas adenosine[21] and reduced glutathione[22] in EBC can be detected by HPLC. pH values in EBC from patients with acute asthma are more than 2 log orders lower than normal and normalize with corticosteroid therapy.[23] Measurement of EBC pH is highly reproducible and could prove to be useful clinically for diagnosis and for monitoring therapy.[24] pH values in EBC from patients with other lung diseases have been reported,[23,25] but the biological significance of these findings is currently unknown.

A wide interindividual variability in the total protein content in EBC (from undetectable to 1.4 mg) has been reported.[26] The reasons for these findings are not known, and efforts should be made to establish the protein concentrations in EBC under standard conditions. In one study, protein concentrations in EBC in 20 healthy subjects averaged 2.3 mg/dl. Amylase concentrations were undetectable in the EBC of five subjects and very low (mean concentration of 4.67 units/ml, or less than 0.01% of that in saliva) in the EBC of the others, indicating little salivary contamination of EBC.[27] Proteins in nasal (collected through a "free touch" technique by negative pressure) and oral EBC were separated by two-dimensional electrophoresis, but they were not identified.[28]

Using immunoassays, cytokines such as inteleukin-1β, tumor necrosis factor-α, interleukin-8, interleukin-4, and interferon-γ[26,29,30] have been measured in EBC in healthy subjects and in patients with different inflammatory airway diseases. However, details on the specificity of the immunoassays that were used in these studies are not available and the measurements still need to be validated by more specific analytical methods. Moreover, concentrations of cytokines in EBC reported in these studies were close to the detection limit of the assay, casting doubts on the reliability of these findings. However, because of its biological importance, the issue of the presence of cytokines in EBC deserves further investigation. One study reported the presence of DNA in EBC in healthy subjects and patients with lung cancer, and proposed the possibility of amplifying DNA by the polymerase chain reaction (PCR).[31] Recently, Vogelberg et al.[32] failed to detect *Pseudomonas aeruginosa* and *B. cepacia* by PCR in the EBC of patients with cystic fibrosis. Whether gene expression analysis in EBC will have diagnostic relevance is unknown.

Comparisons between absolute concentrations of exhaled markers that have been reported by different studies is difficult at present because of (1) differences in the EBC collection procedures and sample handling; (2) differences in the analytical

TABLE 2.1
Markers of Inflammation in EBC

Marker	Analytical Method
Hydrogen ions	pH meter or pH microelectrode[23,24,39]
Electrolytes (sodium, potassium, calcium, magnesium, chloride)	Ion-selective electrodes,[27] ion chromatography[33]

Isoprostanes

8-Isoprostane (8-*iso*-PGF$_{2\alpha}$)	GC/MS,[19] EIA,[13,15,55–57] RIA[35,51–53]

Prostanoids

PGE$_2$	GC/MS,[19] EIA,[36,60] RIA[35,51–53]
PGF$_{2\alpha}$	EIA[36]
PGD$_2$	EIA[36]
Thromboxane B$_2$	EIA,[36] RIA[21,52,61]

Leukotrienes

LTB$_4$	EIA[14,36,55–59,62,63]
LTE$_4$	EIA[36,63]
Cysteinyl-LTs (LTC$_4$/LTD$_4$/LTE$_4$)	EIA[14,55,56,62]

NO-Derived Products

S-Nitrosothiols	Spectrophotometry,[50] fluorometric assay[64]
3-Nitrotyrosine	EIA[14,65]
Nitrite	Spectrophotometry,[29,47,50,66] fluorometric assay[64,65]
Nitrate	Fluorometric assay[64,65]

Others

Hydrogen peroxide	Spectrophotometry,[49,67,68] fluorometric assay,[34,48,69] chemiluminescence[70]
Adenosine	HPLC[21]
Glutathione	HPLC,[22] enzymatic recycling assay[71]
Aldehydes (e.g., malondialdehyde)	GC/MS[20,22]
TBARS	[49]

Cytokines

IL-1β	EIA[26]
TNF-α	RIA[26]
IL-4	ELISA[30]
IL-8	ELISA[29]
Interferon-γ	EIA[30]
DNA	PCR[31]

Abbreviation: EIA, enzyme immunoassay; ELISA, enzyme-linked immunosorbent assay; TBARS, thiobarbituric acid reactive substances.

Source: Montuschi, P., *Nature Reviews Drug Discovery*, Vol. 1, *Indirect Monitoring of Lung Inflammation*, Macmillan Magazines, 2002, pp. 238–242. With permission.

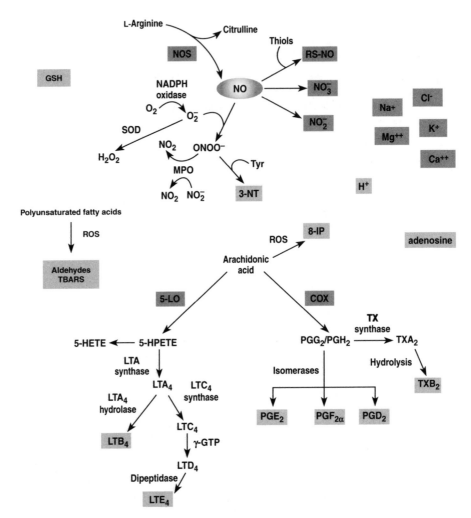

FIGURE 2.3 Biomarkers of airway inflammation and/or oxidative stress that have been measured in EBC in healthy subjects and in patients with airway inflammatory diseases. NO is derived from the amino acid L-arginine by the enzyme nitric oxide synthase NOS. Two isoforms of NOS, constitutive and inducible NOS, have been identified in different cell types within the respiratory tract, including airway and alveolar epithelial cells, macrophages, neutrophils, eosinophils, mast cells, and vascular endothelial and smooth muscle cells. NO in exhaled air is derived mainly from the airways. When free radical production is increased, NO can combine with superoxide anion (O_2^-) to form highly reactive peroxynitrite (ONOO$^-$). This, in turn, can result in nitrosation of either tyrosine or tyrosine residues in proteins to form 3-nitrotyrosine (3-NT). NO can also combine with thiols, such as glutathione or thiol residues in albumin, to produce RS-NO or be metabolized to nitrite (NO_2^-) and nitrate (NO_3^-), which are end-products of NO metabolism. O_2^- can be converted to hydrogen peroxide (H_2O_2) by superoxide dismutase (SOD). 8-Isoprostane (8-IP) is formed by reactive oxygen species (ROS)-catalyzed peroxidation of arachidonic acid. LTs such as LTB_4 and cysteinyl-leukotrienes (LTC_4, LTD_4, and LTE_4) are products of 5-lipoxygenase (5-LO) activity. Prostaglandins (PGE_2, PGD_2, and $PGF_{2\alpha}$) and thromboxane A_2 (TXA_2) are formed by cyclooxygenase (COX). Two COX isoforms (not shown) are known. The pathway leading to PGI_2 synthesis is not shown. PGD_2, $PGF_{2\alpha}$, and TXA_2, the stable hydrolysis product of TXB_2, are only detectable in some healthy subjects and/or patients with asthma and COPD. EBC from patients with acute asthma has a pH over 2 log orders lower than normal. Electrolytes, adenosine, glutathione (GSH), aldehydes, and cytokines (not shown) have been detected in EBC. Abbreviations: -GTP, -glutamyl-transpeptidase; 5-HETE, 5-hydroeicosatetraenoic acid; 5-HPETE, 5-hydroperoxyeicosatetraenoic acid; MPO, myeloperoxidase; NADPH oxidase, reduced nicotinamide adenine dinucleotide phosphate oxidase; TBARS, thiobarbituric acid reactive substances. (Modified from Montuschi, P. and Barnes, P.J., Analysis of exhaled breath condensate for monitoring airway inflammation, in *Trends in Pharmacological Sciences*, Vol. 23, Elsevier, New York, 2002, pp. 232–237. With permission.)

techniques used (enzyme immunoassays, radioimmunoassays, GC/MS, HPLC); (3) incomplete characterization of factors that affect EBC analysis; (4) differences in clinical characteristics of study groups (diagnostic criteria, disease severity, treatment); and (5) interindividual biological variability. Based on electrolyte concentrations, changes in respiratory solutes can also result from variations in the dilution of respiratory droplets, as has been shown in healthy subjects.[27] For this reason, the use of reference indicators such as urea, electrolytes, or conductivity has been proposed.[33]

IV. METHODOLOGICAL ISSUES

To allow comparisons of data from different research centers and to assess the clinical usefulness of EBC analysis, standardization of sample collection and validation of the analytical techniques for measuring each inflammatory biomarker are required. Several methodological issues need to be addressed, including flow dependence, time dependence, and influence of ventilation patterns; origin(s) of exhaled markers; organ specificity of EBC; nasal contamination; saliva and sputum contamination; identification of a dilution marker to ascertain to what extent EBC reflects the composition of airway lining fluid and to adjust for possible variations in the dilution of respiratory droplets; influence of temperature, humidity, and collecting-system materials; reproducibility studies (intrasubject, diurnal variability); comparisons of collection devices; storage issues; the need for sample pretreatment; and the development of sensitive, specific, and reproducible analytical methods to be used routinely.

A. FLOW DEPENDENCE AND INFLUENCE OF VENTILATION PATTERNS

One study has shown that hydrogen peroxide concentrations in EBC depend on expiratory flow rate in healthy adults (n = 15).[34] Mean ± standard error concentrations of hydrogen peroxide in EBC at flow rates of 140, 69, and 48 ml/sec were 0.12 ± 0.02, 0.19 ± 0.02, and 0.32 ± 0.03 µM, respectively, indicating that exhaled hydrogen peroxide levels are flow dependent.[34] In six healthy adults, the concentrations of MDA in EBC collected at flow rates of 200, 150, 100, and 50 ml/sec were similar,[20] indicating that exhaled MDA levels are not flow dependent. In four healthy children, no differences were observed among MDA and glutathione concentrations in EBC samples collected at different flow rates.[22] To study the influence of ventilation patterns on 8-isoprostane, a marker of lipid peroxidation, and PGE_2 concentrations in EBC, we asked 15 healthy adults to breathe at three different expiratory minute ventilations (10, 20, and 30 l/min) for 10, 10, and 5 min, respectively.[35] Mean 8-isoprostane and PGE_2 concentrations in EBC were similar, indicating that the concentrations of these eicosanoids in EBC are not influenced by expiratory minute ventilation.[35] Likewise, leukotriene B4 (LTB_4) (41.2 ± 3.7 vs. 43.9 ± 4.1 pg/ml) and LTE_4 (12.8 ± 1.5 vs. 13.9 ± 2.3 pg/ml) concentrations in EBC were similar in five healthy subjects who breathed at 14 and 28 breaths/min for 15 min, maintaining the same tidal volume.[36] Other researchers have shown that nitrite and total protein concentrations in EBC are unaffected by respiratory pattern[37] and that ethanol levels in EBC samples collected after tidal breathing and deep inspiration and expiration are similar.[38] Taken together, these data indicate that different markers in EBC behave differently regarding flow dependence and ventilation patterns and, therefore, each marker should be considered and studied individually.

For several markers, there are no data on the influence of airflow and/or ventilation patterns on their levels in EBC and additional studies are warranted. Moreover, the influence of airflow and ventilation patterns on the concentrations of EBC markers has been studied in healthy subjects and these data cannot be directly extrapolated to patients with inflammatory lung diseases. Studies on mechanically ventilated patients might clarify the influence of minute ventilation on the concentrations of inflammatory markers in EBC. In one study, the correlation between minute ventilation and 8-isoprostane concentrations in EBC was not significant ($p < .07$).[19] Assessing the flow dependence of different biomarkers is important for the standardization and reproducibility of measurements. On the basis of the flow dependence, EBC sampling will be performed either at a constant flow rate for a fixed time, or at a constant total exhaled volume for a variable time.

The duration of the EBC collection does not influence the concentrations of 8-isoprostane,[19] whereas conflicting results have been reported for MDA. In one study, MDA concentrations in EBC samples collected in 10 and 20 min were similar (16.4 ± 2.4 vs. 17.1 ± 1.7 nmol/L),[20] whereas in another study the MDA levels decreased significantly with prolonged sampling time (5 min, 0.32 pmol/sec vs. 10 min, 0.18 pmol/sec, $p = .020$, vs. 15 min, 0.11 pmol/sec, $p = .0039$).[39] Hydrogen peroxide concentrations in EBC were also reduced as sampling time was prolonged (2 min, 1.2 pmol/sec vs. 4 min, 1.0 pmol/sec vs. 10 min, 0.7 pmol/sec vs. 15 min, 0.6 pmol/sec).[40] EBC concentrations of unstable compounds (e.g., cysteinyl-leukotrienes [cys-LTs] or hydrogen peroxide) are most likely to be affected by sampling time. Additional studies are required to establish the effect of duration of collection on different biomolecules and to establish the ideal sampling time for each of them.

The volume of EBC collected depends on total exhaled volume, ventilation rate, and breath test duration. In healthy subjects, the volumes of EBC collected in a 15-min test were higher at 28 breaths/min compared with those at 14 breaths/min (2.4 ± 0.3 ml vs. 1.4 ± 0.2 ml, $p < .01$).[35] In 10 healthy subjects, there was a correlation between expiratory minute ventilation and EBC volume ($r = 0.7$, $p < .001$), although the condenser efficiency decreased at the higher expiratory minute ventilation values.[37] The mean volume of EBC during 10 and 20 min of tidal breathing was 1.22 ± 0.1 and 2.1 ± 0.1 ml, respectively.[20] The mode of inhalation (oral vs. nasal) does not influence the concentrations of adenosine in EBC in young healthy subjects (8.3 ± 4.3 vs. 7.9 ± 3.9 nM, respectively), whereas the volume of EBC collected is increased when subjects inhale through their noses and exhale through their mouths without wearing a noseclip (2321 ± 736 vs. 1746 ± 400 µl, respectively).[21] This is probably due to an increase in minute ventilation when the sample collection is performed without a noseclip.[21]

B. Origin(s) of Exhaled Markers

There are three aspects related to the origin of markers in EBC: (1) their cellular source(s); (2) the compartment of the respiratory system in which they are primarily produced (airways vs. alveolar region); and (3) the extent to which EBC reflects the composition of airway lining fluid.

EBC analysis is not suitable for studying the inflammatory cells in the respiratory system, and identifying the cellular source(s) of exhaled markers requires invasive techniques such as bronchial biopsies. Indirect information on the cellular source(s) of exhaled biomolecules can be obtained by correlating their concentrations in EBC with inflammatory cell counts in sputum. However, a correlation between an exhaled marker and a cell type does not necessarily indicate that the mediator is released by that cell type. In contrast, a lack of correlation could be due to increased cell activation and consequent enhanced release of mediator without increased cell counts. Flow dependence might provide information on the origin of inflammatory mediators in the respiratory system (airways as opposed to alveolar).[34] If the concentrations of a biomarker in EBC are dependent on expiratory flow rate, this could indicate that the biomarker is mainly produced within the airways, given that flow rate affects the time available for its accumulation in the respiratory tract, and therefore its concentrations in the EBC.[34] In contrast, it is likely that flow rate has a minor role at the level of the alveolar region, so the alveolar contribution to the exhaled markers should not depend on it.[34] Based on these assumptions, hydrogen peroxide in EBC should primarily be derived from the airways,[34] given that it is flow dependent. In contrast, 8-isoprostane,[35] PGE_2,[35,36] aldehydes,[20] and glutathione[22] should be produced mainly within the alveolar region because their concentrations in the EBC are not influenced by expiratory flow. However, these studies were performed in healthy subjects and there is no adequate information for patients with inflammatory lung diseases. In these patients, the increased numbers and/or activation of selective inflammatory cell types in different compartments of the respiratory system (airways vs. alveolar region) might have a different impact on the concentrations of a specific biomarker in EBC compared with healthy subjects. Moreover, the effects of flow rate on the levels of exhaled markers are probably more complex, given that turbulent flow and high current velocity in the airways can facilitate formation of aerosols containing nonvolatile inflammatory mediators (e.g., lipids, proteins) and, therefore, increase their concentrations in the EBC.[16]

Studies of potential flow dependence of breath condensate solutes are more complicated than those pertaining to exhaled nitric oxide because slow or fast flows cannot be maintained easily for the time usually required for EBC collection.[16] The origin of nonvolatile inflammatory mediators, which are probably transported as aerosols (e.g., protein markers) in EBC, can also be studied by identifying cell-specific markers such as surfactant proteins. One study using ethanol as a model compound indicates that both bronchial and alveolar compartments contribute to the formation of EBC, but the ratio between the two compartments depends on ventilation patterns, with an apparent shift toward the alveolar region during forced expiration.[38] Studies on the mechanisms of formation of EBC are necessary to establish to what extent EBC reflects the composition of the airway lining fluid and could be used to investigate lung pathophysiology. The physicochemical properties and mechanism(s) of formation of EBC and its relations with airway lining fluid are discussed in Chapter 3.

C. Organ Specificity of Exhaled Breath Condensate

Whether the concentrations of inflammatory mediators in EBC reflect lung inflammation or overall systemic productions of these compounds is still unknown. It is possible that inflammatory mediators produced at sites remote from the lung could circulate in plasma and enter the pulmonary epithelial lining fluid, particularly under conditions of increased permeability.[19] In this regard, studies aimed at measuring inflammatory mediators in EBC in patients with pathophysiological conditions in which a role for systemic inflammation has been implicated (e.g., systemic lupus erythematosus) might help clarify this question. Comparisons between concentrations of inflammatory markers in EBC and in biological fluids reflecting systemic production of inflammatory mediators such as plasma and/or urine might also be useful.

D. Dilution Reference Indicators

Most EBC collected in cooled condensers is derived from water vapor. However, the presence of nonvolatile compounds in EBC suggests that droplets of the respiratory fluid also have been collected.[27] Calculation of respiratory fluid solute concentrations from EBC requires estimation of the dilution of respiratory droplets by water vapor.[27] Based on condensate EBC electrolyte concentrations, it has been estimated that respiratory fluid represents between 0.01 and 2% of EBC volumes.[27] Although increases in the levels of inflammatory mediators that have been reported in different lung diseases could reflect increases in the concentrations of these markers in the respiratory fluid, they also could reflect increased droplet formation.[33] Part of the variation in nonvolatile compound concentrations in EBC also could be related to differences in the dilution of respiratory droplets by water vapor.[27] However, the selective increase of inflammatory mediators in EBC and the lack of correlation between EBC concentrations of structurally related compounds are not consistent with this evidence. Reference indicators that remain relatively unchanged in the respiratory fluid and, ideally, similar in concentration to those in plasma, are required to estimate the dilution of respiratory droplets in EBC.[33] Recently, it has been shown that measurements of conductivity can be used to estimate airway electrolyte concentrations and the dilution of respiratory droplets by water vapor after most of the ammonia has been removed by lyophilization.[33] This technique provides a reliable method of estimating the total concentrations of ions in EBC and the dilution of respiratory droplets by the water vapor.

E. Nasal Contamination

Inflammatory mediators such as LTs and PGs are formed in the nose and paranasal sinuses under both physiological and pathological conditions (e.g., rhinitis)[41,42] and can enter the oral expiratory air through the posterior nasopharynx. It is important to rule out nasal contamination of EBC samples, which can be achieved by measuring biomarker concentrations in three different experimental settings: inhaling and exhaling without a noseclip, inhaling and exhaling with a noseclip to increase the chance of nasal contamination, and exhaling against a resistance to ensure soft palate closure and minimize nasal contamination. As the concentration of nitric oxide in the nasopharynx might be high relative to that recovered in the lower airways, nasal contamination must be avoided when measuring exhaled nitric oxide. This is generally achieved by exhaling against a resistance to ensure closure of the soft palate. In a similar manner, concentrations of nitric oxide metabolites such as nitrite and nitrate in EBC could be affected by nasal contamination. However, wearing a noseclip during EBC collection to increase the chance of nasal contamination does not affect the concentrations of nitrite and nitrate in this biological fluid.[43] However, collection of EBC when subjects have breathed against a resistance are needed to exclude definitively a possible nasal contribution to nitrite and nitrate concentrations in EBC. In healthy subjects, adenosine, ammonia, and thromboxane B_2 concentrations in EBC are not influenced by the mode of inhalation (oral vs. nasal).[21] Similar results were reported in patients with allergic rhinitis.[21] It is not currently known if the mode of inhalation during the collection of EBC influences the concentrations of other biomolecules.

F. SALIVA CONTAMINATION

Eicosanoids and other biomolecules are present at high concentrations in saliva.[44,45] A simple method to exclude saliva contamination of the EBC consists of measuring amylase concentrations in the samples, with the absence of amylase indicating an absence of saliva.[46] Amylase concentrations were generally undetectable in all or most of the samples tested.[21,27,46–48] In those samples in which amylase concentrations were detectable, they averaged less than 0.01% of those in saliva.[27] In contrast, sodium ion concentrations in EBC averaged 32% of those in saliva.[27] Moreover, adenosine and thromboxane B_2 concentrations in EBC samples obtained through tracheostomy in mechanically ventilated patients or through the mouth in healthy subjects were similar.[21] Taken together, these data indicate that saliva contamination of the EBC, if it occurs, is not a major issue, at least with the solutes discussed above. Relatively few of the droplets captured in the condensate are formed in the mouth; most are presumably formed in the respiratory tract.[26] However, at least three aspects need to be considered: (1) most of the ammonia in the EBC is formed in the mouth, probably as ammonium gas, as indicated by undetectable levels of ammonia in EBC obtained from patients with tracheostomies[27] (these findings indicate that potential saliva contamination of the EBC samples should be considered separately for each marker); (2) the chance of saliva contamination of EBC samples might differ from one condenser to the other (e.g., presence of saliva filters); and (3) for most biomarkers, the concentrations in saliva are much higher than those in EBC, so that even a small saliva contamination might influence their concentrations in EBC. This can be particularly relevant to measurements of LTs, PGs, and isoprostanes in EBC, given that their concentrations are in the range of picograms per milliliter. Measurement of viscosity also can be used to exclude saliva contamination. At present, measurement of amylase concentrations in each EBC sample to exclude gross saliva contamination seems to be a reasonable approach, but more sensitive methods are required to address this point.

G. INFLUENCE OF DIFFERENT FACTORS ON EXHALED MARKERS

There are no data on the influence of temperature and humidity on EBC measurements. Depending on the physical and chemical properties of the different inflammatory mediators, the collecting system materials might affect their concentrations in EBC. After instillation of three concentrations of 8-isoprostane (50, 250, and 500 pg/ml) in a collecting system consisting of Teflon-lined tubing (Tygon®; Norton Performance Plastics, Akron, OH), there was a fractional loss of yield ranging from 24 to 30%, likely due to lipid adsorption to the tubing.[19] However, the linear recovery of 8-isoprostane indicates lack of *ex vivo* lipid peroxidation within the collection system.[19] After nebulization of the same three concentrations of 8-isoprostane, the loss in yield was greater, presumably due both to lipid adsorption to the nebulizer apparatus and incomplete condensation of the airborne droplets.[19] For analysis of eicosanoids, glass or polypropylene collecting systems should be used to avoid adsorption to the containers. A collecting system coated with borosilicate glass seems to be the most suitable for collecting albumin.[17] Smoking affects 8-isoprostane,[15] hydrogen peroxide,[49] and S-nitrosothiols[50] concentrations in EBC. The influence of age, sex, respiratory maneuvers (e.g., spirometry), airway caliber, circadian rhythm, infections, and medications on EBC markers is largely unknown.

H. DIURNAL AND DAY-TO-DAY VARIABILITY OF EXHALED MARKERS

Reproducibility studies are needed to establish intrasubject variability (diurnal and day to day) of biomarker measurements. Hydrogen peroxide shows diurnal variations in healthy subjects.[49] We recently assessed the day-to-day reproducibility of 8-isoprostane and PGE_2 measurements in EBC by collecting three EBC samples on days 1, 3, and 7 from healthy volunteers.[35] 8-Isoprostane and PGE_2 in EBC were measured by radioimmunoassays (RIAs) that were developed in our laboratory and were previously validated by reversed-phase high-performance liquid chromatography (RP-HPLC), providing evidence for their specificity.[51] Measurements of 8-isoprostane (intraclass correlation coefficient = .95) and PGE_2 (intraclass correlation coefficient = .90) in EBC in healthy subjects were highly reproducible.[35] We also assessed day-to-day RIA measurements of 8-isoprostane, PGE_2, and thromboxane B_2 in EBC in 15 children with asthma.[52,53] Repeatability of RIAs was expressed as limits of agreement according to analyses described by Bland and Altman.[54] Day-to-day radioimmunoassay measurements of 8-isoprostane (limits of agreement, 5 and −5 pg/ml) and PGE_2 (limits of agreement, 5.1 and −5.1 pg/ml)[52] in EBC were highly reproducible as well as RIA measurements of thromboxane B_2 (limits of agreement, −3.7 and 4.7 pg/ml),[52] which was detectable only in some asthmatic children. In children with asthma, measurements of LTE_4 and LTB_4 in EBC with commercially available enzyme immunoassays (Cayman Chemicals, Ann Arbor, MI) were less reproducible than RIA for prostanoids as indicated by their limits of agreement (LTE_4, 12.4 and −15.6 pg/ml; LTB_4, 9.8 and −8.4 pg/ml; C. Mondino et al., unpublished data). The mean coefficient of variation for MDA measured in two samples in 8 subjects was 8.2%.[20]

I. SAMPLE HANDLING

There are no studies on the stability of biomolecules in EBC. Information on the stability of the different inflammatory markers in EBC and standardization of sample storage conditions are important for study planning. In particular, the effect of freezing and thawing, temperature, and storage time on the stability of the different compounds should be established.

J. VALIDATION OF ANALYTICAL METHODS

The presence of 8-isoprostane in EBC has been confirmed by stable isotope dilution in conjunction with GC/MS in selected ion mode.[19] The presence of PGE_2 in EBC has also been confirmed by GC/MS but analytical details are not available.[19] We have recently provided evidence for the specificity of 8-isoprostane and PGE_2 measurements in EBC by RIAs developed in our laboratory.[51] In this study, RIAs for 8-isoprostane and PGE_2 were qualitatively validated by RP-HPLC.[51] Because of their biological importance in asthma and other inflammatory airway diseases, there is increasing interest in measuring LTs in EBC. A wide variability in EBC concentrations have been reported for both LTB_4 and cys-LTs even in healthy subjects.[36,55–57] In view of the fact that LTs, particularly cys-LTs, are chemically unstable compounds, part of this variability could be due to collection and/or storage of EBC samples. Efforts should be made to optimize the recovery for LTs in EBC (suitable collecting device material, snap freezing of EBC samples, and storage of EBC samples at $-80°C$ for a short time before measurement). However, part of the variability in LT concentrations in EBC could be related to analytical methods, including specificity, sensitivity, and reproducibility of techniques. In all the studies on LTs in EBC published so far, LTs were measured by commercially available enzyme immunoassays for which robust data on their specificity and reproducibility are not available. We have recently provided evidence for the specificity of a commercially available enzyme immunoassay for LTB_4 by demonstrating identical chromatographic behavior of LTB_4-like immunoreactivity in the EBC with the respective standard.[58] Some studies reported concentrations of LTB_4 and cys-LTs in EBC close to the detection limit of the immunoassays,[56,59] casting doubts on the reliability of these findings and on their interpretation. Enzyme immunoassays for LTs generally work well in buffer, but their behavior in EBC is not known and should be studied carefully. Most of the EBC markers usually have been measured by immunological techniques. Validation by more specific analytical methods (e.g., HPLC, GC/MS, or LC/MS) is critical for providing definitive evidence for the presence of inflammatory biomarkers in EBC and for a more quantitative assessment of their concentrations. Quantitative comparisons between immunoassays and independent assay methods (GC/MS, HPLC) are a prerequisite for large-scale use of immunoassays to measure biomolecules in EBC. Considering that reference analytical techniques such as GC/MS are very expensive, time-consuming, and not suitable for routine use, validation of immunoassays for inflammatory biomarkers may contribute to the development of EBC analysis in respiratory medicine.

V. ADVANTAGES AND LIMITATIONS

Measurements of inflammatory mediators in EBC provide insights into the pathophysiology of inflammatory lung diseases. Because it is completely noninvasive, EBC analysis is well accepted by patients, applicable to children, useful for outpatient or even domiciliary monitoring of lung inflammation as portable and disposable collecting systems will become widely available, suitable for longitudinal studies and patient follow-up, and potentially useful for monitoring drug therapy. Characterization of selective profiles of exhaled markers (e.g., eicosanoids) might be relevant to the differential diagnosis of inflammatory airway diseases. However, EBC analysis requires standardization and validation of the analytical techniques; the origin (airways vs. alveolar region) and cellular sources of exhaled markers are not known; in contrast to sputum induction and BAL fluid, analysis of lung inflammatory cells is not possible; and definite evidence that EBC analysis reflects lung rather than systemic inflammation is required.

VI. CONCLUSIONS AND FUTURE DIRECTIONS

Studies that aim to clarify the methodological issues that are discussed in this chapter are the main priority in this research area. Future research should also include (1) the identification of reference values for the different inflammatory markers in healthy adults and children; (2) large longitudinal studies to ascertain if sequential measurements in the individual patient reflect the degree of lung inflammation and/or disease severity; (3) studies of the relationships between EBC markers and symptoms, lung function, and other indices, and/or methods for quantifying airway inflammation (e.g., sputum and BAL analysis, exhaled nitric oxide); (4) the identification of levels and profiles of exhaled markers in different lung diseases; (5) studies on the relative concentrations of biomarkers in other fluids that reflect lung inflammation (sputum supernatants, BAL fluid); (6) controlled studies to establish the usefulness of EBC analysis for guiding pharmacological treatment in inflammatory airway diseases, given that the available studies on the effects of drugs on EBC markers are mainly cross-sectional; (7) studies to determine the usefulness of EBC analysis for predicting treatment response and assessment of new therapies; (8) the identification of other inflammatory mediators; (9) the possible identification of markers of lung cancer or infectious lung diseases (e.g., proteins, nucleic acids); (10) studies to determine the feasibility of gene expression analysis in EBC; (11) studies on drug disposition in EBC (e.g., antibiotics); and (12) studies on formation of EBC, its origin in the respiratory system, and its relationships with airway lining fluid.

Whether and when EBC analysis will be applicable to the clinical setting is difficult to predict. However, considering the importance of inflammation in the pathophysiology of lung diseases such as asthma and COPD, the relative lack of noninvasive methods for monitoring airway inflammation and therapy, and the relevance of its potential applications, additional research on EBC analysis is warranted. Identification of breath "fingerprints" may open a new era in respiratory medicine. These are the promises. Future research will say if they are reality.

ACKNOWLEDGMENT

Supported by Catholic University of the Sacred Heart, Fondi di Ateneo 2002–2003.

FURTHER READING

1. Wielders, P.L.M.L. and Dekhuijzen, P.N.R., Disease monitoring in chronic obstructive pulmonary disease: is there a role for biomarkers? *Eur. Respir. J.*, 10, 2443, 1997.
2. Barnes, P.J., Chung, K.F., and Page, C.P., Inflammatory mediators of asthma: an update, *Pharmacol. Rev.*, 50, 515, 1998.
3. Suki, B., Lutchen, K.R., Ingenito, E.P., On the progressive nature of emphysema, *Am. J. Respir. Crit. Care Med.*, 168, 516, 2003.
4. Barnes, P.J., Chronic obstructive pulmonary disease, *N. Engl. J. Med.*, 343, 269, 2000.
5. Rutgers, S.R. et al., Markers of active airway inflammation and remodelling in chronic obstructive pulmonary disease, *Clin. Exp. Allergy*, 31, 193, 2001.
6. Adelroth, E., How to measure airway inflammation: bronchoalveolar lavage and airway biopsies, *Can. Respir. J.*, 5, 18A, 1998.
7. Berlyne, G.S. et al., A comparison of exhaled nitric oxide and induced sputum as markers of airway inflammation, *J. Allergy Clin. Immunol.*, 106, 638, 2000.
8. Mutlu, G.M. et al., Collection and analysis of exhaled breath condensate in humans. *Am. J. Respir. Crit. Care Med.*, 164, 731, 2001.
9. Kharitonov, S.A. and Barnes, P.J., Exhaled markers of pulmonary disease, *Am. J. Respir. Crit. Care Med.*, 163, 1693, 2001.
10. Montuschi, P., Indirect monitoring of lung inflammation, *Nat. Rev. Drug Discov.*, 1, 238, 2002.
11. Montuschi, P. and Barnes, P.J., Analysis of exhaled breath condensate for monitoring airway inflammation, *Trends Pharmacol. Sci.*, 23, 232, 2002.
12. Dwyer, T.M., Expired breath condensate (EBC) and the ultimate disposition of airway surface liquid (ASL), *Am. J. Respir. Crit. Care Med.*, 163, A406, 2001.
13. Montuschi, P. et al., Increased 8-isoprostane, a biomarker of oxidative stress, in exhaled condensate of asthma patients, *Am. J. Respir. Crit. Care Med.*, 160, 216, 1999.
14. Hanazawa, T., Kharitonov, S.A., and Barnes, P.J., Increased nitrotyrosine in exhaled breath condensate of patients with asthma, *Am. J. Respir. Crit. Care Med.*, 162, 1273, 2000.
15. Montuschi, P. et al., Exhaled 8-isoprostane as an *in vivo* biomarker of lung oxidative stress in patients with COPD and healthy smokers, *Am. J. Respir. Crit. Care Med.*, 162, 1175, 2001.
16. Hunt, J., Exhaled breath condensate: an evolving tool for non-invasive evaluation of lung disease, *J. Allergy Clin. Immunol.*, 110, 28, 2002.
17. Rosias, P.P.R. et al., Inner coating of condenser systems influences detection of albumin in exhaled breath condensate, *Eur. Respir. J.*, 22, Suppl. 45, 280s, 2003.
18. Gajdocsi, R. et al., The reproducibility and accuracy of on-line hydrogen peroxide bioassay and the decreasing effect of storage on H_2O_2 concentration, *Eur. Respir. J.*, 22, Suppl. 45, 279s, 2003.
19. Carpenter, C.T., Price, P.V., and Christman, B.W., Exhaled breath condensate isoprostanes are elevated in patients with acute lung injury or ARDS, *Chest*, 114, 1653, 1998.
20. Corradi, M. et al., Aldehydes in exhaled breath condensate of patients with chronic obstructive pulmonary disease, *Am. J. Respir. Crit. Care Med.*, 167, 1380, 2003.

21. Vass, G. et al., Comparison of nasal and oral inhalation during exhaled breath condensate collection, *Am. J. Respir. Crit. Care Med.*, 167, 850, 2003.

22. Corradi, M. et al., Aldehydes and glutathione in exhaled breath condensate of children with asthma exacerbation, *Am. J. Respir. Crit. Care Med.*, 167, 395, 2003.

23. Hunt, J.F. et al., Endogenous airway acidification. Implications for asthma pathophysiology, *Am. J. Respir. Crit. Care Med.*, 161, 694, 2000.

24. Vaughan, J. et al., Exhaled breath condensate pH is a robust and reproducible assay of airway acidity, *Eur. Respir. J.*, 22, 889, 2003.

25. Kostikas, K. et al., pH in expired breath condensate of patients with inflammatory airway diseases, *Am. J. Respir. Crit. Care Med.*, 165, 1364, 2002.

26. Scheideler, L. et al., Detection of nonvolatile macromolecules in breath: a possible diagnostic tool?, *Am. Rev. Respir. Dis.*, 148, 778, 1993.

27. Effros, R.M. et al., Dilution of respiratory solutes in exhaled condensates, *Am. J. Respir. Crit. Care Med.*, 165, 663, 2002.

28. Griese, M., Noss, J., and von Bredow, C., Protein pattern of exhaled breath condensate and saliva, *Proteomics*, 2, 690, 2002.

29. Cunningham, S. et al., Measurement of inflammatory markers in the breath condensate of children with cystic fibrosis, *Eur. Respir. J.*, 15, 955, 2000.

30. Shahid, S.K. et al., Increased interleukin-4 and decreased interferon-gamma in exhaled breath condensate of children with asthma, *Am. J. Respir. Crit. Care Med.*, 165, 1290, 2002.

31. Gessner, C. et al., Amplification of DNA from breath condensate of volunteers and patients with non-small cell lung cancer (NSCLC), *Am. J. Respir. Crit. Care Med.*, 163, A482, 2001.

32. Vogelberg, C. et al., Orally and nasally exhaled nitric oxide and nitrite in asthmatic and cystic fibrosis patients, *Eur. Respir. J.*, Suppl. 45, 131s, 2003.

33. Effros, R.M. et al., A simple method for estimating respiratory solute dilution in exhaled breath condensates, *Am. J. Respir. Crit. Care Med.*, 2003 (in press).

34. Schleiss, M.B. et al., The concentration of hydrogen peroxide in exhaled air depends on expiratory flow rate, *Eur. Respir. J.*, 16, 1115, 2000.

35. Montuschi, P. et al., Methodological aspects of exhaled prostanoid measurements, *Eur. Respir. J.*, Suppl. 45, 18s, 2003.

36. Montuschi, P. and Barnes, P.J., Exhaled leukotrienes and prostaglandins in asthma, *J. Allergy Clin. Immunol.*, 109, 615, 2002.

37. McCafferty, J.B. et al., Effect of varying respiratory pattern on exhaled breath condensate collection, *Eur. Respir. J.*, Suppl. 45, 37s, 2003.

38. Rickmann, J. et al., Breath condensate reflects different compartments of respiratory tract depending on ventilation pattern, *Am. J. Respir. Crit. Care Med.*, 163, A407, 2001.

39. Larstad, M., Torén, K., and Olin, A.-C., Influence of sampling time on malondialdehyde levels and pH in exhaled breath condensate, *Eur. Respir. J.*, Suppl. 45, 38s, 2003.

40. Svensson, S., Olin, A.-C., and Torén, K., Sampling time is important for the collection of hydrogen peroxide in exhaled breath condensate (EBC), *Eur. Respir. J.*, Suppl. 45, 78s, 2003.

41. Howarth, P.H., Leukotrienes in rhinitis, *Am. J. Respir. Crit. Care Med.*, 161, S133, 2000.

42. Wang, D.Y., Smitz, J., and Clement, P., Prostaglandin D_2 measurement in nasal secretions is not a reliable marker for mast cell activation in atopic patients, *Clin. Exp. Allergy*, 25, 1228, 1995.

43. Chladék, J. et al., Short-term variation and influence of a nose clip on nitrite and nitrate levels in the exhaled breath condensate, *Eur. Respir. J.*, Suppl. 45, 267s, 2003.

44. Zakrzewski, J.T. et al., Lipid mediators in cystic fibrosis and chronic obstructive pulmonary disease, *Am. Rev. Respir. Dis.*, 136, 779, 1987.

45. McKinney, E.T. et al., Plasma, urinary, and salivary 8-epi-prostaglandin $F_{2\alpha}$ levels in normotensive and preeclamptic pregnancies, *Am. J. Obstet. Gynecol.*, 183, 874, 2000.

46. Montuschi, P. et al., Exhaled 8-isoprostane as a new non-invasive biomarker of oxidative stress in cystic fibrosis, *Thorax*, 55, 205, 2000.

47. Ho, L.P., Innes, J.A., and Greening, A.P., Nitrite levels in breath condensate of patients with cystic fibrosis is elevated in contrast to exhaled nitric oxide, *Thorax*, 53, 680,1998.

48. Ho, L.P. et al., Expired hydrogen peroxide in breath condensate of cystic fibrosis patients, *Eur. Respir. J.*, 13, 103, 1999.

49. Nowak, D. et al., Exhalation of H_2O_2 and thiobarbituric acid reactive substances (TBARs) by healthy subjects, *Free Radic. Biol. Med.*, 15, 178, 2001.

50. Corradi, M. et al., Increased nitrosothiols in exhaled breath condensate in inflammatory airway diseases, *Am. J. Respir. Crit. Care Med.*, 163, 854, 2001.

51. Montuschi, P. et al., Validation of 8-isoprostane and prostaglandin E_2 measurements in exhaled breath condensate, *Inflamm. Res.*, 52, 502, 2003.

52. Montuschi, P.et al., Profile of prostanoids in exhaled breath condensate in childhood asthma, *Eur. Respir. J.*, Suppl. 45, 400s, 2003.

53. Baraldi, E. et al., Increased exhaled 8-isoprostane in childhood asthma, *Chest*, 124, 25, 2003.

54. Bland, M.J., and Altman, D., Statistical methods for assessing agreement between two methods of clinical measurement, *Lancet*, 1, 307, 1986.

55. Antczak, A. et al., Increased exhaled cysteinyl-leukotrienes and 8-isoprostane in aspirin-induced asthma, *Am. J. Respir. Crit. Care Med.*, 166, 301, 2002.

56. Baraldi, E. et al., Cysteinyl leukotrienes and 8-isoprostane in exhaled breath condensate of children with asthma exacerbations, *Thorax*, 58, 505, 2003.

57. Biernacki, W.A., Kharitonov, S.A., and Barnes, P.J., Increased leukotriene B_4 and 8-isoprostane in exhaled breath condensate of patients with exacerbations of COPD, *Thorax*, 58, 294, 2003.

58. Montuschi, P. et al., Validation of leukotriene B_4 measurements in exhaled breath condensate, *Inflamm. Res.*, 52, 69, 2003.

59. Carpagnano, G.E. et al., Increased inflammatory markers in the exhaled breath condensate of cigarette smokers, *Chest*, 124, 1386, 2003.

60. Kostikas, K. et al., Prostaglandin E_2 in expired breath condensate of patients with asthma, *Eur. Respir. J.*, 22, 743, 2003.

61. Huszar, E. et al., Thromboxane in exhaled breath condensate in healthy volunteers and in patients with asthma, *Eur. Respir. J.*, Suppl. 45, 293s, 2003.

62. Csoma, Z. et al., Increased leukotrienes in exhaled breath condensate in childhood asthma, *Am. J. Respir. Crit. Care Med.*, 166, 1345, 2002.

63. Mondino, C. et al., Leukotrienes in exhaled breath condensate in childhood asthma, *Am. J. Respir. Crit. Care Med.*, 167, A445, 2003.

64. Balint, B. et al., Increased nitric oxide metabolites in exhaled breath condensate after exposure to tobacco smoke, *Thorax*, 56, 456, 2001.

65. Balint, B. et al., Increased nitrotyrosine in exhaled breath condensate in cystic fibrosis, *Eur. Respir. J.*, 17, 1201, 2001.

66. Gessner, C. et al., Exhaled breath condensate nitrite and its relation to tidal volume in acute lung injury, *Chest,* 124, 1046, 2003.

67. Dekhuijzen, P.N.R. et al., Increased exhalation of hydrogen peroxide in patients with stable and unstable chronic obstructive pulmonary disease, *Am. J. Respir. Crit. Care Med.*, 154, 813, 1996.

68. Horváth, I. et al., Combined use of exhaled hydrogen peroxide and nitric oxide in monitoring asthma, *Am. J. Respir. Crit. Care Med.*, 158, 1042, 1998.

69. Jöbsis, Q. et al., Hydrogen peroxide in exhaled air of healthy children: reference values, *Eur. Respir. J.*, 12, 483, 1998.

70. Zappacosta, B. et al. A fast chemiluminescent method for H_2O_2 measurement in exhaled breath condensate, *Clin. Chim. Acta*, 310, 187, 2001.

71. Diegel, H. et al., Glutathione in breath condensate samples of healthy individuals and patients with obstructive lung disease, *Am. J. Respir. Crit. Care Med.*, 163, A408, 2001.

3 Exhaled Breath Condensate: Formation and Physicochemical Properties

Richard M. Effros, Julie Biller, Marshall Dunning, and Reza Shaker

CONTENTS

I. BACKGROUND

Approximately 500 mL of water is lost from the body each day in the exhaled air. Until recently, it was assumed that this water was exclusively generated by evaporation from the respiratory surfaces. Water vapor formed in this fashion is a gas, which cannot contain nonvolatile solutes. However, the unexpected observation that the exhaled breath condensate (EBC) does contain nonvolatile solutes indicates that a fraction of the exhaled water must be formed in the respiratory tract as droplets, which deliver these solutes to the condenser.[1] This discovery has attracted considerable attention among pulmonary investigators and clinicians because it seems to offer a new, noninvasive approach for collecting samples of respiratory fluid.[2,3]

Although bronchoalveolar lavage has been used for many years to sample respiratory secretions, it is associated with a number of significant disadvantages. Lavage may be followed by adverse events related to sedation, infections, and impaired gas exchange. In contrast, collection of EBCs is not associated with any appreciable risks and can be repeated as often as needed. Furthermore, artifacts related to the introduction of saline into the airspace are avoided by collecting condensates.[4]

Although a variety of nonvolatile solutes have been found in exhaled condensates, relatively little information has been published concerning the principal osmotic constituents of biological fluids, e.g., the electrolytes and urea. Furthermore, although several groups have made pH measurements in EBCs, there has been little information available concerning the buffer systems that determine the pH of these solutions.

II. DILUTION OF RESPIRATORY SOLUTES
BY CONDENSED WATER VAPOR

On the basis of the extremely low concentration of noninflammatory solutes found in the condensates (see below), we have concluded that more than 99.99% of the EBC is generated as water vapor rather than as respiratory droplets.[5,6] Most of the liquid collected by condensers is formed outside the body, when the exhaled water vapor is cooled. In effect, collection of this excess water can be considered as an artifact, which can be avoided by collecting the respiratory droplets on filters kept at 37°C (see below). The volume of droplets formed in the respiratory tract usually represents less than 0.1 µL in each milliliter of condensate. Furthermore, the fraction of the exhaled water that is formed in this fashion appears to be quite variable between different subjects and even in successive collections in the same individual.[5,6] This is illustrated in Figure 3.1, in which considerable changes in cation concentrations frequently were found when condensates were collected in two consecutive 30-min intervals.

Variability in the fractional contribution of respiratory droplets to the condensate should not be particularly surprising given that the sites and modes of production of water vapor and respiratory droplets are very different. The volume of water vapor exhaled each minute is set by the rate of ventilation and the saturation of the exhaled gas, which is nearly complete. Full saturation of the exhaled air ensures that the respiratory membranes remain moist. High humidity in the exhaled air minimizes the potentially harmful effect of drying on local concentrations of a variety of solutes, including inflammatory mediators. It has been suggested that drying of the airspace surfaces promotes inflammation by increasing the osmolality of the respiratory fluid.[7]

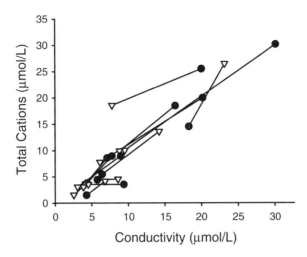

FIGURE 3.1 Considerable variability was found in solute concentrations of EBC, even when consecutive 30-min samples were drawn. These variations appeared real given that changes in conductivity and total cation concentrations were well correlated. Circles represent the first samples and triangles represent the second samples. (From Effros, M. et al. A simple method for estimating respiratory solute dilution in exhaled breath condensates. *Am. J. Respir. Crit. Care Med.,* 168:1500, 2003. With permission.)

The presence of water on the respiratory surfaces also facilitates gas exchange and a variety of aquaporins have been associated with the pulmonary epithelium.[8,9] These presumably allow the movement of water from the pulmonary tissues to the respiratory surfaces, from which evaporation can then occur. This may represent an important role of aquaporins in the lung cells, given that they selectively permit water movement without the corresponding movement of solute.

Although the amount of water vapor that is formed by the lungs each minute is well regulated, there is no obvious reason to believe that the volume of respiratory droplets that are formed within the lungs is kept constant or that it bears a constant relationship to the amount of water vapor that is formed. The discovery that the concentration of electrolytes in the exhaled condensates is variable supports the conclusion that the generation of respiratory droplets within the lungs is not tightly regulated and is not a function of the volume of water vapor that is produced. Respiratory droplets serve no obvious function other than spreading communicable disease within the lungs and to nearby subjects. Nor is it easy to conceive of a mechanism that would ensure that the respiratory droplets would comprise a constant fraction of the exhaled water. Unlike water vapor, which is generated by evaporation from the alveoli as well as the airspaces, the formation of respiratory droplets is presumably related to turbulence within the airways and may be augmented if the airways contain excess secretions or during coughing and forced expiration. These maneuvers would presumably have relatively little effect upon the amount of water that evaporated from the surfaces of the lung.

The observation that the respiratory droplets constitute such a miniscule portion of the exhaled water also is readily understandable given that they presumably represent a very small fraction of the fluid that lines the airways, and the airways represent a small fraction of the respiratory surface of the lungs.

III. RATIONALE FOR REFERENCE INDICATORS OF DILUTION

Our observation that nonvolatile solutes in respiratory droplets are variably diluted by much larger volumes of condensed water vapor led us to conclude that this dilution should be estimated by measuring concentrations of appropriate nonvolatile, noninflammatory solutes in the condensate.[5,6] Although increases in the concentrations of a variety of inflammatory mediators in EBCs have been described in inflammatory diseases, these increases could be due to a number of different factors. This is indicated by the simple equation:

$$[X]_{condensate} = \frac{n[X]_{resp}\,\overline{v}_{droplet}}{n\overline{v}_{droplet} + V_{vapor}} = \frac{[X]_{resp}\,v_{droplet}}{V_{condensate}}$$

An increase in the concentration of the mediator in the condensate ($[X]_{condensate}$) could be due to (1) an increase in respiratory concentrations of X ($[X]_{resp}$), (2) an increase in the number (n) of respiratory droplets, (3) an increase in the average droplet size ($\overline{v}_{droplet}$), and/or (4) a decrease in the volume of water vapor (V_{vapor}) relative to that of the respiratory droplets. The total volume of respiratory droplets (V_{resp}) averages less than 0.01% of the condensate volume ($V_{condensate}$).

Unless dilutional references are used, it is impossible to tell whether reported increases in the condensate concentrations of inflammatory mediators in inflammatory lung diseases reflect true changes in respiratory concentrations or simply an increase in the volume and/or size of respiratory droplets (Figure 3.2). Increases in respiratory droplet production might be expected in patients with rales. It has been suggested that dilutional references are not needed in studies of EBCs, if a comparison is made between different mediators.[10] This is a very risky strategy because an increase in the concentration of one mediator [A] relative to another [B], might indicate an increase in [A] or a decrease in [B]. It obviously would be better to choose a dilutional indicator that is not another inflammatory mediator. A change in the ratio between pairs of reactants (e.g., reduced and oxidized glutathione) could provide useful information regarding redox status of the condensates, though it would not indicate the absolute concentrations of these solutes. The concentrations of several mediators found in condensates have been reported to remain the same in some studies, but even in these studies, remarkable differences are found among normal individuals. The use of reference dilutional indicators could determine whether these differences in condensate mediator concentrations among individuals are related to differences in the number and/or size of respiratory droplets or are due to real differences in respiratory concentrations. Given that there is no obvious reason why the ratio between respiratory droplets and water vapor should remain constant, the unexpected documentation that the concentrations of noninflammatory indicators of

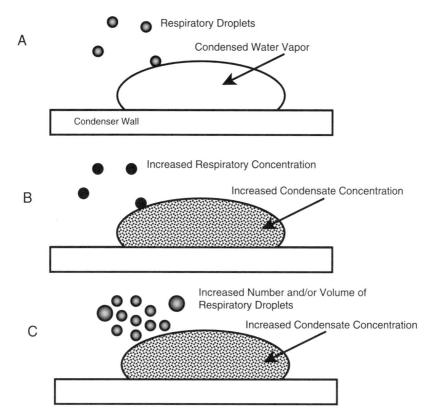

FIGURE 3.2 Increases in the concentration of inflammatory mediators and other solutes in the condensate can be due to either an increase in the concentration of these molecules in the respiratory fluid (B) or an increase in the number and/or volumes of the droplets relative to the amount of condensed water vapor collected in the condenser (C).

dilution remain unchanged in individual subjects would represent an important new observation regarding droplet formation that would deserve further investigation.

IV. SELECTION OF INDICATORS OF DILUTION

We reasoned that it should be possible to estimate the dilution (D) of respiratory droplets and the nonvolatile solutes in these droplets by monitoring the dilution of a suitable reference solute (R). Ideally the concentration of R would be the same in the plasma and the fluid covering the respiratory surfaces. Then:

$$D = \frac{V_{condensate}}{V_{resp.\,droplet}} = \frac{[R]_{resp.}}{[R]_{condensate}} = \frac{[R]_{plasma}}{[R]_{condensate}} \qquad (3.2)$$

where $[R]$ designates the concentrations of the reference indicator in the plasma, respiratory fluid and droplets ("resp"), and the condensate. We initially suggested that the sum of Na^+ and K^+ in the condensate and plasma could be used to estimate the dilution (D) of respiratory solutes by the water vapor present in the condensates:

$$D = \frac{\left[Na^+\right]_{plasma} + \left[K^+\right]_{plasma}}{\left[Na^+\right]_{condensate} + \left[K^+\right]_{condensate}} \tag{3.3}$$

This equation was based upon the assumptions that (1) the respiratory secretions are isotonic relative to plasma, and (2) the sum of Na^+ and K^+ (and associated anions) in the condensates represents most of the osmolality of the respiratory fluid and plasma. Na^+ concentrations could have been used for this purpose, but we found that K^+ concentrations are proportionately greater in the condensates than in the plasma. Some controversy persists regarding the assumption that the respiratory fluids are isotonic, and it is possible that abnormalities in the respiratory osmolality may occur in asthma (osmolality increased) or cystic fibrosis. In theory, this might result in some error in the dilution of the respiratory fluid solutes (see below). Concentrations of Na^+, K^+, and Cl^- were correlated with one another, suggesting that they had all been diluted proportionately by the water vapor.

In this initial study,[5] ion-selective electrodes were used to measure Na^+, K^+, and Cl^- concentrations. In a more recent investigation, we have used an ion chromatograph to measure these concentrations.[6] The sensitivity of this instrument for measurements of electrolytes exceeds that of the ion-selective electrodes by about 10-fold and measurements can also made of other ions, including Ca^{++}, Mg^{++}, SO_4^-, PO_4, NO_2^-, and NO_3^-. Concentrations of Ca^{++} and Mg^{++} were proportionately higher than those found in the plasma, and we therefore included them in estimating the sum of cations in the plasma and condensate:

$$D = \frac{\left[Na^+\right]_{plasma} + \left[K^+\right]_{plasma} + 2\left[Ca^{++}\right]_{plasma} + 2\left[Mg^{++}\right]_{plasma}}{\left[Na^+\right]_{condensate} + \left[K^+\right]_{condensate} + 2\left[Ca^{++}\right]_{condensate} + 2\left[Mg^{++}\right]_{condensate}} \tag{3.4}$$

We had originally hoped that D might be estimated by measuring conductivity of the condensate. The conductivity of extracellular fluids is proportionate to the total concentration of ions and these four cations represent the principal cations in these fluids. The total cation concentration in the condensate is matched by an equivalent concentration of anions, but the anion content of extracellular fluid is more difficult to determine. This effort to use conductivity failed because of the presence of high concentrations of NH_4^+ in normal condensates. Our current measurements of this volatile cation indicate that NH_4^+ represents more than 95% of the cationic content of normal condensates (Figure 3.3). Given that relatively little NH_4^+ was found in patients with tracheotomies, most of the NH_4^+ is generated in the mouth, much of it by bacterial degradation of urea to NH_4^+.[5,6,11] It has been shown that the concentration of NH_3 in the exhaled air can be reduced by 90% after the mouth had been rinsed with acidic fluids, which tend to trap NH_3 as NH_4^+.[12]

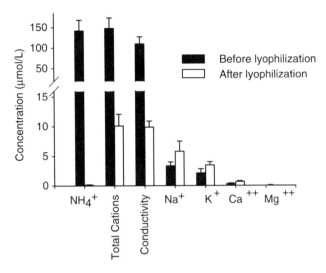

FIGURE 3.3 NH_4^+ is the predominant solute found in normal condensates. Most of this volatile solute is derived from the mouth and can be removed by lyophilization. (From Effros, R. M. et al. A simple method for estimating respiratory dilution in exhaled breath condensates. *Am. J. Respir. Crit. Care Med.*, 168:1500, 2003. With permission.)

We have recently discovered that nearly all of the NH_4^+ can be removed from the condensate samples by lyophilization (freeze drying) at $-100°C$ and a pressure of <2 torr (Figure 3.3)[6] and then rediluting them in ion-free water. Once this is done, the total ionic concentration of the condensate can be accurately estimated from the conductivity of the condensate:

$$D = \frac{\left[Na^+\right]_{plasma} + \left[K^+\right]_{plasma} + 2\left[Ca^{++}\right]_{plasma} + 2\left[Mg^{++}\right]_{plasma}}{[conductivity]_{condensate}} \tag{3.5}$$

where conductivity is expressed in the equivalent concentration of NaCl. The conductivity of lyophilized condensate samples correlates closely with total cation concentrations (Figure 3.4).

There are several important advantages of using conductivity for estimating the dilution of respiratory droplets by condensed water vapor. Conductivity measurements are sensitive, rapidly performed, and do not consume the condensate samples. Furthermore, the equipment needed for these measurements is relatively inexpensive and lyophilization is readily available in most institutions. Lyophilization at low temperatures and under vacuum is frequently used to preserve labile proteins and presumably would be advantageous in processing most mediators. Concentrations of total plasma cations generally are kept within very narrow limits and blood samples probably are unnecessary in many studies. For example, we found that among 50 normal subjects, this parameter averaged 148 ± 2 meq/L (standard deviation) with a coefficient of variation of only 1.2%.

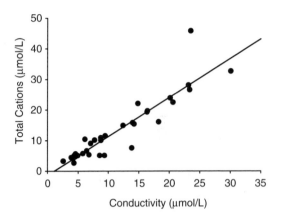

FIGURE 3.4 Total conductivity is well correlated with total cation content of exhaled breath condensates. (From Effros, R. M. et al. A simple method for estimating respiratory dilution in exhaled breath condensates. *Am. J. Respir. Crit. Care Med.*, 168:1500, 2003. With permission.)

V. OSMOLALITY OF THE RESPIRATORY SECRETIONS

Calculation of dilution with Equations 3.2 to 3.5 is based upon the assumption that the osmolality of the respiratory fluid equals that in the plasma. As indicated above, this has been disputed in studies of patients with cystic fibrosis and asthma. On the basis of samples of respiratory fluid collected on small filter strips, Quinton[13] reported that the respiratory fluid is hypotonic among normal subjects and relatively isotonic in patients with cystic fibrosis. This observation has been challenged by other investigators, who found that the respiratory fluid is relatively isotonic among both normal and cystic fibrosis patients.[14] In contrast, evidence has been reported that respiratory fluid becomes hypertonic in patients during asthmatic attacks.[7] Again, this observation remains in dispute.[15] The presence of aquaporins in the airways and airspaces would tend to minimize osmotic gradients between the respiratory fluid and plasma.

We have found evidence that supports the assumption that the respiratory fluid is isotonic in our normal subjects: the average dilution of urea was similar to that of the total cations and conductivity in our subjects.[6] Urea should represent a nearly ideal indicator for dilution because concentrations in the airway fluid and plasma probably are very similar. Urea is a nonvolatile, uncharged molecule that diffuses between the plasma and respiratory fluid more rapidly than do sodium ions.[16] We could find no evidence for either production or consumption of this solute in perfused rat lungs, and there is no evidence for active transport of urea in the lungs. Urea has been used to calculate the dilution of respiratory fluid during bronchoalveolar lavage, but this application is complicated by the observation that urea diffuses from the plasma and tissues into the lavage fluid as the lungs are filled with fluid. This is not a problem in studies of condensates because no fluid is instilled into the lungs: whatever urea is found in the condensates was already present in the fluid lining the airways prior to collection of the condensates. The following equation represents an

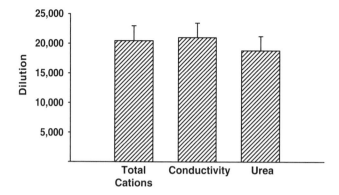

FIGURE 3.5 The average dilution of exhaled respiratory droplets by condensed water vapor is about 1:20,000, regardless of whether this is calculated from the dilution of total cations, conductivity, or urea with Equations 3.4 to 3.6. Means and standard errors of the mean are indicated. (From Effros, R. M. et al. A simple method for estimating respiratory dilution in exhaled breath condensates. *Am. J. Respir. Crit. Care Med.*, 168:1500, 2003. With permission.)

alternative way to calculate the dilution of respiratory droplets by water vapor in condensates:

$$D_{\text{urea}} = \frac{[\text{urea}]_{\text{plasma}}}{[\text{urea}]_{\text{condensate}}} \tag{3.6}$$

Most assays for urea are based upon catalytic degradation by urease to NH_4^+. The advantage of this approach is that it is specific, but the samples must first be lyophilized to remove most of the high concentrations of NH_4^+ that are normally present in condensates. As indicated in Figure 3.5, the average value of D_{urea} agreed well with those obtained with total cations and conductivity. This would suggest that respiratory droplets from these normal subjects are isotonic.

Loss of water by drying of the airway surfaces should increase solute concentrations in the airway fluid if the bronchial circulation is slow or the rate of water passage into the airway fluid did not keep pace with evaporation. This would result in an increase in the concentration of all airway solutes. However, the tendency for urea to diffuse back into the blood would exceed that of the electrolytes, and airway concentrations of urea would therefore be proportionately lower than those of the electrolytes. In other words, the dilution of urea (D_{urea}) would be less than D_{cations} and $D_{\text{conductivity}}$. This was not observed in our studies of normal subjects. Dehydration could presumably increase the concentrations of inflammatory mediators in the respiratory fluid in various illnesses. This might induce a local inflammatory reaction. However, the fractional increase in the concentration of the inflammatory mediator would presumably depend upon how quickly it was produced in the airways and how quickly it diffused back into the plasma.

Although the chemical and physiologic properties of urea would appear to make it a suitable indicator for calculating dilution, concentrations of urea are normally much lower than those of the electrolytes, and analysis is consequently much more difficult. Presumably, this is responsible for the fact that correlation between conductivity and urea was less satisfactory than with the total cations.[6] We were unsuccessful using a high-performance liquid chromatography/mass spectrometry (HPLC/MS) approach to measure urea concentrations, but it is conceivable that an alternative technique might be successful. Another disadvantage of urea is that plasma concentrations are more variable and measurements of plasma urea may be necessary. Furthermore, local urea concentrations could be reduced in infections with bacteria that contain urease.

VI. ALTERNATIVE INDICATORS

It is possible that alternative indicators of dilution can be found. In theory, creatinine, inulin, or ^{99m}Tc-diethylenetriamine pentaacetic acid could be used if these indicators were infused to achieve a constant plasma concentration over the collection period. The best indicators of dilution would be nonvolatile, hydrophilic molecules that equilibrate very rapidly between the plasma and airspaces; e.g., antipyrine might be appropriate in an animal model. Aside from the inconvenience of these infusions, the concentrations of these alternative indicators would have to be exceedingly high in the plasma and/or the analysis exquisitely sensitive to make these measurements. Total protein concentrations might give some information regarding differences in dilution, but the constituents and quantities of proteins in the airspace fluid, many of which are formed in the lungs, differ from those present in the plasma. Concentrations of serum proteins such as albumin in the condensates might be helpful, but local catabolism and transport of these proteins could alter concentrations in the respiratory fluid.

VII. VOLATILE SOLUTES AND THE EFFICIENCY OF COLLECTION WITH CONDENSERS

Although dilutional electrolytes, conductivity, and/or urea can and should be used to calculate the concentrations of nonvolatile mediators in the respiratory fluid, they cannot provide reliable estimates for the dilution of volatile indicators (e.g., NH_4^+, much of which reaches the condensate as NH_3). The absence of appropriate volatile references argues against the use of condensers for collecting volatile or partially volatile solutes. Concentrations of volatile indicators in the condensates are inevitably influenced by the efficiency with which they are extracted from the gaseous phase by water deposited on the condenser walls. Numerous factors can affect the efficiency with which volatile solutes are collected in condensates. These include the temperature and pH of the fluid in the condenser, the design of the condenser, and the pattern and rate of ventilation. Concentrations of volatile solutes found in the condensate might not yield reliable estimates of the corresponding concentrations in the respiratory fluid.

In contrast, the "efficiency" of the condenser in collecting water droplets would have the same effect upon the collection of the dilutional reference solutes as any other nonvolatile solute present in respiratory droplets released from the respiratory surfaces. It would therefore not alter estimates of solute concentrations in the respiratory fluid based upon the dilutional Equations 3.2 to 3.5. The observation (see below) that shortening the tubing between the mouth and condenser increased the recovery of NH_4^+ but had no effect upon concentrations of Na^+ in the condensate is consistent with the conclusion that droplets that contain Na^+ are not selectively fractionated from droplets of water vapor traversing the tubing.[6]

The pattern of respiration might have an important influence upon the sites of respiratory droplet formation within the lungs and consequently might also affect the concentrations of mediators in the condensate. Of course it is important to show that specific mediators and other solutes are not released from or bound to the condenser walls, and that they do not undergo degradation during the collection process.

VIII. HYDROPHOBIC (LIPOPHILIC) SOLUTES

A variety of problems might be associated with studies of lipophilic solutes in condensates. These solutes might become dissolved in surfactant at the surface of the airway droplets. The actual recovery of lipophilic solutes in the condensate might be related in part to the amount of surfactant that is released from the airway surfaces during the formation of respiratory droplets and might not accurately reflect concentrations in the aqueous or surfactant phases of the fluid lining the airways. Care must also be taken that these solutes do not bind to the condenser walls.

IX. SENSITIVITY OF ASSAYS

Documentation of the extreme dilution of exhaled condensates sets certain constraints upon measurements of condensate concentrations. Before embarking upon studies of mediators in exhaled condensates, investigators should be certain that the sensitivity of their assays is sufficient to allow measurements of condensate concentrations of these substances. An estimate of the anticipated concentrations of condensate can be made from reported concentrations of these mediators in sputum and bronchoalveolar lavage. Condensate concentrations of nonvolatile mediators should average about 0.01% of those in sputum[6] and 1% of those in bronchoalveolar lavage.[4]

X. pH AND BUFFERS IN NORMAL EXHALED
BREATH CONDENSATES

The extreme dilution of respiratory secretions also complicates measurements of the pH of EBCs. Evidence has been reported that condensates are relatively acidic in a variety of inflammatory lung disorders.[17–20] It was concluded that acidification of the condensates is due to acidification of the fluid lining the respiratory tract. Although it is possible that the condensates and respiratory secretions are both acidified in these conditions, it is by no means clear that these phenomena are directly linked or that condensate acidification provides a reliable index of the pH of the respiratory surfaces.

Because NH_4^+ represents more than 95% of the cations in the condensates, it is the principal cationic buffer in normal condensate samples. Most of this NH_4^+ is produced in the mouth, by either degradation of urea by bacterial urease or release of NH_4^+ from glutamine by tissue glutaminase. Proof of an oral source for NH_4^+ is provided by (1) studies that show that NH_4^+ concentrations are much lower when collected from patients with tracheostomies or endotracheal tubes, and (2) evidence that the rate of NH_3 excretion can be reduced by 90% after washing the mouth with acidic solutions, which trap NH_3 as NH_4^+.[5,6,11,12]

Because the concentrations of NH_4^+ in the mouth are nearly 100 times greater than those in the blood and 10 times those in the condensates, it is possible that some of the NH_4^+ found in the condensates represents direct contamination of the condensates with macroscopic or microscopic droplets of saliva. However, direct oral contamination with NH_4^+ should be associated with the presence of other cations that are present in even higher concentrations in the oral cavity (e.g., K^+). Given that NH_4^+ concentrations in the condensates are considerably greater than those of K^+, it can be concluded that the delivery of NH_4^+ must have been primarily diffusive (as NH_3 gas) rather than convective (in oral droplets). Evidence for diffusion was provided by the observation that acidification of the condensate lining the condenser with 5% CO_2 increased the recovery of NH_4^+ in the condensate.[5] Acidification of the water lining the condenser enhances production of NH_4^+ from NH_3 in accordance with the equation:

$$\frac{\left[NH_4^+\right]_{condensate}}{\left[NH_4^+\right]_{oral}} = \frac{\left[H^+\right]_{condensate}}{\left[H^+\right]_{oral}} \qquad (3.7)$$

The remarkable efficiency with which NH_3 is trapped in the condensate is related to the fact that the distribution coefficient of NH_3 and NH_4^+ between the aqueous and gaseous phases favors solution in water at a pH 7.4 by a factor of about 50,000 at 5 to 10°C (the usual temperature of the exhaled air emerging from the condenser). NH_4^+ concentrations in the collected samples can be reduced by 95% if the exhaled air is collected on filters kept at 37°C, to minimize condensation of water vapor (Figures 3.6 and 3.7).

The success with which droplets can be collected on these filters indicates that filters should not be used between the mouth and the condensers in the collection of condensates, a practice that was used to minimize contamination of condensates with saliva.[17] Collection of saliva can be minimized by increasing the distance between the mouthpiece and condenser and placing a saliva trap in this line.

We also found that concentrations of NH_4^+ in the condensate could be increased by shortening the dead space tubing between the mouth and condenser.[5] We concluded that NH_3 had exchanged with water droplets on the walls of the tubing and consequently did not reach the condenser. Shortening the tubing had no effect upon the concentrations of Na^+ in the condensates. These observations also suggest that smaller tidal volumes also would decrease NH_4^+ concentrations in EBCs. Furthermore, it is likely that concentrations of NH_4^+ in condensates will be increased when

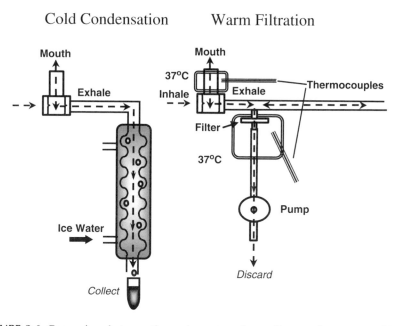

FIGURE 3.6 Comparison between the equipment used to collect condensates at cold temperatures and to collect filtrands at body temperature. Condensation is accomplished with a conventional glass condenser. In the filtration studies, the exhaled air is suctioned from a length of respiratory tubing through a 0.4-µm-diameter filter. The filter is kept at 37°C to minimize condensation. Respiratory droplets that land on the filter are subsequently washed off with 3 mL of deionized water. Filtration at body temperature avoids collection of large volumes of exhaled water vapor. This in turn minimizes the amount of NH_4^+ collected in the exhaled samples.

collected in some commercial devices that do not allow fluid to drain from the condensers until the end of the collection period.

XI. THE EFFECTS OF INFLAMMATORY LUNG DISEASES ON EXHALED BREATH CONDENSATE BUFFERS AND pH

Concentrations of NH_4^+ in condensates appear to be decreased in exacerbations of bronchial asthma.[20] Hunt et al[20] detected glutaminase in the lungs and concluded that decreases in exhaled NH_3 might be due to reduced concentrations of glutaminase and NH_4^+ production in these patients. Although it is possible that glutaminase levels are lower in asthmatics, it is difficult to understand why this would have any measurable effect upon collection of NH_4^+ in the condensates, most of which is derived from the mouth. Furthermore, most of the NH_3 formed in the body is generated in the liver and kidneys and is delivered to the lungs in the blood.[21] The alveolar capillary barrier is extremely permeable to NH_3,[22] and most of the NH_3 released from the lungs probably is derived from the blood traversing the pulmonary and bronchial capillaries.

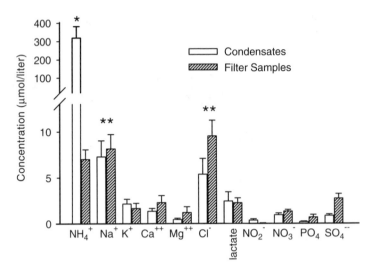

FIGURE 3.7 Condensates were collected from 13 normal subjects and filtrands were collected from 15 normal subjects. One-hour collection periods were used in each set of studies. It will be noted that NH_4^+ concentrations collected from filtrands were considerably less (<5%) than those collected in condensate samples (* $p < .01$). Na^+ and Cl^- were the principal electrolytes in both the condensates and filtrands (** $p < .05$). Means and standard errors of the mean are indicated.

Hunt et al.[20] also proposed that NH_4^+ produced in the lungs normally plays an important role in buffering the respiratory fluids. This also seems unlikely, given that concentrations of NH_4^+ in most biological fluids are less than 0.1% of those of HCO_3^- and are considerably less important than protein in buffering these solutions. A third proposal by these authors is that acidification of the lining of the airways acts to slow the release of NH_3 from the airways. It is true that abrupt acidification of the airways would result in transient trapping of NH_3 as NH_4^+, but in the steady-state, the presence of increased NH_4^+ in the airway fluid should enhance the excretion of NH_3 gas (Figure 3.8). A similar process of facilitated diffusion has been described for the effect of HCO_3^- upon the excretion of CO_2.[23]

In view of the fact that most of the NH_4^+ collected in normal subjects is derived from the mouth, it seems much more likely that decreased production or exchange of NH_4^+ in the mouth is responsible for reduced NH_4^+ concentrations in condensates collected from patients with asthma and other inflammatory lung diseases. Decreases in NH_4^+ concentrations could also contribute to the low pH observed in these patients. Drying of the oral membranes and pharmacologic agents (including aerosolized bronchodilators and antibiotics) might alter concentrations of NH_4^+ and NH_3 in the mouth. Furthermore, alterations in the pattern of ventilation could affect the efficiency of exchange in both the mouth (where the NH_3 is generated) and the condenser (in which it is trapped). As indicated above, the discovery that shortening of the dead space tubing increases condensate NH_4^+ concentrations indicates that a decrease in tidal volume should decrease the amount of NH_3 that actually reaches the condenser. The physiologic dead space of the lungs characteristically is increased in

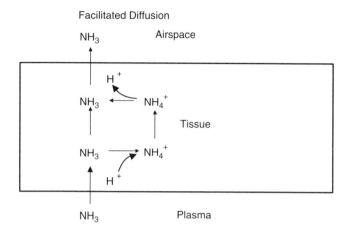

FIGURE 3.8 Facilitated diffusion. The accumulation of NH_4^+ in the respiratory fluid is enhanced if this fluid is acidic. Although there is a very transient decline in the amount of NH_3 exhaled, subsequent loss of NH_3 is actually enhanced by parallel movement of NH_4^+ in the tissue fluid.

patients with acute and chronic airway obstruction. Increased dead space results in a decrease in end tidal PCO_2. As noted above, such a reduction in PCO_2 in asthmatics should increase the pH of the droplets lining the condenser walls and reduce trapping of NH_3 as NH_4^+ by the condenser. The effect of CO_2 in the mouth would be less pronounced because oral secretions are much better buffered than the extremely dilute solutions that become deposited on the walls of the condensers.

XII. CONDENSATE ANIONS AND THE ROLE OF HCO_3^-

The requirement for electroneutrality in bulk solutions mandates the presence of one or more anions in condensates at concentrations equivalent to those of NH_4^+. As indicated in Figure 3.7, concentrations of the measured nonvolatile anions (Cl^-, PO_4, and SO_4^-) were very low compared with those of NH_4^+. NO_2^- and NO_3^- concentrations also were much lower than those of NH_4^+. We have not found concentrations of organic anions comparable to those of NH_4^+ in normal subjects. The observation that lyophilization eliminates more than 95% of the NH_4^+ indicates that the missing anion(s) must be volatile. Lyophilization under the conditions we used does not appreciably reduce NH_4^+ concentrations from solutions of NH_4Cl (which contain the nonvolatile anion, Cl^-) but does remove nearly all of the NH_4^+ from solutions of NH_4OH (which contain HCO_3^- after equilibration with the air). It can be calculated readily that the concentrations of CO_2 in the air (0.033% and increasing) are sufficient to increase HCO_3^- levels in condensates to values comparable to those of NH_4^+. Because the mobile phase in the ion chromatograph contains HCO_3^-, it is not possible to measure this constituent with the ion chromatogram, and alternative measurements of HCO_3^- with sufficient sensitivity are difficult. Nevertheless, at the pH of normal condensates, HCO_3^- presumably represents most of the unmeasured anion.

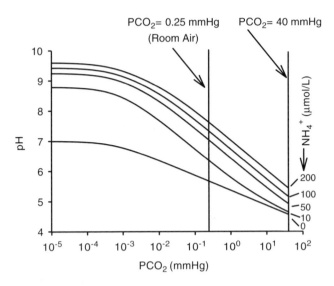

FIGURE 3.9 The pH values of solutions containing different concentrations of NH₄OH are plotted against the PCO₂ of these solutions. At physiologic PCO₂, theses solutions are acidic. When PCO₂ is reduced, the solutions become more alkaline. However, CO₂ continues to influence pH even at ambient CO₂ concentrations. For example, the pH of water left in room air is about 5.75. Removal of all CO₂ should increase the pH of exhaled breath condensates (which normally contain about 200 μM/L of NH₄⁺) to more than 9.5. Failure to observe pH values this high suggests that some CO₂ persists despite purging with inert gases. These graphs were calculated using the Stewart approach.[24]

In an attempt to eliminate the influence of exhaled CO₂ upon the pH of the condensates, Hunt et al.[17] introduced the practice of purging their samples with argon until the pH appeared to stabilize. It is difficult to eliminate all of the CO₂ from these samples. More than an hour may be needed to fully purge CO₂ from condensates.[28] The criteria used for stabilization are not indicated and a recording of this approach of pH to a steady value would be helpful. As indicated in Figure 3.9, it would be necessary to reduce PCO₂ concentrations by 2 orders of magnitude below those found in the atmosphere to eliminate the effect of CO₂, and special anaerobic chambers presumably would be necessary for this purpose. Furthermore, the pH should have stabilized even if room air containing CO₂ rather than argon was used to purge the samples. Removal of CO₂ from the samples initially results in the conversion of HCO₃⁻ to CO₃²⁻ followed by the formation of OH⁻. In the absence of any CO₂, the pH of solutions containing NH₄⁺ at concentrations found in condensates should increase to more than 9, a value never reported in the literature (Figure 3.9). This indicates that some residual CO₂ or some other anion must remain in the condensate. Purging condensates with inert gases should be discouraged because of uncertainty regarding residual PCO₂ and the failure of this approach to remove NH₄⁺. Furthermore, although purging condensates with inert gases for short intervals has little effect upon NH₄⁺ concentrations, it might reduce concentrations of other volatile buffers that are derived from the lungs. Purging with compressed gases might also cool the samples and produce turbulence and pressure changes that can also alter pH measurements. The gases used for purging the samples are usually dry and the samples might therefore become concentrated by dehydration. These considerations suggest that more effective methods should be used to remove both CO_2 and NH_3 from the condensates (e.g., lyophilization).

It has been reported that the pH of condensates obtained from the mouth and endotracheal tubes are similar despite the presence of more NH_4^+ in oral samples.[29] This led Vaughan et al.[29] to conclude that NH_3 has little influence on condensate pH. However, as indicated in Figure 3.9, changes in NH_4^+ concentrations have relatively little effect on pH unless nearly all of the NH_4^+ is removed. This can be attributed to the fact that the amount of ambient CO_2 trapped as HCO_3^- decreases as NH_4^+ concentrations fall. Concentrations of NH_4^+ and HCO_3^- represent the principal buffers in both oral and endotracheal condensate samples collected from normal subjects.

XIII. WHAT DETERMINES THE pH OF EXHALED CONDENSATES?

The volatile ions, NH_4^+ (measured) and HCO_3^- (calculated from the pH and ambient PCO_2), are clearly the predominant buffers in normal condensates and they effectively determine the pH of these solutions in normal condensates. Concentrations of all other ions (and buffers) in normal condensates are generally less than 10% of those of NH_4^+ and HCO_3^- and cannot significantly influence the pH of these solutions (Figure 3.10). Note that a relatively strong acid (lactic acid, pKa = 3.0) has little

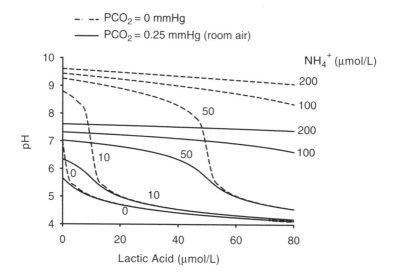

FIGURE 3.10 The effect of increasing the concentration of lactate upon pH is shown at different concentrations of NH_4OH in the presence and absence of ambient CO_2. Note the profound effect of PCO_2 to acidify condensate pH. The presence of a relatively strong acid (lactic acid) does not have an appreciable effect upon pH until concentrations of this acid approach those of NH_4^+.

effect on pH at the concentrations present in normal condensates (about 30% of those of Na^+). These graphs are calculated using the strong ion equations of Stewart.[24,25] This analytic approach calculates the pH of solutions on the basis of (1) the assumption of electroneutrality, (2) conservation of acids and bases, (3) the strong ion difference between the strong cations and strong anions, and (4) knowledge of the concentrations and dissociation constants of each of the constituents of the solutions. Given that most of the NH_4^+ in the condensates is derived from the mouth and all of the HCO_3^- in the samples that have been exposed to air is derived from ambient CO_2, it is unlikely that the pH of normal condensates is influenced significantly by events in the respiratory tract.

XIV. DOCUMENTATION OF AIRWAY ACIDIFICATION WITH EXHALED BREATH CONDENSATES

It is probable that the pH of normal condensates is determined by the presence of NH_3 from the mouth and CO_2 from the ambient air. However, it is possible that acidification of condensates in asthma and other diseases is due the presence of acids (probably anions) in concentrations that approach or exceed those of NH_4^+ and HCO_3^-. Vaughan et al.[26] reported that concentrations of acetate (pKa = 4.75) exceed 100 millimoles/L in the condensates of some patients with severe asthma.

Ambient CO_2 is responsible for the fact that the pH of "pure" rainwater is 5.6 rather than 7.0.[27] Alternatively, it is possible that acidification of the EBC is due to acid reflux, which is prevalent in patients with obstructive lung diseases. Aerosolization of even a minute quantity of gastric fluid (pH 1 to 2) in the stomach or pharynx could acidify exhaled condensates and would be difficult to recognize or prevent.

Given that the pH of condensates is normally governed by the concentrations of NH_4^+ and HCO_3^- rather than nonvolatile buffers in respiratory droplets, it would be preferable to remove these volatile constituents by lyophilization before measuring pH. However, it is difficult to measure the pH of solutions that contain the extremely low concentrations of nonvolatile buffers found in normal condensates. This is illustrated in Figure 3.11. Dilution of conventional nonvolatile buffers to the range observed in normal subjects results in a convergence of pH toward the pH of the deionized water at ambient CO_2 tensions that was used for dilution. The pH of the deionized water is itself dependent upon ambient CO_2 tension. At a typical pH of about 6.1, the concentration of CO_2 and HCO_3^- are each about 7 micromoles/L. The concentrations of CO_2/HCO_3^- buffer pair frequently are greater than that of any nonvolatile buffers found in normal condensates (Figure 3.7), and care must be taken to avoid exposure to ambient air following lyophilization. The pH of the condensates might also be influenced by the containers in which they are stored.[27]

Errors are inevitable if differences in the ionic strength of the conventional pH standards and the condensates are not appreciated. The ionic strength (μ) of a solution is calculated from the concentrations (c_i) of all of the ions with the equation:

$$\mu = \frac{1}{2}\sum_i c_i z_i^2 \tag{3.8}$$

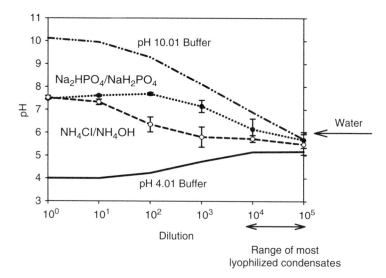

FIGURE 3.11 Dilution of conventional buffers to the extent found in most lyophilized condensates results in the convergence of pH close to that of water at ambient PCO_2.

where c_i is the concentration and z_i is the valence of the ith ion in the solution. The ionic strength of condensates is frequently more than 10,000 times lower than that of the standard pH reference solutions. These differences can result in changes in the junction potential of the reference electrode and errors in pH measurements.[25] The ionic strength of the buffers should be reduced to that of the condensates (a practice used by hydrologists for pH measurements of rain water). It should be noted that the presence of salts in aqueous solutions also alters the activity of both H^+ and OH^-, resulting in small changes in pH.[25]

Conventional glass electrodes (Figure 3.12) are not well suited for measuring pH in extremely dilute solutions such as lyophilized condensates because the resistances of the glass and reference system are too high. The resistance of the reference electrode is due in large part to the resistance of the liquid junction of the ceramic plug that separates the outer reference solution of the electrode from that of the EBC sample. This increases as the concentration and conductivity of this solution decreases and equilibration times may exceed 30 min. Electrodes with low internal resistance are available for measuring the pH of very dilute aqueous solutions (e.g., the Aquatorode, Metrohm, Herisau, Switzerland).

Mention should be made of an alternative method of detecting airway acidification with EBCs. The distribution of pH indicators (e.g., salicylates, barbiturates, and nicotine) between the plasma and airway fluid would be influenced by differences between the pH of these compartments.[28,29] Alterations in the relative concentrations of comparable indicators in the condensates, in theory, could be used to estimate the pH of the respiratory droplets.

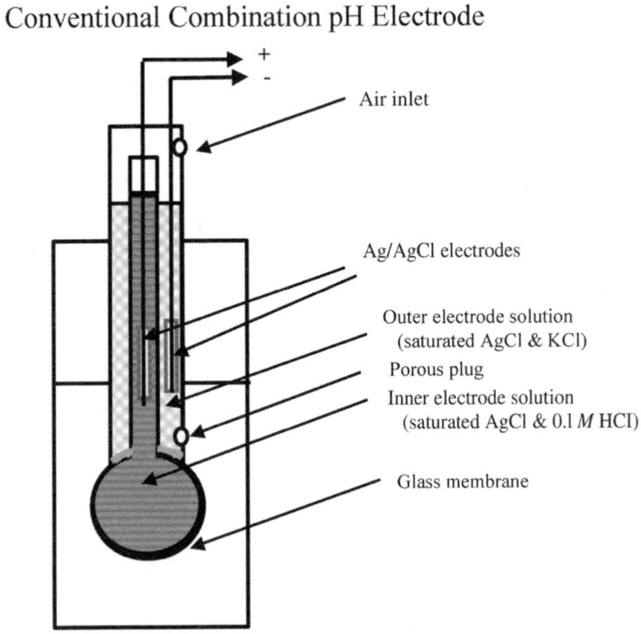

Conventional Combination pH Electrode

+

−

Air inlet

Ag/AgCl electrodes

Outer electrode solution
(saturated AgCl & KCl)
Porous plug
Inner electrode solution
(saturated AgCl & 0.1 M HCl)

Glass membrane

FIGURE 3.12 The resistance of pH combination electrodes is related primarily to the resistance of the H⁺ selective glass and the ceramic plug through which electrolytes are conducted. Specialized electrodes for measuring pH in dilute solutions are constructed with decreased resistance at each of these sites. Means and standard errors of the mean are indicated.

XV. THE FUTURE OF EXHALED BREATH CONDENSATES

New diagnostic approaches often are welcomed with an initial enthusiasm that subsequently subsides when the limitations of the procedures are better understood. Much has been learned about the normal constituents of the condensates. These solutions are remarkably dilute, containing primarily NH_4^+ (most of which is derived from the mouth) and HCO_3^- (which is set by the ambient CO_2 in the atmosphere) and the concentration of NH_4^+ in the condensate. Only trace concentrations of other extracellular solutes are present in this fluid, and less than 0.1 μL of respiratory fluid is present in each milliliter of water vapor that is collected by the condensers. Furthermore, there is no reason to believe that the volume of respiratory droplets formed each minute bears any constant relationship to the amount of water vapor that is lost from the airway surfaces. Significant variability is observed when samples are collected sequentially from the same individual. This variability is related in large part to differences in the volume of droplets formed.

Fortunately, it is possible to correct for variations in respiratory droplet formation by using dilutional reference indicators. Conductivity of lyophilized samples appears to be particularly promising because it can be measured rapidly with inexpensive equipment that does not consume the sample. Introduction of reference indicators in EBC studies may prove as valuable as calculation of clearance has been in studies of urinary excretion of solutes. Not only does it allow calculation of respiratory fluid concentrations from those found in the condensates, but it also provides information regarding the influence of both physiologic and pathologic processes upon the production of respiratory droplets. This new conceptual framework regarding EBCs also sets limits on the use of the condensate approach, which should be reserved for the analysis of nonvolatile, preferably hydrophilic solutes.

Additional progress in the EBC approach will depend upon a variety other factors including the development of more sensitive assays for both the reference and test solutes and procedures for enhancing the generation of respiratory droplets. However, it is also possible that "dry, warm" methods of collecting respiratory droplets may prove more useful than "wet, cold" condensation. These could include filtration, impaction, and electrostatic precipitation, all of which could minimize both water and NH_4^+ accumulation.

ACKNOWLEDGMENTS

We would like to thank the following individuals who helped make these studies possible: Kelly Hoagland, Mark Bosbous, Daniel Castillo, Bradley E. Foss, Wen Lin, Feng Sun, Maier Gare, and Mike Bregantini. Supported by NIH grants HL60057 and DC03191.

FURTHER READING

1. Scheideler, L. et al., Detection of nonvolatile macromolecules in breath. A possible diagnostic tool?, *Am. Rev. Respir. Dis.*, 148, 778, 1993.
2. Kharitonov, S.A. and Barnes, P.J., Exhaled markers of pulmonary disease, *Am. J. Respir. Crit. Care Med.*, 163, 1693, 2001.
3. Mutlu, G.M. et al., Collection and analysis of exhaled breath condensates in humans, *Am. J. Respir. Crit. Care Med.*, 164, 731, 2001.
4. Feng, N.H., Hacker, A., and Effros, R.M., Solute exchange between the plasma and epithelial lining fluid of rat lungs, *J. Appl. Physiol.*, 72, 1081, 1992.
5. Effros, R.M. et al., Dilution of respiratory solutes in exhaled condensates, *Am. J. Respir. Crit. Care Med.*, 165, 663, 2002.
6. Effros, R.M. et al., A simple method for estimating respiratory solute dilution in exhaled breath condensates, *Am. J. Respir. Crit. Care Med.*, 168, 1500, 2003.
7. Anderson, S.D. et al., Sensitivity to heat and water loss at rest and during exercise in asthmatic subjects, *Eur. J. Respir. Dis.*, 63, 459, 1982.
8. Borok, Z. and Verkman, A.S., Lung edema clearance: 20 years of progress. Role of aquaporin water channels in fluid transport in lung and airways, *J. Appl. Physiol.*, 93, 2199, 2002.
9. Effros, R.M. et al., Water transport and the distribution of Aquaporin 1 in the pulmonary airspaces of rats, *J. Appl. Physiol.*, 83, 1002, 1997.
10. Gaston, B., Breath condensate analysis: perhaps worth studying, after all, *Am. J. Respir. Crit. Care Med.*, 167, 292, 2003.
11. Vass, G. et al., Comparison of nasal and oral inhalation during exhaled breath condensate collection, *Am. J. Respir. Crit. Care Med.*, 167, 850, 2003.

12. Norwood, D.M. et al., Breath ammonia depletion and its relevance to acidic aerosol exposure studies, *Arch. Environ. Health*, 47, 309, 1992.
13. Quinton, P.M., Physiological basis of cystic fibrosis: a historical perspective, *Physiol. Rev.*, 79, S3, 1999.
14. Verkman, A.S., Lung disease in cystic fibrosis: is airway surface liquid composition abnormal?, *Am. J. Physiol. Lung Cell Mol. Physiol.*, 281, L306, 2001.
15. Kotaru, C. et al., Desiccation and hypertonicity of the airway surface fluid and thermally induced asthma, *J. Appl. Physiol.*, 94, 227, 2003.
16. Effros, R.M. et al., Kinetics of urea exchange in air-filled and fluid-filled rat lungs, *Am. J. Physiol. Lung Cell Mol. Physiol.*, 263, L619, 1992.
17. Hunt, J. et al., Endogenous airway acidification: implications for asthma pathophysiology, *Am. J. Respir. Crit. Care Med.*, 161, 694, 2000.
18. Kostikas, K. et al., pH in expired breath condensate of patients with inflammatory airway diseases, *Am. J. Respir. Crit. Care Med.*, 165, 1364, 2002.
19. Tate, S., et al., Airways in cystic fibrosis are acidified: detection by exhaled breath condensate, *Thorax*, 57, 926, 2002.
20. Hunt, J.F. et al., Expression and activity of pH-regulatory glutaminase in the human airway epithelium, *Am. J. Respir. Crit. Care Med.*, 165, 101, 2002.
21. Huizenga, J.R., Gips, C.H., and Tangerman, A., The contribution of various organs to ammonia formation: a review of factors determining the arterial ammonia concentration, *Ann. Clin. Biochem.*, 33, 23, 1996.
22. Effros, R.M. et al., Resistance of the pulmonary epithelium to movement of buffer ions, *Am. J. Physiol. Lung Cell Mol. Physiol.*, 285, L476, 2003.
23. Gros, G. and Moll, W., Facilitated diffusion of CO_2 across albumin solutions, *J. Gen. Physiol.*, 64, 356, 1974.
24. Stewart, P.A., *How to Understand Acid-Base. A Quantitative Acid-Base Primer for Biology and Medicine*, Elsevier, New York, 1981.
25. Harris, D.C., *Quantitative Analysis*, 4th ed., W.H. Freeman and Co., New York, 1995.
26. Vaughan, W. et al., Acetic acid contributes to breath condensate acidity in asthma, *Eur. Respir. J.*, 18, 463S, 2001.
27. Story, D.A., Thistlethwaite, P., and Bellomo, R., The effect of PVC packaging on the acidity of 0.9% saline, *Anaesth. Intensive Care*, 28, 287, 2000.
28. Effros, R.M. and Chinard, F.P., The *in vivo* pH of the extravascular space of the lung, *J. Clin. Invest.*, 49, 1983, 1969.
29. Effros, R.M., Corbeil, N., and Chinard, F.P., Arterial pH and the distribution of barbiturates between pulmonary tissue and blood, *J. Appl. Physiol.*, 33, 656, 1972.

4 Isoprostanes, Prostanoids, and Leukotrienes in Exhaled Breath Condensate

Paolo Montuschi

CONTENTS

I. INTRODUCTION

Eicosanoids are lipid mediators that include leukotrienes (LTs), prostaglandins (PGs), and thromboxane A_2 (TXA_2). LTC_4, D_4, and E_4, known as cysteinyl-leukotrienes (cys-LTs), contract airway smooth muscle, increase vascular permeability, stimulate mucus secretion, and decrease mucociliary clearance.[1] These effects may be relevant to bronchial obstruction in patients with asthma, and selective cys-LT_1 receptor antagonists are currently used in asthma therapy.[2] LTB_4 is a potent chemoattractant of neutrophils, enhances neutrophil-endothelial interactions, and stimulates neutrophil activation.[2] LTB_4 has weak effects on smooth muscle, but it may contribute to airway narrowing by producing local edema and by increasing mucus secretion.[2] The importance of LTB_4 in causing asthmatic airway inflammation is not known, although this compound could play a role particularly during some exacerbations or severe persisting asthma, which is associated with increased neutrophils in the airways.[3,4] LTB_4 and cys-LTs are detectable in sputum in patients with chronic bronchitis.[5,6] The concentrations of LTB_4 in serum are increased in patients with chronic obstructive pulmonary disease (COPD)[7] and release of LTB_4 by alveolar macrophages is increased in α_1-antitrypsin deficiency.[8] Because of its chemoattractant activity of neutrophils, LTB_4 could have an important pathophysiological role in COPD, which is characterized by increased numbers and activation of neutrophils. Leukotriene pathway inhibitors are under development for the treatment of COPD.[9]

Prostaglandins have both deleterious and beneficial effects on the lung. PGD_2 and $PGF_{2\alpha}$ cause bronchoconstriction in patients with asthma but not in healthy subjects.[10,11] Inhaled PGE_2 attenuates allergen-induced airway responses and airway inflammation in patients with asthma.[12] TxA_2 is a potent bronchoconstrictor and causes airway smooth muscle hyperplasia, a characteristic feature of asthmatic airways *in vitro*.[13] Sputum levels of PGE_2, $PGF_{2\alpha}$, 6-oxo-$PGF_{1\alpha}$, and TxB_2 have been detected in patients with COPD but their effects are unknown.[6] Isoprostanes or isoeicosanoids are prostaglandin-like compounds that are produced *in vivo* independently of cyclooxygenase (COX) enzymes, primarily by free radical-induced peroxidation of arachidonic acid.[14] F_2-Isoprostanes, a group of 64 compounds isomeric in structure to COX-derived $PGF_{2\alpha}$, are currently considered among the best available biomarkers of oxidative stress status and lipid peroxidation *in vivo*.[15] Measurement of F_2-isoprostanes in tissues and/or biological fluids has several advantages over other quantitative markers of oxidative stress because they are chemically stable, are specific products of endogenous peroxidation, are formed *in vivo*, and are present in detectable amounts in all normal tissues and biological fluids, thus allowing the definition of a normal range.[15] Measurement of F_2-isoprostanes provides a uniquely valuable new approach to the quantification of oxidative stress as well as a biochemical basis for assessing therapeutic intervention and establishing effective antioxidant regimens.[15] Isoprostanes are not only biomarkers of oxidative stress, but also have numerous biological effects in the respiratory system such as contraction of human bronchial smooth muscle *in vitro*[16] and airflow obstruction and plasma exudation in guinea pigs *in vivo*,[17] suggesting that they might also function as pathophysiologic mediators of oxidant injury in the lung.

Most of the studies investigating the role of eicosanoids in inflammatory airway diseases have used invasive techniques such as bronchoalveolar lavage[18,19] or have measured these compounds in plasma or urine remote from the site of production.[20]

Leukotrienes and prostanoids also have been detected in sputum in healthy subjects and patients with inflammatory airway diseases. However, sputum induction is a semi-invasive technique that is not well accepted by patients and causes inflammation as it increases neutrophil counts in sputum after repeated induction within short intervals.[21]

Recently, attention has focused on the measurement of LTs, prostanoids, and isoprostanes in exhaled breath condensate (EBC), which is a completely noninvasive technique to sample secretions from the airways[22,23] (Figure 4.1). In view of the important role of eicosanoids in airway inflammation and the possibility of collecting several samples, this approach might be particularly useful for quantifying lung inflammation and monitoring pharmacological therapy. However, several methodological issues need to be addressed before this method can be considered in the clinical setting, as discussed in Chapter 2. This chapter summarizes the current

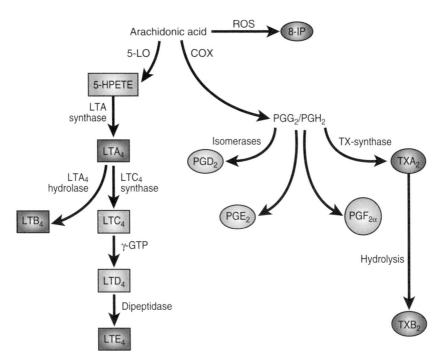

FIGURE 4.1 Arachidonic acid products which have been detected in EBC in healthy subjects and patients with airway inflammatory diseases. LTs such as LTB_4 and cysteinyl-leukotrienes (LTC_4, LTD_4, and LTE_4) are products of 5-lipoxygenase (5-LO) activity. Two COX isoforms (not shown) are known to act on arachidonic acid to lead, eventually, to the formation of PG, E_2, D_2, $PGF_{2\alpha}$, and TXA_2. PGE_2 is always detectable in EBC. PGD_2, $PGF_{2\alpha}$, and TXA_2 are detectable in EBC only in some healthy patients and/or patients with asthma and chronic obstructive pulmonary disease. The pathway leading to PGI_2 synthesis is not shown. Isoprostanes are PG-like compounds that are produced *in vivo* independently of COX enzymes, primarily by free radical-induced peroxidation of arachidonic acid. Abbreviations: 8-IP, 8-isoprostane; γ-GTP, γ-glutamyl-transpeptidase; 5-HPETE, 5-hydroperoxyeicosatetraenoic acid; ROS, reactive oxygen species. (Modified from Montuschi, P., *Nature Reviews Drug Discovery, Vol. 1, Indirect Monitoring of Lung Inflammation*, Macmillan Magazines, 2002, pp. 238–242. With permission.)

knowledge on the measurement of LTs, prostanoids, and isoprostanes in EBC. Studies on the measurement of isoprostanes will be presented first, given that the analytical evidence for these compounds in EBC is more convincing.

II. MEASUREMENT OF EICOSANOIDS IN EXHALED BREATH CONDENSATE: ANALYTICAL METHODS

Isoprostanes and PGE_2 have been detected in EBC by using gas chromatography/ mass spectrometry (GC/MS), the reference analytical method, which demonstrated their presence in this biological fluid.[24] Radioimmunoassays for 8-isoprostane and PGE_2 in EBC also are available and they have been qualitatively validated by reversed-phase high-performance liquid chromatography (RP-HPLC).[25] Day-to-day radioimmunoassay measurements of 8-isoprostane and PGE_2 in EBC in healthy subjects are highly reproducible.[26] In most of the published studies, 8-isoprostane,[27–37] LTs,[38–46] and prostanoids[31,38,47] have been measured in EBC by using commercially available enzyme immunoassays, which need to be validated by independent analytical methods such as liquid chromatography/mass spectrometry (LC/MS). Conflicting results have been reported on the measurement of 8-isoprostane in EBC with a commercially available enzyme immunoassay kit (Cayman Chemical, Ann Arbor, MI).[48,49] Studies on the intrasubject reproducibility of measurements of LTs in EBC are required. Some studies reported 8-isoprostane,[32,33,36,37] cys-LTs,[33] or LTB_4[32,44] concentrations in EBC of few picograms per milliliter that were close to the detection limit of the enzyme immunoassay, or even below.[33] At these concentrations, the analytical variability is very high, raising substantial questions about the reliability of measurements, the interpretation of results, and the biological significance of differences in eicosanoid levels among study groups.

A. ISOPROSTANES

Isoprostanes have been measured in EBC by GC/MS,[24] enzyme immunoassays,[27–37] and a radioimmunoassay.[25,26,50,51]

8-Isoprostane, a compound that belongs to the F_2 class of isoprostanes and is the most studied isoprostane, has been detected in EBC in healthy subjects using stable isotope dilution methods in conjunction with GC/MS.[24] This study provided the first and definitive evidence for the presence of 8-isoprostane in EBC. Samples were collected from 10 patients without lung disease who were intubated while undergoing minor surgical procedures, and from 22 patients with acute respiratory distress syndrome (ARDS)/acute lung injury (ALI).[24] The collecting system consisted of Tygon® (Norton Performance Plastics, Akron, OH) tubing submerged in an ice bath in line with the expiratory limb of the ventilator circuit.[24] The presence of 8-isoprostane in the EBC was demonstrated by a peak in the EBC samples that co-eluted with the internal standard.[24] A selected ion current profile was used for the quantification of 8-isoprostane. The peak co-eluting with the internal standard represents the endogenously formed 8-isoprostane as indicated by the linear recovery of 8-isoprostane after instillation and nebulization of three concentrations of this eicosanoid (50, 250, and 500 pg/ml) in the Tygon tubing.[24] This experiment excludes *ex vivo* production of 8-isoprostane in the collecting system.[24]

Recently, we have qualitatively validated a radioimmunoassay for 8-isoprostane in EBC developed in our laboratory by using RP-HPLC.[25] Validation of the EBC analysis was sought by two different criteria: RP-HPLC purification of a pool of EBC samples with subsequent radioimmunoassays of the eluted fractions for 8-isoprostane, and simultaneous measurements of unextracted EBC samples with two anti-8-isoprostane sera with different cross-reactivities.[25] A single peak of 8-isoprostane-like immunoreactivity co-eluting with the 8-isoprostane standard (retention time: 13 min) was identified by radioimmunoassay. Testing with two antisera showed similar results (limits of agreement, 4.5 and –4.1 pg/ml; $n = 12$).[25] This study provides evidence for the specificity of this radioimmunoassay for 8-isoprostane in EBC.

However, quantitative comparisons between radioimmunoassay and GC/MS measurements are required. In most studies, 8-isoprostane in EBC was measured by using a commercially available enzyme immunoassay kit (Cayman Chemical).[27–37] This enzyme immunoassay for 8-isoprostane has been validated by GC/MS in plasma and urine,[52] but not in EBC. Moreover, data on the day-to-day reproducibility of 8-isoprostane measurements in EBC with this enzyme immunoassay are inadequate and conflicting.[48,49]

B. PROSTANOIDS

Prostaglandin E_2 has been measured by GC/MS in EBC but analytical details are not available.[24] We measured PGE_2 in EBC by a radioimmunoassay developed in our laboratory.[25] As with 8-isoprostane, we demonstrated identical chromatographic behavior of PGE_2-like immunoreactivity in EBC with authentic PGE_2. We characterized PGE_2-like immunoreactivity by RP-HPLC and found a single peak co-eluting with the reference standard.[25] The validity of radioimmunoassay measurements for PGE_2 in EBC was reinforced by the simultaneous use of different antisera to measure unextracted samples, given that every antiserum has a unique profile of cross-reactivity. Similar concentrations of PGE_2-like immunoreactivity (limits of agreement, 6.1 and –6.1 pg/ml) were measured in unextracted EBC samples using either antiserum.[25] Taken together, these findings provide evidence for the specificity of our radioimmunoassay for PGE_2 in EBC. However, this method needs to be validated by GC/MS. PGE_2 also has been measured in EBC by a commercially available enzyme immunoassay (Cayman Chemical)[31,38] as well as $PGF_{2\alpha}$ and PGD_2-methoxime, a stable derivative of PGD_2.[38]

TxB$_2$ has been measured in EBC by an enzyme immunoassay (Cayman Chemical)[38] and by two radioimmunoassays.[53,54] By using the commercially available enzyme immunoassay for TxB_2, we were able to measure this compound in EBC in 7 of 15 adult asthmatic patients (9.1 ± 0.5 pg/min)[38]; TxB_2 in EBC was below the sensitivity of the assay in the other patients with asthma and in the healthy subjects.[38] Likewise, by using a radioimmunoassay for TxB_2 that we developed,[54] this eicosanoid was detectable at low concentrations only in few asthmatic and healthy children.[51] In contrast, by using a different radioimmunoassay (Izotop, Institute of Isotopes Co., Ltd., Budapest, Hungary),[53] other authors reported concentrations of TxB_2 in EBC that were detectable in most healthy subjects[53] and patients with asthma.[55] However, details on this radioimmunoassay, such as sensitivity, specificity, intra- and interassay coefficients of variation, are not available. Interindividual variability of TxB_2 concentrations in EBC was high, as indicated by the standard error of the means (SEM).[55]

C. LEUKOTRIENES

In all published studies, LTs (LTB_4, cys-LTs, LTE_4) have been measured in EBC using commercially available enzyme immunoassay kits.[31–33,38–46] These results need to be validated by more specific analytical techniques, such as HPLC or LC/MS. Using HPLC, we have recently shown that LTB_4-like immunoreactivity in EBC has identical chromatographic behavior with the respective standard, providing evidence for the specificity of the enzyme immunoassay that we used (Cayman Chemical).[39] However, the definitive evidence for the presence of LTs in EBC and a quantitative assessment of their concentrations in this biological fluid by a reference analytical method are still lacking. There are few data on the intrasubject reproducibility of LTB$_4$ and LTE$_4$ in both adults[38] and children (Mondino et al., unpublished data) with asthma, but this issue needs to be addressed formally. A wide variability in both LTB$_4$ and cys-LTs concentrations in EBC in patients with airway inflammatory diseases of similar severity and even in healthy subjects has been reported in different studies.[31–33,38,40–42,45] This might be explained partly by the chemical structure of LTs. These eicosanoids, particularly cys-LTs, are highly unstable compounds and different collection procedures, handling, and storage of EBC samples might result in highly different concentrations of LTs in EBC. Moreover, because they are sticky compounds, the concentrations of LTs in EBC might depend on the collecting system material, resulting in a variable recovery in the EBC. Efforts should be made to identify the most suitable material(s) for collecting LTs in EBC samples and for establishing their stability in this biological fluid. However, part of the variability in LT concentrations in EBC is probably related to the enzyme immunoassays, which usually work well in buffer, but less so in EBC. Because of the lack of standardized procedures for collecting and handling EBC samples, comparisons between results obtained in different research centers at present are difficult.

III. EICOSANOIDS IN EXHALED BREATH CONDENSATE IN INFLAMMATORY LUNG DISEASES

A. ISOPROSTANES

8-Isoprostane is detected in EBC from healthy subjects and indicates the presence of physiological levels of oxidant stress.[24,28] Measurements of 8-isoprostane using GC/MS and an enzyme immunoassay provided comparable baseline values (7 ± 3.8 pg/ml and 11 ± 0.8 pg ml/ml, respectively [mean ± SEM]).[24,28] Compared with healthy subjects, 8-isoprostane in EBC is increased in adults with stable asthma, with the increase correlating with the severity of the disease and the degree of inflammation.[27] Despite treatment with oral and/or high doses of inhaled corticosteroids, patients with severe asthma had the highest concentrations of exhaled 8-isoprostane (49 ± 5.0 pg/ml).[27] Compared with healthy subjects (20 ± 7 pg/ml, mean ± standard deviation), other authors reported a similar increase in 8-isoprostane concentrations in EBC in patients with stable moderate asthma who were either steroid-naïve or treated with inhaled glucocorticosteroids (40 ± 9 pg/ml), although subanalysis for the effects of inhaled glucocorticosteroids was not presented.[34] In one study, 8-isoprostane concentrations in EBC were measured in patients with aspirin-sensitive asthma, in patients with aspirin-tolerant asthma, and in healthy subjects.[31] Asthmatic patients were either steroid-naïve or treated with inhaled or oral corticosteroids. Aspirin-sensitive (90.0 ± 19.0 pg/ml; $p < .05$) and aspirin-tolerant patients with asthma (79.2 ± 19.5 pg/ml; $p < .05$) had higher 8-isoprostane concentrations in EBC compared with healthy subjects (21.9 ± 4.5 pg/ml).[31] There was no difference in

8-isoprostane levels between the two groups of patients with asthma.[31] 8-Isoprostane was detectable in the EBC of healthy children (34.2 ± 4.5 pg/ml), and its concentrations were increased in both steroid-naïve asthmatic children (56.4 ± 7.7 pg/ml; $p < .01$) and steroid-treated asthmatic children (47.2 ± 2.3 pg/ml; $p < .05$).[50] 8-Isoprostane concentrations in EBC were higher than those reported in asthmatic adults.[27] This might be explained partly by differences in the collecting system (homemade device vs. ECoScreen) and in the analytical method (radioimmunoassay vs. enzyme immunoassay). There was no difference in 8-isoprostane concentrations in EBC between the two groups of children with asthma ($p = .14$).[50]

Taken together, these findings indicate that oxidative stress is elevated in both adults and children with stable asthma, as reflected by increased 8-isoprostane concentrations in EBC; this increase seems to be relatively resistant to steroid therapy. This hypothesis is further supported by a study showing that, in healthy subjects, pretreatment with a high dose of the inhaled corticosteroid budesonide (1600 mg/day for 14 days) had no effect on the increase in 8-isoprostane in EBC induced by short-term exposure to ozone (400 ppb).[30] Compared with healthy children (2.6 pg/ml; range, 2.1 to 3), median and interquartile range, 8-isoprostane concentrations were increased in children with asthma exacerbations before steroid treatment (12.0 pg/ml; range, 9.4 to 29.5; $p < .001$).[33] Note that 8-isoprostane concentrations in healthy children are lower than the detection limit of the enzyme immunoassay (6 pg/ml; Cayman Chemical). Details on how the authors improved the sensitivity the immunoassay are not provided. After oral prednisone at a dose of 1 mg/kg/day for 5 days, there was a decrease in 8-isoprostane (8.4 pg/ml; range, 5.4 to 11.6; $p = .04$), but 8-isoprostane concentrations remained higher than controls ($p < .001$).[33] The slight effect (mean difference, 3.6 pg/ml) of glucocorticoid treatment on 8-isoprostane in EBC reported in this study might be due to the different route of administration of glucocorticoids (oral vs. inhaled) and/or different effects of glucocorticoids in stable or exacerbated asthma. In any case, interpretation of these findings is difficult because the concentrations of 8-isoprostane in asthmatic children were close to the detection limit of the enzyme immunoassay. At these concentrations, measurements are much less reliable. Additional controlled studies are required to establish how glucocorticoids modulate 8-isoprostane concentration in EBC in patients with asthma and other inflammatory lung diseases.

8-Isoprostane in EBC also is increased in current and ex-smokers with stable COPD (45 ± 3.6 and 40 ± 3.1 pg/ml, respectively) and, to a lesser extent, in healthy smokers (24 ± 2.6 pg/ml), compared with healthy nonsmokers (11 ± 0.8 pg/ml).[28] The similar levels of 8-isoprostane in the EBC of current and ex-smokers with COPD might indicate that oxidative stress caused by chronic smoking reaches a point at which smoking cessation has little, if any, effect.[28] In another study, the mean concentration of 8-isoprostane in EBC was elevated in patients with COPD (47 pg/ml; 95% confidence interval [CI]; 41 to 53 pg/ml, $p < .0001$) compared with that of the control group (29 pg/ml; 95% CI, 25 to 33 pg/ml).[35] Concentrations of 8-isoprostane in EBC were increased in patients with COPD exacerbations (13.0 ± 9.0 pg/ml; $p < .005$) compared with healthy subjects (6.2 ± 0.4 pg/ml) and were reduced after antibiotic treatment (9.0 ± 0.6 pg/ml; $p < .0001$).[32] However, although this difference represents a 41% reduction of mean 8-isoprostane concentrations in

EBC after antibiotic treatment, an absolute reduction of 4 pg/ml of 8-isoprostane levels could be of limited biological relevance. 8-Isoprostane concentrations in EBC are also increased in patients with cystic fibrosis (43 ± 4.5 pg/ml)[29] and more markedly in patients with ALI/ARDS (87 ± 27.6 pg/ml), which reflects the severe oxidant damage associated with this syndrome.[24] There is no correlation between exhaled 8-isoprostane and lung function in patients with asthma[27] or COPD,[28] whereas exhaled 8-isoprostane levels correlate negatively with forced expiratory volume in 1 second (FEV_1) in cystic fibrosis patients.[29] These differences might be explained partly by the different biological significance of exhaled 8-isoprostane and FEV_1 and partly by differences in the pathophysiology of these lung diseases. 8-Isoprostane can be formed by the activity of COX-1 and/or COX-2 in isolated cells and, to some extent, in healthy subjects.[56] This does not occur in patients with COPD because nonselective inhibition of COX does not affect concentrations of 8-isoprostane in EBC[57] or urine.[58] 8-Isoprostane concentrations in EBC were found to be higher in patients with obstructive sleep apnea (9.5 ± 1.9 pg/ml; $p < .0001$) than in healthy obese subjects (6.7 ± 0.2 pg/ml).[37] In patients with obstructive sleep apnea, a reduction was seen after continuous positive airway pressure therapy (7.7 ± 0.9 vs. 9.6 ± 1.7 pg/ml; $p < .005$).[37] Although highly statistically significant, it is unlikely that an absolute mean reduction of 1.9 pg/ml of 8-isoprostane concentrations in EBC has biological significance, particularly because of the high analytical variability at these low concentrations.

B. PROSTANOIDS

Little is known about the prostanoids in EBC. The presence of PGE_2 in the EBC of healthy subjects has been demonstrated by GC/MS.[24] Compared with healthy subjects (median, 44.3 pg/ml; range, 30.2 to 52.1 pg/ml), PGE_2 is increased in steroid-naïve (98.0 pg/ml; range 57.0 to 128.4 pg/ml; $p < .001$) and steroid-treated patients with stable COPD (93.6 pg/ml; range, 52.8 to 157.0 pg/ml; $p < .001$).[40] In both groups of patients, exhaled PGE_2 concentrations correlate with exhaled LTB_4,[40] indicating that the greater the lung inflammation, the higher the production of an endogenous anti-inflammatory mediator such as PGE_2. There was no difference in PGE_2 concentrations in EBC between steroid-naïve and steroid-treated patients with COPD ($p = .59$). Nonselective inhibition of COX by oral ibuprofen reduces exhaled PGE_2 in COPD patients (from 98 ± 8.5 to 18 ± 2.4 pg/ml).[57] Considering the protective role of PGE_2 in the lungs, this effect might be relevant to the modulation of airway inflammation in COPD. Preliminary data indicate that rofecoxib, a selective COX-2 inhibitor, has no effect on PGE_2 and LTB_4 concentrations in EBC and might be better tolerated than nonselective nonsteroidal anti-inflammatory drugs in patients with COPD, which is characterized by increased lung inflammation.

Impaired production of PGE_2 has been implicated in the pathogenesis of asthma.[59] Our findings do not seem to support this hypothesis given that exhaled PGE_2 concentrations in adults with mild asthma who were not treated with corticosteroids (47.7 ± 2.9 pg; 95% CI, 41.5 to 53.9) and in healthy adults (45.6 ± 3.9 pg; 95% CI, 37.0 to 54.1) were similar.[38] Likewise, PGE_2 concentrations in EBC in healthy children (46.8 ± 5.3 pg/ml; 95% CI, 35.1 to 58.5), in steroid-naïve children with asthma (44.6 ± 5.0 pg/ml; 95% CI, 35.5 to 55.7), and in steroid-treated children with asthma (51.5 ± 4.0 pg/ml; 95% CI, 43.3 to 59.6) were similar ($p = .56$).[50] In patients with asthma, PGE_2 concentrations in EBC were increased in current smokers but not in nonsmokers, whereas healthy smokers and healthy nonsmokers had similar PGE_2 levels in EBC.[47]

TxB$_2$, a potent bronchoconstrictor, was detected in EBC in 7 of 15 adults with mild asthma[38] who were steroid-naive, whereas it was undetectable in either patients with COPD or healthy subjects.[40] Other authors reported detectable concentrations of TxB_2 in most of the healthy subjects.[53] Patients with allergic rhinitis, atopic asthma, and nonatopic asthma had TxB_2 concentrations in EBC similar to those in healthy subjects.[55]

Other prostanoids that cause bronchoconstriction, such as PGD_2 and $PGF_{2\alpha}$, were detected in some healthy and asthmatic adults. In those subjects in whom PGD_2 and $PGF_{2\alpha}$ were measurable, there was no difference in the concentrations of these prostanoids between the two groups.[38] The biological significance of these findings is still unclear.

C. LEUKOTRIENES

LTB$_4$ and cys-LTs have been detected in the EBC of healthy subjects[31,38,41] and are increased in adults with stable, moderate to severe asthma.[41] In adults with mild asthma, both increased[38] and similar[41] concentrations of exhaled LTE$_4$ and LTB$_4$ have been reported. Differences in airway hyperresponsiveness between patients, as shown by different reactivities to methacholine, might partly explain these discrepancies. In one study, the baseline concentrations of exhaled cys-LTs in steroid-naive, aspirin-sensitive asthma patients (152.3 ± 30.4 pg/ml; $p < .05$) were higher than those in steroid-naïve, aspirin-tolerant asthmatics (50.7 ± 15.7 pg/ml).[31] Both groups of patients with asthma had higher concentrations of exhaled cys-LT than healthy subjects (19.4 ± 2.8 pg/ml).[31] Steroid-naïve and steroid-treated patients with aspirin-tolerant asthma had similar cys-LT concentrations in EBC (50.7 ± 15.7 vs. 36.6 ± 7.1 pg/ml), whereas steroid treatment was associated with lower levels of cys-LTs in patients with aspirin-sensitive asthma (152.3 ± 30.4 vs. 55.2 ± 10.1 pg/ml; $p < .05$).[31] These findings indicate that cys-LT concentrations in EBC in patients with aspirin-tolerant asthma are relatively resistant to corticosteroids. However, because of the observational study design, the different route of administration of corticosteroids (oral vs. inhaled), and the limited number of patients, definitive conclusions are not possible. There is no correlation between exhaled LTs and lung-function tests in patients with asthma.[31,38,41]

NO synthase (NOS) activity seems to maintain LTB$_4$ synthesis in patients with asthma because exhaled LTB$_4$ is reduced compared with basal values 1 h after inhibition of NOS.[44] Compared with controls (15.9 ± 2.2 pg/ml; 95% CI, 10.2 to 21.5), LTE$_4$ concentrations in EBC were increased about 2-fold in both steroid-naïve (30.5 ± 2.8 pg/ml; $p < .05$; 95% CI, 24.7 to 36.3) and steroid-treated children with stable asthma (31.8 ± 4.9 pg/ml; $p < .05$; 95% CI, 20.7 to 43.0) who had normal lung function.[43] We also measured exhaled NO in the same study groups as an independent marker of airway inflammation. Compared with healthy children (6.3 ± 1.1 ppb; 95% CI, 3.6 to 8.9), exhaled NO levels were increased in steroid-naïve asthmatic children (28.3 ± 5.9 ppb; $p < .004$; 95% CI, 14.7 to 41.8), but not in steroid-treated asthmatic children (9.4 ± 3.0 ppb; 95% CI, 1.7 to 17.1).[43] LTB_4 concentrations in EBC were similar in the three study groups ($p = .15$).[43] This study indicates that LTE_4 concentrations in EBC are elevated in asthmatic children with normal lung function; in contrast to exhaled NO, exhaled LTE_4 seems to be resistant to inhaled corticosteroids, although controlled studies are required; measurement of LTE_4 in EBC might be useful for identifying those children with asthma who are most likely to benefit from LT receptor antagonists. In another study, cys-LTs and LTB_4 in EBC were found to be elevated in asthmatic children with mild persistent asthma who were receiving low-dose inhaled steroids and in children with moderate persistent asthma who were receiving high-dose inhaled steroids, but not in steroid-naïve children with mild intermittent asthma.[42] These findings are partly in contrast with our study, which showed elevated levels of LTE_4 in mild asthmatic children with normal lung function. This discrepancy might be explained partly by methodological differences and/or a different degree of airway inflammation in asthmatic children with similar lung function and symptoms.

Cys-LT concentrations in EBC have found to be increased in children with asthma exacerbations (median, 12.7 pg/ml; interquartile range, 5.4 to 15.6), compared with healthy children (median, 4.3 pg/ml; interquartile range, 2.0 to 5.7).[33] After 5 days of therapy with oral prednisone (1 mg/kg/day) there was a reduction in cys-LT concentrations in EBC in children with asthma exacerbations (5.2 pg/ml; 3.9 to 8.8; $p = .005$).[33] These findings indicate a reduction of 60% of median exhaled cys-LT concentrations in children with asthma exacerbations after oral corticosteroids. However, 9 of 15 children with an asthma exacerbation had cys-LT concentrations in EBC before treatment that were lower than 15 pg/ml. At these concentrations, it is difficult to interpret the biological significance of variations in exhaled cys-LT concentrations because the variability of the immunoassay is very high. In one study, levels of cys-LTs in EBC in adults with asthma were undetectable.[60]

In contrast to exhaled LTE_4, exhaled LTB_4 is increased in steroid-naïve (median, 100.6 pg/ml; range, 73.5 to 145.0 pg/ml; $p < .001$) and steroid-treated patients with stable COPD (median, 99.0 pg/ml; range, 57.9 to 170.5 pg/ml) who were ex-smokers compared with healthy subjects (median, 38.1 pg/ml; range, 31.2 to 53.6 pg/ml).[40] Both groups of COPD patients had similar concentrations of LTB_4 in EBC ($p = .43$). In patients with COPD,[40] the profile of LTs is different from that in patients with asthma.[38] LTE_4 in EBC is selectively increased in patients with asthma,[38] whereas exhaled LTB_4 is increased more markedly in patients with COPD.[40] In patients with COPD exacerbations, LTB_4 concentrations were reduced 2 weeks after treatment with antibiotics (15.8 ± 1.1 vs. 9.9 ± 0.9 pg/ml; $p < .0001$) and this effect was maintained after 2 months (8.5 ± 0.8 pg/ml; $p < .005$).[32] The increase in LTB_4 concentrations in EBC in healthy smokers (9.4 ± 0.4 pg/ml) compared with healthy nonsmokers (6.1 ± 0.3 pg/ml; $p < .001$)[45] is unlikely to have any biological relevance because the mean increase is small (3.3 pg/ml) and the analytical variability at concentrations close to the detection limit of the immunoassay is very high. LTB_4

concentrations in EBC are increased in patients with bronchiectasis (80 ± 8.4 pg/ml) compared with healthy subjects (35 ± 2.4 pg/ml) and in steroid-naive patients with stable cystic fibrosis (76 ± 9.7 pg/ml), whereas exhaled LTE_4 is not (P. Montuschi, unpublished data). LTB_4 concentrations in EBC are also increased during exacerbations of cystic fibrosis (31.1 ± 4.4 pg/ml) and are reduced after 2 weeks of antibiotic treatment (18.8 ± 0.8 pg/ml; $p < .001$).[46] This is consistent with the central role of neutrophils in the pathophysiology of these lung inflammatory diseases.

IV. CONCLUSIONS

Measurements of LTs, prostanoids, and isoprostanes in EBC might provide insights into the pathophysiology of lung diseases. Selective eicosanoid profiles in EBC might prove to be important for differentiating between inflammatory lung diseases. Because it is completely noninvasive, this approach is potentially useful for quantifying lung inflammation and monitoring pharmacological therapy, even in children. EBC analysis of eicosanoids and isoprostanes might be suitable for testing novel pharmacological therapies in pulmonary diseases and might clarify the effects of glucocorticoids on lung inflammation and oxidative stress, providing a more rational pharmacological basis for their administration in inflammatory airway diseases. Measurement of LTE_4 or cys-LTs in EBC might be useful for identifying those patients with asthma who are most likely to benefit from LT receptor antagonists. However, because of the lack of a standardized procedure for EBC analysis of eicosanoids and the current methodological limitations, comparisons of results from different laboratories are difficult. At present, this method is limited to research purposes. Several important methodological issues need to be addressed before analysis of eicosanoids in the EBC can be considered for clinical applications.

Robust analytical methodology usually precedes the application of a new technique. In the case of EBC, the initial enthusiasm, the search for new biomolecules in this biological fluid, and the availability of immunoassays for several inflammatory mediators led researchers to overlook a rigorous analytical approach, leaving open the question of the specificity and reliability of these immunoassays. Convincing analytical evidence should be the basis, and not the consequence, of the widespread use of immunoassays for EBC analysis. The time has come for a different approach to be followed.

ACKNOWLEDGMENT

Supported by Catholic University of the Sacred Heart, Fondi di Ateneo 2002–2003.

FURTHER READING

1. Busse, W.W., Leukotrienes and inflammation, *Am. J. Respir. Crit. Care Med.*, 157, S210, 1998.
2. Drazen, J.M., Israel, E., and O'Byrne, P.M., Treatment of asthma with drugs modifying the leukotriene pathway, *N. Engl. J. Med.*, 340, 197, 1999.

3. O'Byrne, P.M., Why does airway inflammation persist? Is it leukotrienes?, *Am. J. Respir. Crit. Care Med.*, 161, S186, 2000.

4. Jatakanon, A. et al., Neutrophilic inflammation in severe persistent asthma, *Am. J. Respir. Crit. Care Med.*, 160, 1532, 1999.

5. Hill, A.T., Bayley, D., and Stockley, R.A., The interrelationship of sputum inflammatory markers in patients with chronic bronchitis, *Am. J. Respir. Crit. Care Med.*, 160, 893, 1999.

6. Zakrzewski, J.T. et al., Lipid mediators in cystic fibrosis and chronic obstructive pulmonary disease, *Am. Rev. Respir. Dis.*, 136, 779, 1987.

7. Seggev, J.S., Thornton, W.H., and Edes, T.E., Serum leukotriene B_4 levels in patients with obstructive pulmonary disease, *Chest*, 99, 289, 1991.

8. Hubbard, R.C. et al., Neutrophil accumulation in the lung in α_1-antitrypsin deficiency: spontaneous release of leukotriene B_4 by alveolar macrophages, *J. Clin. Invest.*, 88, 891, 1991.

9. Kilfeather, S., 5-Lipoxygenase inhibitors for the treatment of COPD, *Chest*, 121, 197S, 2002.

10. Hardy, C.C. et al., The bronchoconstrictor effect of inhaled prostaglandin D_2 in normal and asthmatic men, *N. Engl. J. Med.*, 311, 209, 1984.

11. Mathe, A.A. and Hedqvist, P., Effect of prostaglandin $F_{2\alpha}$ and E_2 on airway conductance in healthy subjects and asthmatic patients, *Am. Rev. Respir. Dis.*, 111, 313, 1975.

12. Gauvreau, G.M., Watson, R.M, and O'Byrne, P.M. Protective effects of inhaled PGE_2 on allergen-induced airway responses and inflammation, *Am. J. Respir. Crit. Care Med.*, 159, 31, 1999.

13. Noveral, J.P. and Grunstein, M.M., Role and mechanism of thromboxane-induced proliferation of cultured airway smooth muscle cells, *Am. J. Physiol.*, 263, L555, 1992.

14. Morrow, J.D. et al., A series of prostaglandin F_2-like compounds are produced *in vivo* in humans by a non-cyclooxygenase, free radical-catalyzed mechanism, *Proc. Natl. Acad. Sci. USA*, 87, 9383, 1990.

15. Roberts, L.J. and Morrow, J.D., Measurement of F_2-isoprostanes as an index of oxidative stress *in vivo*, *Free Radic. Biol. Med.*, 28, 505, 2000.

16. Kawikova, I. et al., 8-Epi-$PGF_{2\alpha}$, a novel noncyclooxygenase-derived prostaglandin, constricts airways *in vitro*, *Am. J. Respir. Crit. Care Med.*, 153, 590, 1996.

17. Okazawa, A. et al., 8-Epi-$PGF_{2\alpha}$ induces airflow obstruction and airway plasma exudation *in vivo*. *Am. J. Respir. Crit. Care Med.*, 155, 436, 1997.

18. Wenzel, S.E. et al., Effect of 5-lipoxygenase inhibition on bronchoconstriction and airway inflammation in nocturnal asthma, *Am. J. Respir. Crit. Care Med.*, 152, 897, 1995.

19. Asano, K. et al., Diurnal variation of urinary leukotriene E_4 and histamine excretion rates in normal subjects and patients with mild-to-moderate asthma, *J. Allergy Clin. Immunol.* 96, 643, 1995.

20. Kumlin, M., Measurement of leukotrienes in humans, *Am. J. Respir. Crit. Care Med.*, 161, S102, 2000.

21. Nightingale, J.A., Rogers, D.F, and Barnes P.J., The effect of repeated sputum induction on cell counts in normal volunteers, *Thorax*, 53, 87, 1998.

22. Montuschi, P., Indirect monitoring of lung inflammation, *Nat. Rev. Drug Discov.*, 1, 238, 2002.

23. Montuschi, P. and Barnes, P.J., Analysis of exhaled breath condensate for monitoring airway inflammation, *Trends Pharmacol. Sci.*, 23, 232, 2002.

24. Carpenter, C.T., Price, P.V, and Christman, B.W. Exhaled breath condensate isoprostanes are elevated in patients with acute lung injury or ARDS, *Chest*, 114, 1653, 1998.

25. Montuschi, P. et al., Validation of 8-isoprostane and prostaglandin E_2 measurements in exhaled breath condensate, *Inflamm. Res.*, 52, 502, 2003.
26. Montuschi, P. et al., Measurements of exhaled prostanoids: reproducibility and flow-dependence, *Am. J. Respir. Crit. Care Med.*, 167, A752, 2003.
27. Montuschi, P., et al., Increased 8-isoprostane, a marker of oxidative stress, in exhaled condensate of asthma patients, *Am. J. Respir. Crit. Care Med.*, 160, 216, 1999.
28. Montuschi, P. et al., Exhaled 8-isoprostane as an *in vivo* biomarker of lung oxidative stress in patients with COPD and healthy smokers, *Am. J. Respir. Crit. Care Med.*, 162, 1175, 2000.
29. Montuschi, P. et al., Exhaled 8-isoprostane as a new non-invasive biomarker of oxidative stress in cystic fibrosis, *Thorax*, 55, 205, 2000.
30. Montuschi, P. et al., Ozone-induced increase in exhaled 8-isoprostane in healthy subjects is resistant to inhaled budesonide, *Free Rad. Biol. Med.*, 33, 1403, 2002.
31. Antczak, A. et al., Increased exhaled cysteinyl-leukotrienes and 8-isoprostane in aspirin-induced asthma, *Am. J. Respir. Crit. Care Med.*, 166, 301, 2002.
32. Biernacki, W.A., Kharitonov, S.A., and Barnes, P.J., Increased leukotriene B_4 and 8-isoprostane in exhaled breath condensate of patients with exacerbations of COPD, *Thorax*, 58, 294, 2003.
33. Baraldi, E. et al., Cysteinyl leukotrienes and 8-isoprostane in exhaled breath condensate of children with asthma exacerbations, *Thorax*, 58, 505, 2003.
34. Kostikas, K. et al., pH in expired breath condensate of patients with inflammatory airway diseases, *Am. J. Respir. Crit. Care Med.*, 165, 1364, 2002.
35. Kostikas, K. et al., Oxidative stress in expired breath condensate of patients with COPD, *Chest*, 124, 1373, 2003.
36. Carpagnano, G.E. et al., Increased 8-isoprostane and interleukin-6 in breath condensate of obstructive sleep apnea patients, *Chest*, 122, 1162, 2002.
37. Carpagnano, G.E. et al., 8-Isoprostane, a marker of oxidative stress, is increased in exhaled breath condensate of patients with obstructive sleep apnea after night and is reduced by continuous positive airway pressure therapy, *Chest*, 124, 1386, 2003.
38. Montuschi, P. and Barnes, P.J., Exhaled leukotrienes and prostaglandins in asthma, *J. Allergy Clin. Immunol.*, 109, 615, 2002.
39. Montuschi, P. et al., Validation of leukotriene B_4 measurements in exhaled breath condensate, *Inflamm. Res.*, 52, 69, 2003.
40. Montuschi, P. et al., Exhaled leukotrienes and prostaglandins in COPD. *Thorax*, 58, 585, 2003.
41. Hanazawa, T., Kharitonov, S.A., and Barnes, P.J., Increased nitrotyrosine in exhaled breath condensate of patients with asthma, *Am. J. Respir. Crit. Care Med.*, 162, 1273, 2000.
42. Csoma, Z. et al., Increased leukotrienes in exhaled breath condensate in childhood asthma, *Am. J. Respir. Crit. Care Med.*, 166, 1345, 2002.
43. Mondino, C. et al., Leukotrienes in exhaled breath condensate in childhood asthma, *Am. J. Respir. Crit. Care Med.*, 167, A445, 2003.
44. Montuschi, P. et al., Nitric oxide synthase inhibition decreases exhaled leukotriene B_4 in patients with asthma, *Am. J. Respir. Crit. Care Med.*, 163, A594, 2001.
45. Carpagnano, G.E. et al., Increased inflammatory markers in the exhaled breath condensate of cigarette smokers, *Chest*, 124, 1386, 2003.
46. Carpagnano, G.E. et al., Increased leukotriene B_4 and interleukin-6 in exhaled breath condensate in cystic fibrosis, *Am. J. Respir. Crit. Care Med.*, 167, 1109, 2003.
47. Kostikas, K. et al., Prostaglandin E_2 in expired breath condensate of patients with asthma, *Eur. Respir. J.*, 22, 743, 2003.

48. van der Meer, R., et al., Levels of 8-isoprostane in exhaled breath condensate are not reproducible in asthmatic and normal subjects, *Am. J. Respir. Crit. Care Med.*, 165, A14, 2002.

49. Anderson, D.G. et al., Biomarker reproducibility study in exhaled breath and induced sputum in non-smokers, smokers and COPD patients, *Eur. Respir. J.*, 22, Suppl. 45, 77s, 2003.

50. Baraldi, E., et al., Increased exhaled 8-isoprostane in childhood asthma, *Chest*, 124, 25, 2003.

51. Montuschi, P., et al., Profile of prostanoids in exhaled breath condensate in childhood asthma, *Eur. Respir. J.*, Suppl. 45, 400s, 2003.

52. Wang, Z. et al., Immunological characterization of urinary 8-epi-prostaglandin $F_{2\alpha}$ excretion in man, *J. Pharmacol. Exp. Ther.*, 275, 94, 1995.

53. Vass, G. et al., Comparison of nasal and oral inhalation during exhaled breath condensate collection, *Am. J. Respir. Crit. Care Med.*, 167, 850, 2003.

54. Patrono, C. et al., Radioimmunoassay of serum thromboxane B_2: a simple method of assessing pharmacologic effects on platelet function. *Adv. Prostaglandin Thromboxane Res.*, 6, 187, 1980.

55. Huszar, E. et al., Thromboxane in exhaled breath condensate in healthy volunteers and in patients with asthma, *Eur. Respir. J.*, Suppl. 45, 293s, 2003.

56. Klein, T. et al., Generation of the isoprostane 8-epi-prostaglandin $F_{2\alpha}$ *in vitro* and *in vivo* via the cyclooxygenases, *J. Pharmacol. Exp. Ther.*, 282, 1658, 1997.

57. Montuschi, P. et al., Non selective cyclo-oxygenase inhibition decreases exhaled prostaglandin E_2 in patients with chronic obstructive pulmonary disease, *Am. J. Respir. Crit. Care Med.*, 163, A908, 2001.

58. Pratico, D. et al., Chronic obstructive pulmonary disease is associated with an increase in urinary levels of isoprostane $F_{2\alpha}$-III, an index of oxidant stress, *Am. J. Respir. Crit. Care Med.*, 158, 1709, 1998.

59. Pavord, I.D. and Tattersfield, A.E., Bronchoprotective role for endogenous prostaglandin E_2, *Lancet*, 334, 436, 1995.

60. Sandrini, A. et al., Effect of montelukast on exhaled nitric oxide and nonvolatile markers of inflammation in mild asthma, *Chest*, 124, 1334, 2003.

5 Hydrogen Peroxide in Exhaled Breath Condensate

Wendy J.C. van Beurden and P.N. Richard Dekhuijzen

CONTENTS

I. HYDROGEN PEROXIDE

Oxidative stress is known to play an important role in the pathophysiology of several pulmonary diseases. Oxidative stress can be defined as increased exposure to oxidants and/or decreased antioxidant capacities. Cigarette smoke is a rich source of oxidants. The tar component contains an estimated 10^{18} radicals per gram. Oxidants are also produced by inflammatory cells, mainly neutrophils, macrophages, and eosinophils.[1]

Activated inflammatory cells respond with a "respiratory burst," which results in the production of reactive oxygen species (ROS). Naturally occurring free radicals have an oxygen- or nitrogen-based unpaired electron. Classical examples are superoxide anion (O_2^-), hydroxyl radical ($\bullet OH^-$), and nitric oxide (NO). O_2^- is formed from oxygen. The reaction of O_2^- and hydrogen peroxide (H_2O_2) in the presence of transition metal produces $\bullet OH$. When catalyzed by neutrophil myeloperoxidase (MPO), H_2O_2 and a chloride form hypochlorous acid (HOCl) (Figure 5.1).[1] H_2O_2 acts as a central precursor. H_2O_2 levels reflect the underlying state of oxidative stress in the lungs.

II. MEASURING EXHALED HYDROGEN PEROXIDE

H_2O_2 is a volatile oxidant that passes the alveolar membrane and can be measured in exhaled air. Analysis of H_2O_2 requires cooling of the expired breath, which results

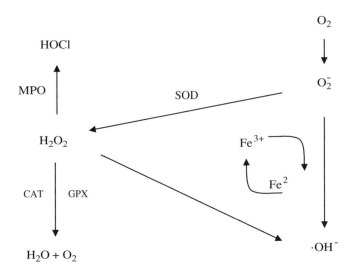

FIGURE 5.1 The formation of hydrogen peroxide (H_2O_2) and other ROS. CAT, catalase; Fe^{2+}, ferrous ion; Fe^{3+}, ferric ion; GPX, glutathione peroxidase; O_2^-, superoxide anion; •OH^-, hydroxyl radical; SOD, superoxide dismutase; HOCl, hypochlorous acid.

in condensation. Cooling of the exhaled air in a tube can be achieved by using wet or dry ice or liquid nitrogen.

The patient is instructed to breathe tidally directly into the tubing or through a mouthpiece connected to the tubing (Figure 5.2).[2] It takes about 5 to 10 minutes to collect 1 to 5 ml in adults. Given that most substances are present not only in the lower airways but throughout the respiratory tract, including the nasal passages, it is important to prevent contamination of the exhaled breath. Contamination with saliva should also be prevented because it contains high levels of H_2O_2.

Methods of H_2O_2 measurement in exhaled breath condensate (EBC) are based on the ability of H_2O_2 to react with suitable substrates, leading to the release of color, light, or fluorescence. Two methods of analysis have been used most: the spectrophotometric method according to Gallati and Pracht and the fluorimetric method according to Hyslop and Sklar or to Ruch.[3] In the first method the EBC is mixed with 3'3'5'5'-tetramethylbenzidine and horseradish peroxidase and the reaction is stopped by adding sulfuric acid. In the other methods the EBC is mixed with *p*-hydroxyphenylacetic acid and horseradish peroxidase. The reaction products are measured with a spectrophotometer or a fluorimeter.

A. PRACTICAL ASPECTS OF MEASURING EXHALED HYDROGEN PEROXIDE

The concentration in normal individuals is almost undetectable and in many diseases the levels found are at the lower detection limit of the assays employed. The collection and storage of the samples is also a source of errors. Samples (after adding the reagents) should be frozen rapidly because H_2O_2 changes back into its volatile form. Furthermore, the H_2O_2 concentration is not only determined by the airway inflammation — other factors also appear to influence the concentration.

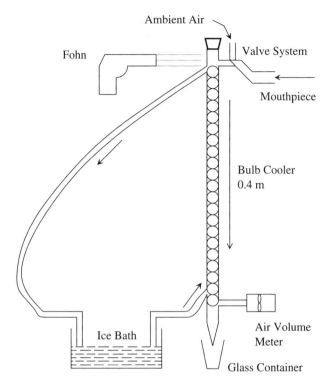

FIGURE 5.2 An example of an EBC collecting device. The patient breathes tidally into the mouthpiece and the exhaled air goes down the tube while countercurrent ice water cools the air; condensation water can be collected in the container.

First, smoking influences the H_2O_2 concentration in EBC, not only because cigarette smoke contains many oxidants, but also because smoking stimulates airway inflammation. There are other complicating factors. Exercise appears to increase the production of oxidants and could thus influence the H_2O_2 concentration in the breath condensate. Food and beverage intake might also influence the H_2O_2 concentration, possibly due to oxidants and/or antioxidants in some products.[4,5] Schleiss[6] and van Beurden[7] observed rather high variations within repeated measurements (variation coefficient 60 to 80%). It is therefore important to measure subjects at the same time of the day and under similar conditions when exhaled H_2O_2 is used to study patients or healthy subjects.

III. RESULTS IN DIFFERENT SUBJECTS

Several groups have explored the value of H_2O_2 measurement in different groups of subjects such as smokers and patients with asthma or chronic obstructive pulmonary disease (COPD). In general, it is difficult to compare different studies because of differences in procedures and analysis techniques. Moreover, most studies were performed with a small study population.

In healthy, young, nonsmoking subjects, exhaled H_2O_2 levels range from 0.01 to 0.09 µmol/l. However, van Beurden et al.[7] measured exhaled H_2O_2 in elderly healthy persons, all smokers or ex-smokers, and found a higher H_2O_2 concentration (0.21 µmol/l). Nowak et al.[8] found higher levels of exhaled H_2O_2 in healthy smokers compared with nonsmokers.

Few investigators studied exhaled H_2O_2 levels in COPD patients. Two cross-sectional studies showed an increased concentration of exhaled H_2O_2 in stable COPD patients compared with healthy subjects. Exhaled H_2O_2 levels appeared to be lower in current smokers in the study by Dekhuijzen et al.,[9] whereas Nowak et al.[10] found no difference between current and ex-smokers. The concentration was further increased in COPD patients with an exacerbation. In contrast, van Beurden et al.[7] did not find a difference in levels of exhaled H_2O_2 between stable COPD patients and elderly healthy smokers, which could be explained by a possible effect of age and smoking history on exhaled H_2O_2. The exhaled H_2O_2 concentration appeared to be the same in current smokers and ex-smokers, though the subgroups were small.

Most studies measuring exhaled H_2O_2 have been performed in asthma patients.[11-13] Exhaled H_2O_2 levels were increased in asthmatic children and adults. There was an inverse correlation between H_2O_2 concentration and forced expiratory volume in 1 second (FEV_1) percentage of predicted, and exhaled H_2O_2 concentration was related to the number of sputum eosinophils and airway hyperresponsiveness in asthma of different severity.

Few intervention studies have been performed investigating the effect of treatment on the H_2O_2 concentration. Recently, Ferreira et al.[14] treated 20 stable COPD patients (mean FEV_1 55% predicted) for 2 weeks with beclomethasone (500 µg bid or placebo). The baseline H_2O_2 concentration did not change after treatment. Van Beurden et al.[15] performed a cross-over study in which COPD patients were treated for 4 weeks with beclomethasone-hydrofluoroalkane-134a (800 µg bid) or fluticasone (750 µg bid) and found a reduction (0.1 and 0.2 µmol/l, respectively) in exhaled H_2O_2 level in both treatment groups. The difference in effect could be explained by the longer treatment period in this study. Kasielski et al.[16] performed an intervention study with N-acetyl-L-cysteine (NAC; 600 mg daily), which is an antioxidant, and placebo in 44 stable COPD patients for a period of 1 year. The exhaled H_2O_2 concentration was significantly lower in patients treated with NAC compared with placebo after 9 and 12 months.

In asthma patients ($n = 17$) one intervention study has been performed comparing the effect of a 4-week treatment with inhaled corticosteroids on the H_2O_2 concentration and placebo.[17] The baseline concentration was significantly higher in asthmatic patients than in normal subjects. The H_2O_2 concentration decreased significantly after treatment and was significantly lower than that in the placebo group.

In summary, levels of exhaled H_2O_2 are higher in stable COPD patients compared with young, healthy, nonsmoking controls. When H_2O_2 levels of stable COPD patients are compared with controls of the same age and smoking status, there seems to be no difference. In healthy persons, exhaled H_2O_2 levels are higher in current smokers, whereas in COPD patients levels seem to be the same in current smokers and ex-smokers. One study has shown that exhaled H_2O_2 is increased further during exacerbation. Inhaled corticosteroids could have an effect on the exhaled H_2O_2

concentration after a longer treatment period. One study has suggested that antioxidant therapy reduces exhaled H_2O_2 levels. In asthma patients, the exhaled H_2O_2 concentration is higher than in COPD patients and is reduced after treatment with inhaled corticosteroids. Measuring exhaled H_2O_2 is not yet standardized and there seems to be quite a large intraindividual variability.

IV. CLINICAL USE OF EXHALED HYDROGEN PEROXIDE

There is an increasing interest in noninvasive biomarkers, which can be used to investigate the pathophysiology, treatment, and prognosis of COPD. H_2O_2 is biomarker that can be measured in a relatively simple way and noninvasively. However, the procedure of measuring H_2O_2 in EBC is not yet standardized and few randomized studies have been performed.

It is important to use an efficient, sensitive, and reproducible procedure for measuring H_2O_2 in EBC. Given that the mean H_2O_2 concentration in EBC in stable COPD patients is low (0.2 µmol/l), it is also important to have a low detection limit.

Several studies have shown that the H_2O_2 concentration increases significantly during the day in both COPD patients and healthy controls. The cause of this increase is still unclear, but it is possible that exhaled H_2O_2 levels are influenced by the intake of food and drinks or exercise. It is therefore very important to perform H_2O_2 measurements in follow-up studies at the same time of day under the same conditions.

It is not clear whether COPD patients produce higher levels of exhaled H_2O_2 than healthy persons. This means that exhaled H_2O_2 levels cannot be used to differentiate COPD patients from healthy persons. On the other hand, asthma patients have significantly higher levels of exhaled H_2O_2 than healthy persons and COPD patients. The H_2O_2 concentration in EBC is more elevated during exacerbations and decreases after treatment in asthma patients. In COPD patients this seems to be less obvious, although inhaled corticosteroids reduce the H_2O_2 concentration in stable COPD patients.

Additional studies are needed to establish the clinical usefulness of measuring hydrogen peroxide in EBC.

Further Reading

1. Repine, J.E., Bast, A., and Lankhorst I., Oxidative stress in chronic obstructive pulmonary disease, *Am. J. Crit. Care Med.*, 156, 341, 1997.
2. van Beurden, W.J.C. et al., An efficient and reproducible method for measuring hydrogen peroxide in exhaled breath condensate, *Respiration*, 96, 196, 2002.
3. Kharitonov, S.A. and Barnes, P.J., Exhaled markers of pulmonary disease, *Am. J. Respir. Crit. Care Med.*, 163, 1693, 2001.
4. Halliwell, B., Clement, M.V., and Long, L.H., Hydrogen peroxide in the human body, *FEBS Lett.*, 486, 10, 2000.
5. Heunks, L.M.A. et al., Xanthine oxidase is involved in exercise-induced oxidative stress in chronic obstructive pulmonary disease, *Am. J. Physiol.*, 277, R1697, 1997.

6. Schleiss, M.B. et al., The concentration of hydrogen peroxide in exhaled air depends on expiratory flow rate, *Eur. Respir. J.*, 16, 1115, 2000.

7. van Beurden, W.J.C. et al., Variability of exhaled hydrogen peroxide in stable COPD patients and matched healthy controls, *Respiration*, 69, 211, 2002.

8. Nowak, D. et al., Exhalation of hydrogen peroxide and thiobarbituric acid-reactive substances (TBARS) by healthy subjects, *Free Rad. Biol. Med.*, 30, 178, 2001.

9. Dekhuijzen, P.N.R. et al., Increased exhalation of hydrogen peroxide in patients with stable and unstable chronic obstructive pulmonary disease, *Am. J. Respir. Crit. Care Med.*, 154, 813, 1996.

10. Nowak, D., et al., Increased content of thiobarbituric acid-reactive substances and hydrogen peroxide in the expired breath condensate of patients with stable chronic obstructive pulmonary disease: no significant effect of cigarette smoking, *Respir. Med*, 93, 389, 1999.

11. Antczak, A., et al., Increased hydrogen peroxide and thiobarbituric acid-reactive products in expired breath condensate of asthmatic patients, *Eur. Respir. J.*, 10, 1235, 1997.

12. Jobsis, Q. et al., Hydrogen peroxide in exhaled air is increased in stable asthmatic children, *Eur. Respir. J.*, 10, 519, 1997.

13. Dohlman, A.W., Black, H.R., and Royall, J.A., Expired breath hydrogen peroxide is a marker of acute airway inflammation in pediatric patients with asthma, *Am. Rev. Respir. Dis.*, 148, 955, 1993.

14. Ferreira Martens, I. et al., Exhaled nitric oxide and hydrogen peroxide in patients with chronic obstructive pulmonary disease (effects of inhaled beclomethasone), *Am. J. Respir. Crit. Care Med.*, 164, 1012, 2001.

15. van Beurden, W.J.C., Effects of inhaled corticosteroids with different lung deposition on exhaled hydrogen peroxide in stable COPD patients, *Respiration*, 70, 242, 2003.

16. Kasielski, M. and Nowak, D., Long-term administration of N-acetylcysteine decreases hydrogen peroxide exhalation in subjects with chronic obstructive pulmonary disease, *Respir. Med.*, 95, 448, 2001.

17. Antczak, A. et al., Inhaled glucocorticosteroids decrease hydrogen peroxide level in expired air condensate in asthmatic patients, *Respir. Med.*, 94, 416, 2000.

6 Measurement of Exhaled Breath Condensate pH: Implications for Pathophysiology and Monitoring of Inflammatory Airway Diseases

Benjamin Gaston and John F. Hunt

CONTENTS

I. INTRODUCTION

A variety of biochemical processes relevant to airways disease are pH dependent. Evidence is accumulating that airway pH may be low in a variety of airway diseases ranging from viral respiratory infections to asthma exacerbations. It now appears that airway pH is regulated to prevent cytotoxicity and to enhance innate host defense. Acid stress, like oxidant stress, is an important pathologic mechanism of airway disease. Thus, understanding the mechanisms involved in airway pH regulation has become an area of interest for researchers studying the pathophysiology of airways diseases, the development of new treatment modalities, and noninvasive mechanisms for measuring and monitoring airway inflammation.

II. ABNORMAL AIRWAY pH: IMPLICATIONS FOR DISEASE PATHOPHYSIOLOGY

pH ($-\log$ [H^+]) is carefully regulated in all living systems. Certain mammalian organs (for example, the kidney and stomach) will set pH in a particular compartment at a value substantially different from that of blood; this benefits the organism as a whole. It is increasingly appreciated that mammalian airway pH is also exquisitely well-regulated and can experience deviations from normal in order to respond to environmental insults such as infections. These recent observations suggest that there may be exciting opportunities for monitoring and treating airway disease based on our improved understanding of the role of pH regulation in the airway epithelium.

It is difficult to measure airway pH directly *in vivo*. Different methods give substantially different results, depending on the type of pH probe, the mechanism for grounding the reference electrode, and the use of acidifying topical anesthetics (such as lidocaine).[1-4] Methods involving removal of airway lining fluid for pH measurement are also imperfect because the fluid layer is only microns deep[5]; efforts to remove a sample are invariably complicated by the uncertainty principle, which holds that to make a measurement, one must change the composition of that which is being measured.

However, *in vivo* and *ex vivo* measurements of airway pH in normal humans, ferrets, rats, rabbits, and cows have been made. Secretions suctioned from the tracheobronchial tree in 126 humans revealed a mean pH of 7.73 ± 0.54.[6] These data are quite comparable to exhaled breath condensate (EBC) pH measurements from healthy subjects (7.65 ± 0.20).[7] The *ex vivo* tracheal pH of ferrets measured by pH probe, is ~ 7.0.[8] The *in vivo* tracheal pH has been shown to be 7.42 to 7.57 in rats,[9] 7.7 in rabbits,[10] and 7.67 to 8.27 in cows.[11]

Both indirect and direct measures of lung water pH suggest that airway proton concentrations may be high in airways disease, and that pH decreases in proportion to the acuity and/or severity of obstruction. EBC[7] pH decreases by more than 2 log orders of magnitude during acute asthma exacerbations. It also decreases, but generally not as much, in normal subjects who have viral respiratory infections.[12] Peak expiratory flow and airway pH measured by trans-cricoid pH probe concurrently decrease in subjects with asthma during episodes of gastroesophageal reflux.[4] There are reports that the pH of nasal secretions decreases during allergic and viral rhinitis episodes, but not during bacterial rhinitis[13]; these issues have not been fully clarified. Expectorated sputum in subjects with asthma has been reported to be acidic.[14,15] Breath condensate pH also has been reported to be low in subjects with chronic obstructive pulmonary disease (COPD), cystic fibrosis, bronchiectasis, and acute lung injury (ALI).[16-19]

A recent study of the asthmatic lung using hyperpolarized helium magnetic resonance imaging has provided a remarkable visualization of reversible airflow obstruction in asthma,[20] and reveals what our intuition has known all along: that asthmatic airway anatomy and functional disturbances are patchy — irregular and rapidly changing. It can be anticipated that airway biochemical disturbance likewise might be patchy. Airway pH might be abnormal in one location and not in another, and pH abnormalities might be transient. To date there exist no studies invasively mapping airway pH in disease, and such studies might well be limited by the inability to access peripheral airways for invasive measurement.

A. POTENTIAL CAUSES OF A DECREASE IN AIRWAY pH

Though it is an imperfect analogy, we find it helpful to conceptualize the regulation of airway pH in the context of the regulation of urine pH. In this analogy, the alveolus equates to the glomerulus, and the airway equates to the nephron. In the nephron, filtrate in need of pH regulation is produced in the glomerulus; a variety of different enzyme systems then modulate the luminal pH in the proximal and distal tubules. In the normal airway, a variety of different factors might favor acidification of airway lining fluid in the alveolus. Perhaps the most important of these is the low pH[3,4] of lamellar bodies secreted by alveolar type 2 cells.[21] These lamellar bodies are acidified before excretion by vacuolar ATPases (VATPases) in the lamellar body membrane. The teleology of this low lamellar body pH is incompletely understood but may involve alveolar host defense and maintenance of surfactant proteins B and C in a favorable state for activity before excretion (analogous to maintenance of stable procaspases in the acidic mitochondrial intermembrane space).[22] Whatever the reason for this acidification, continuous excretion of lamellar bodies into the alveolus is likely to promote acidification. In addition, the normal alveolus contains large numbers of macrophages that also contain acidic granules such as lysosomes.[23] Necrosis of these macrophages might also contribute to alveolar acidification. Finally, the pCO_2 is higher in the alveolus than in any other part of the airway. Indeed, indirect preliminary evidence (unpublished) based on nitrite inhalation suggests that the alveolus is somewhat acidic in normal subjects. We believe that this somewhat acidic distal airway fluid becomes more alkaline as it works its way proximally. The known mechanisms for this proximal alkalinization appear to involve airway epithelial cell enzyme systems, including carbonic anhydrases[24] and glutaminase,[25] in addition to ion channel activity (Na^+/H^+ exchange systems and HCO_3^-/Cl^- channels)[26] and the presence of buffering proteins such as albumin in the airway lining fluid.

In disease states, the situation becomes more complex. Conceptually, we believe that the more proximal airway becomes more acidic as a result of inflammatory processes. Teleologically, this effect may serve to protect the airway against infection (analogous to gastric acidification) as a mechanism of innate host defense. For example, Th1 cytokines can activate at least three acidifying processes in the airway. First, it has been appreciated recently that airway epithelial cells have nicotinamide adenine dinucleotide phosphate (NADPH) oxidase-like activity[27] that could be primed by inflammation.[28] Activation of epithelial NADPH oxidase not only produces superoxide but also could result in proton production and excretion into the lumen.[27,29] Indeed, it is even hypothesized that the NADPH oxidase protein might serve as a proton channel. Second, Th1 cytokine stimulation inhibits airway epithelial glutaminase activity, preventing excretion of buffering ammonia and bicarbonate into the airway lumen.[25,30] Third, cytokine stimulation recruits and activates macrophages and neutrophils in the airway lumen; necrosis of these inflammatory cells is acidifying. In addition to these nonspecific inflammatory responses, there might also be disease-specific acidifying mechanisms. For example, the cystic fibrosis transmembrane regulatory protein (CFTR) can regulate HCO_3^- efflux into the airway,[31,32] and defective airway alkalinization has been proposed to be involved in the pathophysiology of cystic fibrosis.[33]

B. AIRWAY EFFECTS OF ACIDIFICATION

Inhalation of acidic droplets in the form of air pollution or acid challenges (classically, citric acid) causes a variety of adverse effects on lung health and recapitulates many aspects of asthmatic airways disease. Clinical features resulting from acid inhalation include airway inflammation, bronchial hyperreactivity, reversible airway obstruction, mucus overproduction, and cough. Observations associated with airway epithelial cell acidification *in vitro* include impaired ciliary motility,[34] increased mucus viscosity,[11,35] augmentation of neurogenic bronchoconstriction,[36,37] enhanced necrosis of inflammatory cells such as eosinophils with release of cytotoxic mediators,[7] and enhancement of the cytotoxicity of potential inflammatory mediators such as nitrite, peroxynitrite, and superoxide.[38,39] Peroxynitrite stability and cytotoxicity are pH dependent (pKa 6.8). Nitrite (pKa 3.4), once protonated, will form NO through nitrous acid. Furthermore, hypochlorous acid (HOCl), which mediates oxidative damage both to the host and to invading microorganisms, has pKa very close to neutral and its toxicity, following formation by myeloperoxidase, is enhanced by acidification.

All of these untoward effects might contribute to the pathophysiology of airways disease. As noted above, exogenous acidification mimics many effects of asthma, COPD, and cystic fibrosis. Indeed, it can be argued that low airway pH not only results from chronic neutrophilic inflammation in bronchiectasis, but might also promote airway stasis and injury associated with the development of bronchiectasis. In addition, there is evidence that the pH of respiratory mucus is low in subjects with impending ventilator-associated pneumonia, and this decline in pH occurs prior to the appearance of other clinical evidence.[40]

In summary, increasing evidence suggests that airway pH is carefully regulated—both in health and disease—by a variety of different mechanisms. Th1 cytokines and inflammation appear to be associated with a decrease in airway pH that might have a role both in host defense and in acute and chronic airway injury. There is evidence that this airway acidification mechanism might contribute to the pathophysiology of airway disease in acute viral infections, asthma, COPD, cystic fibrosis, bronchiectasis, and ALI.

III. EXHALED BREATH CONDENSATE ASSAYS

Several groups have reported that pH is low in the EBC of patients with inflammatory airways diseases such as asthma, cystic fibrosis, COPD, bronchiectasis, and

ALI.[7,16–19] This "acidopnea" is extraordinarily reproducible, is unrelated to hyper- or hypoventilation, is present when the upper airway is bypassed by endotracheal intubation, and is accentuated and stabilized—but not dependent upon—removal of CO_2 from the sample.[41] More importantly, it is highly reproducible and informative with regard to disease severity; i.e., it is inversely associated with airway inflammatory cells and directly associated with forced expiratory volume in 1 second (FEV_1).[16] In addition, EBC pH normalizes with therapy.[7,17,18] The process of collection and measurement of EBC pH also is extremely simple, an important feature that should not be underestimated. In this section, we provide general comments regarding measurement techniques for EBC pH.

The pH of EBC seems predominantly determined by the volatile water-soluble constituents, as opposed to nonvolatiles that have evolved by aerosolization from the airway wall. As such, a low pH in the EBC is a reflection of enhanced exhalation of water-soluble volatile acids and/or decreased exhalation of water-soluble volatile bases. In an acidic source fluid (in our case, the airway lining fluid), volatile bases are trapped as nonvolatile ions, whereas acids are protonated to neutral molecules and therefore may become volatile. Thus, acidic EBC reflects airway lining fluid acidification. The caveat is important: In disease, the airway is acidified somewhere, and to some degree, but the extent and precise location of the acidification is not assessed in EBC assays. Given the lack of homogeneity in asthmatic airway obstruction and inflammation, it would not be surprising to find that airway pH is likewise patchy. It is important to emphasize that breath condensate pH reflects at least the concentrations, pKAs, volatility, and solubility of acids and bases in the airways and lungs in addition to the determinants of the relative amounts of vapor and droplets, including Reynold's number and the surface tension at different airway levels.

It also is important to emphasize that the solute determinants (acids and bases) of acidopnea have not all been determined. Having low ammonium concentration in the condensate is necessary, but not sufficient, to explain low pH in subjects with asthma. In most of the data, there is a fascinating gap between pH 7.4 and 7.5 (in mild asthmatic subjects) in which there are no data points. This likely reflects "silent buffers" slightly above and below this range. As the composition of these condensates is determined, we hope to accumulate substantially more knowledge about the pathophysiology of inflammatory lung disease.

A. Equipment Issues

Several important issues must be considered when the measurements are made. First, the collection system needs to be free of soluble acids and buffers. We have found that a variety of different collection tube materials give the same pH result (aluminum, Tygon, Teflon, polypropylene, glass, and stainless steel, for example) as long as the entire system is rinsed with deionized water and blown dry. The system should be sealed before use so that environmental pollutants do not lodge in the lumen. Second, it might be important to eliminate salivary contamination. Measurements of salivary amylase activity are not necessarily satisfactory to rule out the possibility of salivary contamination because the protein is subject to proteolysis during its storage, and commercial assays are not sensitive enough to detect small amounts of saliva. A gravity-based salivary trap or drain may not prevent microcontamination because airflow might carry saliva into the collector. A 0.2- to 0.3-μm filter can be used to help minimize salivary contamination. Data to date support that use of such a filter does not affect pH measurement, a finding consistent with the volatility of the compounds determining pH. A filter might affect concentrations of nonvolatile solutes, however. For ease of use, it is ideal to have a system that will enable an adequate sample to be obtained in as short a time as possible. With regard to temperature of collection, if a condenser is very cold, it will collect EBC in the form of a solid (snow). We believe that EBC pH is controlled by water-soluble volatiles, and these volatiles might not be as well trapped when EBC is collected at too low a temperature. Although condenser temperatures down to –40°C have been found to provide EBC pH values identical to those at temperatures of +10°C,[41] suggesting that EBC pH is not affected by collection temperature, these studies have been limited to healthy volunteers. We currently recommend condenser temperatures be maintained in the range of 0 to +10°C, which avoids this theoretical concern while keeping the system simple and highly flexible for use in a variety of settings, including the home.

B. Patient Issues

EBC can be collected in almost any environment. The technique lends itself to use in the operating room, the intensive care unit, clinic, pulmonary function laboratory, worksite, and to the home. Unlike other assays in EBC, pH measurement also is suitably simple to be done at home. It is desirable to minimize sampling time, and the EBC pH measurement has proven to be independent of duration of collection between 2 and 7 minutes. The pH of EBC is not an artifact of oral contamination because EBC pH is the same in consecutive samples obtained orally and subsequently through an endotracheal tube ($n = 32$).[41] These data obviate any argument that oral ammonia is the principal determinant of EBC pH.[42] Indeed, although ammonia concentration can vary widely in EBC (same-subject intraweek coefficient of variation [CV], ~50%), EBC pH varies little (intraweek CV, <4%). Ammonia is found in low concentrations in EBC samples that have low pH. However, the converse is not necessarily true: EBC pH can be normal despite low ammonia levels. In this regard, it seems that low ammonia levels in EBC reflect not only production of ammonia in the airway, but also trapping of ammonia (as ammonium) when the airway lining fluid is acidic.

Although patients with obstructive lung disease are often hypoxic, and therefore hyperventilate to some extent, the data demonstrate that spontaneous and dramatic changes in minute ventilation (resulting in changes in end-tidal CO_2 values between 25 and 47) do not affect breath condensate pH at all.[41] In analysis of more than 4000 samples collected from 160 subjects in one study, we identified no effects of age or sex on EBC pH values. The effects of pregnancy or ovulatory cycle have not been examined.

Ingestion of foods and drinks that contain volatile acids within 30 minutes of sample collection may cause artifact. We have found this to be true predominantly for foods containing vinegar (acetic acid). We recommend that sample be collected

1 hour or more after eating. Other than this one instruction, it does not appear to be necessary to provide specific controls on how a patient breathes when providing a sample for EBC pH assay. Duration of collection, depth of breathing, frequency of breathing, and nasal air entrainment do not affect the results.

C. ASSAY ISSUES

Measurement of EBC pH, when deaerated with argon gas, has proven to be a remarkably simple, reproducible, and robust assay. There are several key advantages to the EBC pH measurement. First, the assays employed are completely suitable for the fluid and readily able to distinguish normal from abnormal. When measuring pH, we are not dealing with tiny concentrations of unstable molecules. Second, the timing of the assay is not critical. It can be done immediately or years later. Third, the coefficient of variation between same sample pH measurements divided into aliquots and measured concurrently, or years apart, approaches zero. Fourth, the assay is very inexpensive. Fifth, the standard concerns regarding uncertain degree of dilution of EBC biomarkers do not directly apply. As a ratio of acid to base, pH serves as its own internal standard. Keep in mind that the sample storage container (often a microcentrifuge tube) should be inert and free of any acids, bases, or buffers, and should be cleaned, dried, and preserved just like the collection system. Duration of storage in −4 to −80°C temperatures does not alter the EBC pH.[41]

As a general rule, we recommend deaerating samples for 5 to 10 minutes with an inert gas. This rapidly moves CO_2 out of the EBC — essentially standardizing the assay by preventing ambient CO_2 from affecting the results. The deaerated sample provides a pH measurement that is completely stable, and that can be reassayed years later to provide precisely the same value.[41] However, it is important that the deaerating gas contain no acids or bases. We use argon to deaerate the sample because it is very inexpensive and it is heavier than air, thus protecting the sample from reabsorbing atmospheric CO_2 while the pH is measured. A simple assay to ensure that the deaeration gas contains no volatile acids (such as CO_2) is to apply the deaeration system to deionized water: if the deaeration results in a decline in pH, it is not satisfactory.

IV. ACIDOPNEA: THE CHICKEN AND THE EGG

The technique of pH measurement in EBC has been used successfully by many research groups to identify and follow lung inflammation. In one study, along with tight correlations of EBC pH with eosinophilic and neutrophilic sputum cell counts, there was a correlation between EBC pH and FEV_1.[16] This is consistent with FEV_1 decline caused either by the inflammation or more directly by the airway acidification altering bronchial muscle tone. The order of the chicken and egg becomes unclear here. Although it is entirely clear that EBC pH decline is not caused by airflow obstruction itself — given that methacholine-induced obstruction does not alter EBC pH[41] — it remains uncertain if airway acidification is secondary to inflammation or is the principal initiator of inflammation. Perhaps shedding some light on this, EBC pH declines within 2 hours after nasal inoculation with a common cold virus (rhinovirus), long before cellular inflammation or clinical symptoms become evident.[12] This acidification is the first identifiable abnormality that occurs with rhinovirus infection, and provides strong evidence that airway pH homeostasis is disturbed as a primary event in the inflammatory process.

V. IMPLICATIONS OF ACIDOPNEA FOR DISEASE MONITORING

Experimental infection with human rhinovirus (HRV) results in a decrease in EBC pH, both in asthmatic and control subjects,[12] adding to the data implicating a lower respiratory response to the common cold. The mechanism may be neuronal — particularly cholinergic. There is evidence that the decrease in EBC pH is associated with an increase in EBC acetic acid levels,[43] in addition to virally induced Th1 cytokine effect that causes an inhibition of airway epithelial glutaminase. With regard to longitudinal assessment, it is also of interest that there is a biphasic decrease in condensate pH that might be related to cycles of viral replication in the nose, followed by a long, gradual normalization during several days. Because most acute asthma exacerbations that require hospitalization follow intercurrent, community-acquired viral respiratory infections, it is possible that decreased airway pH in these asthmatic subjects is related, at least in part, to virus-induced acidification. In addition to following resolution of virally associated asthma exacerbations, assessment of breath condensate pH might be useful as a noninvasive marker for the presence or resolution of a viral illness in children with school obligations or adults with work obligations.

EBC pH is low in subjects with moderate and severe asthma and is even lower in subjects with acute asthma exacerbations.[7,16] The pH values in EBC are proportional to markers of airway obstruction such as FEV_1 and increase with anti-inflammatory therapy. Importantly, decreases in EBC pH are more common in asthmatics being withdrawn from fluticasone therapy than in controls. Because breath condensate pH can be measured at home, it is conceivable that exacerbations could be predicted based on EBC measurements. This would be particularly true for exacerbations precipitated by viral illnesses. The decease in EBC pH occurs within hours of infection with rhinovirus, and precedes development of not only asthma symptoms, but also the symptoms of the cold itself, thus providing an opportunity for earlier and perhaps briefer intervention with anti-inflammatory therapy.

The role of EBC pH measurement in cystic fibrosis, COPD, and bronchiectasis remains to be defined. Although it is appreciated that increasing severity of these lung diseases is associated with a lower baseline EBC pH, and that therapies aimed at treating exacerbations of these diseases improve EBC pH,[16,17] longitudinal data suggesting that outcomes can be predicted based on the measurements are not available.

In the case of ALI, EBC pH might be useful for diagnosis and anticipatory management. In this regard, EBC can be readily obtained from intubated subjects. In particular, patients who have undergone operative lobectomy — who might be at risk for a long ventilator course/ALI — have a lower EBC pH, on the average, than patients at lower risk following coronary artery bypass graft.[44] Because there are interventions that might prevent acute respiratory distress syndrome (ARDS)/ALI if it can be anticipated before it develops into a full syndrome, EBC pH might have a role in the management of these patients and other at-risk patients (such as lung transplantation patients). Additional studies will need to be done to define the precise clinical role of these assays in this setting.

Perhaps the most interesting of all potential applications of EBC pH analysis to lung injury is to consider the potential therapeutic implications. Ahmed et al.[45,46] have shown that nebulization of a base (sodium bicarbonate) substantially improves peak flows in asthmatic subjects. Similarly, many authors have reported that systemic use of proton pump inhibitors results in improvement in asthma outcomes for many patients. It is assumed that this improvement is associated with treatment of gastroesophageal reflux — likely related to decreased microaspiration of acid — but it conceivably also involves inhibition, to some extent, of endogenous airway acidification mechanisms. Our preliminary data suggest that inhalation of buffers decreases expired NO and might improve lung function in subjects with obstructive disease. These and related data suggest that the identification of patients with low EBC pH might enable targeted drug delivery to alkalinize the airway, providing another treatment option for patients with asthma, COPD, cystic fibrosis, and ALI.

As a corollary, airway acidification might have evolved for the purpose of preventing microbial growth. Survival of bacteria (including *Mycobacterium tuberculosis* and other Mycobacterium),[47–49] rhinovirus,[50,51] and other organisms is impeded by low pH. Interestingly, *M. tuberculosis* requires exogenous ammonia[52,53] (in addition to a neutral pH environment) to survive. Inhibition of glutaminase might prevent survival of the organism following initial inhalation into the airway, before phagocytosis by macrophages. Thus, airway acidification might be an important modality to augment airway defense in certain situations. Speculatively, EBC pH might identify effects of severe acute respiratory syndrome (SARS), as well as biological warfare agents.

VI. SUMMARY

Airway acidification might occur endogenously, perhaps as an innate immune response to invading microorganisms. In certain settings, this protective acidification response, or other causes of airway acidification such as aspiration of gastric acid, might lead to pathological consequences, and thus be considered acid stress. Acid stress injures the airway, causing inflammation and the symptoms of obstructive airway disease. Exhaled breath condensate pH measurement is a simple modality to identify abnormal acidic load in the airway, whether it is an appropriate immune response, or a pathologic process. The technique is very hardy, simple, well studied technically, inexpensive, and useful. The likelihood of EBC pH becoming a clinical diagnostic and management tool in the near future is high.

ACKNOWLEDGMENTS

Supported by United States National Institutes of Health (NIH) grants R01 HL 69170, RO1 HL 59337, and R01 HL72429-01, and an NIH Asthma Center grant 1U19-A134607.

FURTHER READING

1. McShane, D. et al., Airway surface pH in subjects with cystic fibrosis, *Eur. Respir. J.*, 21, 37, 2003.

2. Guerrin, F. et al., Bronchial pH measurement in situ. Effects of metabolic acidosis, *J. Physiol. (Paris)*, 62, Suppl. 2, 282, 1970.

3. Guerrin, F. et al., Apport de la pH metrie bronchique in situ, *Prog. Respir. Res.*, 6, 372, 1971.

4. Jack, C.I. et al., Simultaneous tracheal and oesophageal pH measurements in asthmatic patients with gastro-oesophageal reflux, *Thorax*, 50, 201, 1995.

5. Widdicombe, J.H. et al., Regulation of depth and composition of airway surface liquid, *Eur. Respir. J.*, 10, 2892, 1997.

6. Metheny, N.A. et al., pH and concentration of bilirubin in feeding tube aspirates as predictors of tube placement, *Nurs. Res.*, 48, 189, 1999.

7. Hunt, J.F. et al., Endogenous airway acidification. Implications for asthma pathophysiology, *Am. J. Respir. Crit. Care Med.*, 161, 694, 2000.

8. Kyle, H., Ward, J.P., and Widdicombe, J.G., Control of pH of airway surface liquid of the ferret trachea in vitro, *J. Appl. Physiol.*, 68, 135, 1990.

9. Gatto, L.A., pH of mucus in rat trachea, *J. Appl. Physiol.*, 50, 1224, 1981.

10. Gatto, L.A., pH of mucus in rabbit trachea: cholinergic stimulation and block, *Lung*, 163, 109, 1985.

11. Holma, B., Lindegren, M., and Andersen, J.M., pH effects on ciliomotility and morphology of respiratory mucosa, *Arch. Environ. Health*, 32, 216, 1977.

12. Ngamtrakulpanit, L. et al., Exhaled breath condensate acidification during rhinovirus cold, *Am. J. Respir. Crit. Care Med.*, 167, A446, 2003.

13. Small, P.A., 1999. Rapid diagnostic method for distinguishing allergies and infections. US Patent 5,910,421.

14. Ryley, H.C. and Brogan, T.D., Variation in the composition of sputum in chronic chest diseases, *Br. J. Exp. Pathol.*, 49, 625, 1968.

15. Shimura, S. et al., Chemical properties of bronchorrhea sputum in bronchial asthma, *Chest*, 94, 1211, 1988.

16. Kostikas, K. et al., pH in expired breath condensate of patients with inflammatory airway diseases, *Am. J. Respir. Crit. Care Med.*, 165, 1364, 2002.

17. Antczak, A., and Gorski, P., Endogenous airway acidification and oxidant overload in infectious exacerbation of COPD, *Am. J. Respir. Crit. Care Med.*, 163, 725A, 2001.

18. Tate, S. et al., Airways in cystic fibrosis are acidified: detection by exhaled breath condensate, *Thorax*, 57, 926, 2002.

19. Gessner, C. et al., Airway acidification in artificial ventilated patients, *Eur. Respir. J.*, 18, Suppl. 33, 480s, 2001.

20. Samee, S. et al., Imaging the lungs in asthmatic patients by using hyperpolarized helium-3 magnetic resonance: assessment of response to methacholine and exercise challenge, *J. Allergy Clin. Immunol.*, 111, 1205, 2003.

21. Wadsworth, S.J., Spitzer, A.R., and Chander, A., Ionic regulation of proton chemical (pH) and electrical gradients in lung lamellar bodies, *Am. J. Physiol.*, 273, L427, 1997.

22. Mannick, J.B. et al., *S*-Nitrosylation of mitochondrial caspases, *J. Cell Biol.*, 154, 1111, 2001.

23. Heilmann, P. et al., Intraphagolysosomal pH in canine and rat alveolar macrophages: flow cytometric measurements, *Environ. Health Perspect.*, 97, 115, 1992.

24. Swenson, E.R., Robertson, H.T., and Hlastala, M.P., Effects of carbonic anhydrase inhibition on ventilation-perfusion matching in the dog lung, *J. Clin. Invest.*, 92, 702, 1993.

25. Hunt, J.F. et al., Expression and activity of pH-regulatory glutaminase in the human airway epithelium, *Am. J. Respir. Crit. Care Med.*, 165, 101, 2002.

26. Dudeja, P.K. et al., Expression of the Na+/H+ and Cl-/HCO-3 exchanger isoforms in proximal and distal human airways, *Am. J. Physiol.*, 276, L971, 1999.

27. Schwarzer, C. et al., Expression of NADPH oxidase homologs and proton secretion in human airway epithelia, *FASEB J.*, 17, A819, 2003.

28. Miesel, R., Kurpisz, M., and Kroger, H., Suppression of inflammatory arthritis by simultaneous inhibition of nitric oxide synthase and NADPH oxidase, *Free Radic. Biol. Med.*, 20, 75, 1996.

29. Fischer, H., Widdicombe, J.H., and Illek, B., Acid secretion and proton conductance in human airway epithelium, *Am. J. Physiol. Cell Physiol.*, 282, C736, 2002.

30. Griffith, O.W., Glutaminase and the control of airway pH: yet another problem for the asthmatic lung?, *Am. J. Respir. Crit. Care Med.*, 165, 1, 2002.

31. Ballard, S.T. et al., CFTR involvement in chloride, bicarbonate, and liquid secretion by airway submucosal glands, *Am. J. Physiol.*, 277, L694, 1999.

32. Choi, J.Y. et al., Aberrant CFTR-dependent HCO3- transport in mutations associated with cystic fibrosis, *Nature*, 410, 94, 2001.

33. Coakley, R.D. and Boucher, R.C., Regulation and functional significance of airway surface liquid pH, *J.O.P.*, 2, Suppl. 4, 294, 2001.

34. Luk, C.K. and Dulfano, M.J., Effect of pH, viscosity and ionic-strength changes on ciliary beating frequency of human bronchial explants, *Clin. Sci.*, 64, 449, 1983.

35. Holma, B. and Hegg, P.O., pH- and protein-dependent buffer capacity and viscosity of respiratory mucus. Their interrelationships and influence on health, *Sci. Total Environ.*, 84, 71, 1989.

36. Ricciardolo, F.L.M. et al., Bronchoconstriction induced by citric acid inhalation in guinea pigs: role of tachykinins, bradykinin, and nitric oxide, *Am. J. Respir. Crit. Care Med.*, 159, 557, 1999.

37. Bevan, S. and Geppetti, P., Protons: small stimulants of capsaicin-sensitive sensory nerves, *Trends Neurosci.*, 17, 509, 1994.

38. Gaston, B. and Stamler, J.S., Nitrogen oxides, in *The Lung: Scientific Foundations*, Crystal, R.G., ed., 2nd ed., Lippincott-Raven, Philadelphia, 1997, pp. 239–253.

39. Crow, J.P. et al., On the pH-dependent yield of hydroxyl radical products from peroxynitrite, *Free Radic. Biol. Med.*, 16, 331, 1994.

40. Karnad, D.R., Mhaisekar, D.G., and Moralwar, K.V., Respiratory mucus pH in tracheostomized intensive care unit patients: effects of colonization and pneumonia, *Crit. Care Med.*, 18, 699, 1990.

41. Vaughan, J. et al., Exhaled breath condensate pH is a robust and reproducible assay of airway acidity, *Eur. Respir. J.*, 22, 889, 2003.

42. Effros, R.M. et al., Dilution of respiratory solutes in exhaled condensates, *Am. J. Respir. Crit. Care Med.*, 165, 663, 2002.

43. Vaughan, J.W. et al., Acetic acid contributes to exhaled breath condensate acidity in asthma, *Eur. Respir. J.*, 18, Suppl. 33, 463, 2001.

44. Moloney, E.D. et al., Exhaled breath condensate detects markers of acute lung injury after cardiothoracic surgery, *Am. J. Respir. Crit. Care Med.*, 2004 (in press).

45. Ahmed, T., Iskandrani, A., and Uddin, M.N., Sodium bicarbonate solution nebulization in the treatment of acute severe asthma, *Am. J. Ther.*, 7, 325, 2000.

46. Ahmed, T., Ali, J.M., and al-Sharif, A.F., Effect of alkali nebulization on bronchoconstriction in acute bronchial asthma, *Respir. Med.*, 87, 235, 1993.

47. Crowle, A. J. et al., Evidence that vesicles containing living, virulent *Mycobacterium tuberculosis* or *Mycobacterium avium* in cultured human macrophages are not acidic, *Infect. Immun.*, 59, 1823, 1991.

48. Gomes, M.S. et al., Survival of *Mycobacterium avium* and *Mycobacterium tuberculosis* in acidified vacuoles of murine macrophages, *Infect. Immun.*, 67, 3199, 1999.

49. Portaels, F. and Pattyn, S.R., Growth of mycobacteria in relation to the pH of the medium, *Ann. Microbiol. (Paris)*, 133, 213, 1982.

50. Hughes, J.H. et al., Acid lability of rhinovirus type 14: effect of pH, time, and temperature, *Proc. Soc. Exp. Biol. Med.*, 144, 555, 1973.

51. Hughes, J.H. et al., Acid lability of rhinoviruses: loss of C and D antigenicity after treatment at pH 3.0, *J. Immunol.*, 112, 919, 1974.

52. Gordon, A.H., Hart, P.D., and Young, M.R., Ammonia inhibits phagosome-lysosome fusion in macrophages, *Nature*, 286, 79, 1980.

53. Harth, G., Clemens, D.L., and Horwitz, M.A., Glutamine synthetase of *Mycobacterium tuberculosis*: extracellular release and characterization of its enzymatic activity, *Proc. Natl. Acad. Sci. U.S.A.*, 91, 9342, 1994.

7 Nitric Oxide-Derived Markers in Exhaled Breath Condensate

Sergei A. Kharitonov

CONTENTS

0-415-32465-3/05/$0.00+$1.50
© 2005 by CRC Press LLC

I. INTRODUCTION

Nitric oxide (NO) plays an important role in pulmonary diseases and the high intensity of nitrosative stress significantly contributes to the pathogenesis and clinical outcome of asthma and chronic obstructive pulmonary disease (COPD).[1] Nitration of proteins might be responsible for steroid resistance in asthma and the ineffectiveness of steroids in COPD, supporting the potential role of future therapeutic strategies aimed at regulating NO synthesis in asthma and COPD, and the importance of NO monitoring.[2]

The need to monitor inflammation and nitrosative stress in the lungs has led to the exploration of exhaled breath condensate (EBC), which might assist in monitoring pulmonary diseases, assessing disease severity, and assessing response to treatment.[1,3,4]

A. THE IMPORTANCE OF MONITORING LOCAL NITROSATIVE STRESS IN THE LUNG

The complexity of NO as a physiological messenger and cytotoxic or cytoprotective effector molecule is based on its biosynthesis (which includes transcriptional, translational, and posttranslational regulatory mechanisms) and its concentration, site of production, and association with other molecules or proteins.

NO binds to a variety of proteins (for example, cytochrome P450, the primary O_2-reducing protein) and inhibits its activity without being reduced.[5] This process allows O_2 to be reduced exclusively in the presence of NO but independently of NO, perhaps explaining the existence of discrepancies between the levels of oxidative stress and exhaled NO in more severe asthma[6] and COPD.[7]

1. Nitration of Proteins

Reactive nitrogen species (RNS) modify proteins in asthma and COPD, and the magnitude of this modification correlates with the degree of oxidative and nitrosative stresses. Protein nitration is unique among posttranslational modifications in its dependency on reactivity of tyrosine residues in the protein target. It might be achieved by peroxynitrite (formed from the reaction between NO and $O_2^{\cdot-}$), through the reaction of NO with protein tyrosyl radicals, or by the reaction of nitrite with peroxidases.[8]

Nitration of proteins by peroxynitrite is a dose-dependent process related to formation of two distinctive forms of nitrated proteins: stable 3-nitrotyrosine (nitration) and labile S-nitrosocysteine (S-nitrosation).[9] Both of these nitrated proteins can be further enzymatically modified by glutathione S-transferase or glutathione peroxidase via converting NO_2^- to NH_2^- in tyrosine residues; denitrating NO_2^- directly/indirectly in tyrosine residues; or changing S-nitrosothiol (SNO) to SH^- in cysteine residues, or denitrosation.

Nitration of mitochondrial proteins might change the activity of several enzymes involved in energy production (glutamate dehydrogenase), or in the electron transport chain (cytochrome oxidase and adenosine triphosphatase [ATPase]), or energy distribution (creatine kinase).[10] In fact, both energy production and apoptosis are affected by NO and related oxides[11] and are different in asthma and COPD. The susceptibility of asthmatic bronchial epithelium to oxidant-induced apoptosis is greater than normal,[12] but alveolar macrophages and bronchial epithelial cells from smokers have reduced cell death.[13] The activity of enzymes in the central bronchial epithelium that protect cells against oxidative damage[10] is low due to their nitration in patients with COPD.[14]

Protein nitration might be beneficial. Thus, it has been shown that surfactant protein A (SP-A), a product of tyrosine nitration of human pulmonary surfactant, downregulates T-cell-dependent alveolar inflammation and protects against idiopathic pneumonia injury.[15] Tyrosine nitration in proteins is also sufficient to induce an accelerated degradation of the modified proteins by the proteasome, which might be critical for the removal of nitrated proteins *in vivo*.[16]

2. Tyrosine

Tyrosine nitration, a covalent posttranslational and reversible[17] protein modification, occurs in basal and/or inflammatory diseases and changes protein function. It may occur through either a peroxynitrite-dependent (interaction of peroxynitrite either with $O_2^{\cdot-}$ or CO_2) or peroxynitrite-independent pathway. The latter involves tyrosine nitration by myeloperoxidase,[18] eosinophil peroxidase, tyrosyl radicals, or by reaction of NO with a tyrosyl radical.[8]

Nitration of tyrosine residues in tyrosine kinase substrates might prevent phosphorylation and, therefore, inhibit tyrosine kinase function in cellular signaling.[17] This may represent a novel mechanism of NO interaction with tyrosine kinase signaling, although the inhibition of tyrosine phosphorylation by tyrosine nitration remains highly speculative.

3. Nitrotyrosine

Nitrotyrosine can be formed when nitrite (NO_2^-) or NO are oxidized to nitrogen dioxide or peroxynitrite that couple with the tyrosyl radical to form a weak complex, which re-aromatizes to nitrotyrosine. A peroxynitrite-independent mechanism of nitrotyrosine formation is through the direct reaction of NO with a tyrosyl radical,[8] when NO can form an unstable complex with the tyrosyl residue of prostaglandin

H synthase-2, and this complex can be oxidized to form a nitrotyrosine. Alternatively, free tyrosine can act as a cosubstrate in myeloperoxidase-mediated tyrosine nitration.

Nonasthmatic lungs showed little or no nitrotyrosine staining, whereas lungs of patients who died of status asthmaticus have a high presence of nitrotyrosine in both the airways and lung parenchyma. We have identified an increased bronchial inducible NOS (iNOS) activity and nitrotyrosine formation in mild asthma[19] and elevated levels of free nitrotyrosine in EBC during asthma exacerbations,[6] although nitrotyrosine formation in airway epithelial and inflammatory cells is significantly higher in COPD than in asthma.[20]

Despite the recent discovery of enzymatic nitrotyrosine dinitrase activity in lung homogenates,[21] suggesting the potential role of nitration (and dinitration) as a signaling mechanism, it remains to be established whether nitrotyrosine is merely a biomarker of increased nitrosative stress or whether it actively contributes to cellular dysfunction and development of the airway inflammatory processes in asthma or COPD.

4. Prostacyclin Synthase

Both NOS and prostacyclin synthase maintain a balance of vasodilators and vasoconstrictors. This balance might be disrupted by oxidative stress and/or by prostaglandin synthase nitration by peroxynitrite, resulting in reduced prostacyclin-mediated vasodilation,[22] and elevated levels of proinflammatory prostanoids, such as prostaglandin (PG) E_2 and $PGF_{2\alpha}$, in EBC in COPD,[1] but not in asthma.

Pulmonary hypertension is a complication of severe COPD that is associated mostly with remodeling of the pulmonary arterial walls. Currently, prostacyclin derivatives, endothelin antagonists, and NO donors[23] have been used effectively in patients with primary pulmonary hypertension. We speculate that iNOS inhibitors might be also effective in treatment of secondary pulmonary hypertension by reducing or reversing arterial wall and airway remodeling in COPD.

5. Surfactant

Nitration of pulmonary SP-A diminishes its protective role against the collapse of small airways. It can be speculated that SP-A might have impaired function in chronic smokers and patients with COPD as a result of peroxynitrite formation.

Interestingly, it has been shown that males with alleles of loci flanking SP-B had more severe COPD (forced expiratory volume in 1 second/forced vital capacity [FEV_1/FVC] ratio 40%),[24] indicating that the surfactant protein alleles might be useful in COPD by either predicting the disease in a subgroup and/or by identifying disease subgroups that might be used for therapeutic intervention.

6. Superoxide Dismutase

Superoxide dismutase (SOD) activity is reduced in asthma and COPD. Reactive nitrogen species impair the crucial antioxidant enzymes, such as SOD, catalase (CAT), and glutathione peroxidase (GPX) in a donor-specific and dose-dependent manner.[25] Peroxynitrite specifically nitrates only one tyrosine residue, Tyr34, located near the bound manganese of SOD that might cause mitochondrial dysfunction in asthma and COPD.

7. S-Nitrosylation

Nitrosylation is a chemical and not an enzymatically catalyzed reaction that depends on the local concentration of NO and superoxide radicals and heme proteins. There is some specificity in nitrosylation, however; not every protein with available cysteine residues becomes nitrosylated.[17] SNO protein levels might be influenced by either the activity of iNOS and/or cnNOS (constitutive, neuronal).[26] This suggests that SNO protein modification may serve as a major effector of NO-related bioactivity within human lung, both in NOS-containing cells and during NO-derived intercellular signaling.

Expression of some regulatory proteins, such as glyceraldehyde 3-phosphate dehydrogenase (GAPDH) and β-actin mRNA, is 10 times lower in both broncho-alveolar lavage (BAL) fluid cells and biopsy tissue in steroid-naïve asthmatic vs. healthy individuals.[27] NO can reversibly nitrosylate cysteine residue in the active site of the caspase enzyme,[17] reducing cell survival, but treatment with the caspase inhibitor prevents septal cell apoptosis and emphysema development.[28]

The delayed apoptosis of eosinophil in the bronchial mucosa in asthma and macrophages in COPD[13] has been indicated as a novel mechanism by which these cells accumulate in the airways. This reduced airway macrophage apoptosis in COPD is linked to cytoplasmic expression of p21 proteins, and their nitrosylation by NO results in activation of activity instead of inhibition.

Therefore, treatment with NO donors might restore the lack of tracheal S-nitro-sothiols, which are endogenous bronchodilators, in acute severe asthma,[29] or might restore the delayed cell apoptosis in COPD.

8. Histones

Chemical nitration of histones has been demonstrated previously *in vitro* and recently *in vivo*.[30] In NO-exposed cytoplasmic proteins were nitrated after only 1 day of exposure, although nitration of histones was not apparent until 3 days and then it increased with time, reaching a maximum at about 6 days.[30] Therefore, the delay in histone nitration might be due to the relative inaccessibility of nuclei to the nitrating RNS, suggesting that histones are appreciably more stable than the average cellular protein and their slower turnover may permit them to accumulate 3-nitrotyrosine more than high-turnover proteins. Hence, the presence of nitrated histones in tissues may reflect the long-term exposure to RNS.[6]

Inducible NOS and other nuclear factor kappa B (NF-κB)-dependent genes involved in inflammation might be regulated by the specific recruitment of histone deacetylase (HDAC)-2 to NF-κB at target promoters and the consequent effects on their acetylation status,[31] which might further enhance cytokine induction of both the iNOS and the NF-κB.

HDAC activity and expression are reduced in bronchial biopsy samples obtained from mild asthmatics[32] compared with normal subjects, but might be restored by steroids that activate histone acetyltransferases.[32] It has been shown that in subjects with severe asthma and COPD with reduced HDAC activity, the ability of inhaled steroids to control inflammation might be lost.[32]

II. EXHALED BREATH CONDENSATE

EBC is collected by cooling or freezing exhaled air and is totally noninvasive. Although the collection procedure has not been standardized, there is strong evidence that abnormalities in condensate composition might reflect biochemical changes of airway lining fluid.[33] Potentially, EBC can be used to measure the targets of modern therapy in clinical trials and monitor asthma and COPD in the clinic.

A. FACTORS AFFECTING NO-DERIVED MARKERS IN EXHALED BREATH CONDENSATE

1. Instability of NO in Aqueous Solutions

NO gas is difficult to measure in aqueous solutions because it is a free radical that reacts rapidly with reactive oxygen species (ROS) in aqueous solution to form oxides of nitrogen (NOx). Some NOx metabolites, such as peroxynitrite ($OONO^-$) or peroxynitrous acid, are unstable intermediates that then decompose, forming nitrite (NO_2^-), a weak base with a short lifetime in aqueous solution, and nitrate (NO_3^-), which is a stable bioactive oxidative end product of NO metabolism. Therefore, the measurement of NOx in airway fluids is normally expressed as NO_2^- or as NO_3^- levels,[34] unless novel methods of real-time $ONOO^-$ measurements are applied.[35]

2. Smoking

Exhaled NO concentrations are significantly reduced in smokers, with a strong relation between the exhaled NO and cigarette consumption.[36] One of the mechanism of this reduction is that the smoke extract decreases NO by decreasing iNOS mRNA transcription in lung epithelial cells.[37] No difference in the levels of nitrite, nitrite/nitrate, S-nitrosothiols, and nitrotyrosine in the EBC, however, were seen between smokers and nonsmokers.[38] After subjects smoke two cigarettes, however, nitrite/nitrate levels might be significantly but transiently increased, with no changes in the levels of NO in exhaled air and nitrite, S-nitrosothiols, or nitrotyrosine in the EBC 30 and 90 minutes after smoking. These findings suggest that acute smoking can increase the level of nitrate, but not nitrite, S-nitrosothiols, or nitrotyrosine in breath condensate.[38]

3. Nitrate in the Diet

The presence of high concentrations of nitrite/nitrate from the diet may potentially affect exhaled NO[39] and NO-related markers in condensate. It is therefore important to minimize and monitor salivary contamination. Perhaps each subject should rinse his or her mouth before collection and keep the mouth dry by periodically swallowing the saliva.

4. Intravenous or Digested L-Arginine

Intravenous, inhaled,[40] or digested L-arginine,[41] the substrate for NOS, increases exhaled NO levels in normal and asthmatic subjects and might, potentially, affect NO markers in EBC.

5. NOS Inhibitors

Nebulized L-NMMA and L-NAME, nonspecific inhibitors of NOS, reduced exhaled NO[42,43] and nasal NO.[44,45] Inhalation of aminoguanidine, an iNOS inhibitor, significantly decreased exhaled NO and ONOO⁻ in EBC.[35] In a randomized, double-blind, placebo-controlled, crossover trial, we have demonstrated that a single oral dose of a specific iNOS inhibitor rapidly (within 15 minutes) and dramatically reduced exhaled NO in both normal subjects and asthmatics for at least 72 h.[46]

6. Environmental Factors

Environmental factors, such as NO, ozone, and chlorine dioxide, are known to increase exhaled NO levels.[47] No influence of low levels of ambient NO upon nitrite in EBC of healthy children was found,[48] although their EBC H_2O_2 levels were increased.

B. NO-Derived Markers in Exhaled Breath Condensate

A significant proportion of NO is consumed by chemical reactions in the lung, leading to formation of nitrite, nitrate, and S-nitrosothiol in the lung epithelial lining fluid. In contrast to decreased S-nitrosothiols in tracheal aspirates from children with asthmatic respiratory failure,[29] increased nitrotyrosine in asthmatic airway epithelium has been inferred from immunostaining of lung biopsies,[19] and elevated levels of free nitrotyrosine have been observed in EBC in asthma.[6]

NO reacts with superoxide to yield peroxynitrite, can be trapped by thiol-containing biomolecules, such as cysteine and glutathione, to form S-nitrosothiols or can be oxidized to nitrate and nitrite.[49] Nitrogen intermediates (for example, peroxynitrite) can induce a number of covalent modifications in various biomolecules, such as nitroso- and nitro-adducts. One such modification yields 3-nitrotyrosine, and detection of this adduct in proteins is now commonly used as a diagnostic tool to identify involvement of NO-derived oxidants in many disease states.[50] The balance among nitrite/nitrate, S-nitrosothiols, and nitrotyrosine in lung epithelial lining fluids, as reflected by EBC, gives insight into NO synthesis and short- and long-term changes in NO production.

NO_3^- is detectable in the majority of healthy nonsmoking subjects,[34] and is elevated in smokers and in mild steroid-naïve asthmatic patients (Table 7.1). Patients with mild COPD, however, might have normal NO_3^- (Table 7.2), which corresponds to their normal exhaled NO levels.[7] Patients with severe COPD have elevated exhaled NO,[7] as well as increased iNOS activity and elevated NO_2^-/NO_3^- in sputum.[20] Severe COPD patients have significantly higher numbers of iNOS⁺ cells in alveolar walls.[51]

TABLE 7.1
Biomarkers of NO-Derived Markers in Exhaled Breath Condensate in Asthma

Biomarker	Control[0]	Asthma — Mild[1] (Steroid-Naïve)	Moderate[2]	Severe[3]	Effect of Disease	Effect of Steroids	Collection/ Analysis	Reference
SNO (µM)	0.11 (0.02)	0.08 (0.01)		0.81 (0.06)	636% ↑ [0-3]		G/CA/SPh	74
SNO (µM)		1 (0.5–1.5)–0.5(0.2–0.7)[Bud 400]				50% ↓ [Bud 400]	G/ELISA	59
		0.9 (0.5–1) –1(0.5–1)[Bud 100]				No effect		
		0.8 (0.1–1)–0.5(0.2–1)[Placebo]				No effect		
NT (ng/ml)	6.3 (0.8)	15.3 (2.0)	5.0 (0.6)	3.3 (0.6)	142% ↑ [0-1]	67% ↓ [1-2]	Es/EIA	6
						78% ↓ [1-3]		
NO$_3^-$ (µM)	9.6 (2.6–119.4)	68 (25.8–194.6)			608% ↑ [0-1]	No effect	G/C	35

Note: The effect of disease or steroids is expressed as the comparison between, for example, control ([0]) and mild asthma ([1]) = [0-1]; [Bud 400, 100, placebo] = before and after treatment with 400 or 100 µg budesonide (Bud) or placebo. Data are mean ± (standard error of the mean), or [SD], or (95% confidence interval).

Abbreviations: NT, nitrotyrosine; SNO, *S*-nitrosothiols; Es, EcoScreen condenser; G, glass condenser; CA, colorimetric assay; SPh, spectrophotometry; ELISA, enzyme-linked immunosorbent assay; EIA, specific enzyme immunoassay.

TABLE 7.2
Biomarkers of NO-Derived Markers in Exhaled Breath Condensate in COPD

Biomarker	Control (Nonsmokers)[0]	Control (Smokers)[1]	COPD Mild[2]	Moderate[3]	Severe[4]	Effect of Disease/Smoking	Effect of Steroids	Collection/ Analysis	Reference
SNO (µM)	0.1 (0.1)	0.5 (0.2)				No effect[0-1]	Not studied	G/F	39
SNO (µM)	0.11 (0.02)	0.46 (0.09)		0.24 (0.04) 43% on ICS		318%↑[0-1] 118%↑[0-3]	Possible effect (↓)	G/CA/SPh	74
NT (ng/ml)	6.3 (0.8)	7.2 (1.3)				No effect[0-1]	Not studied	G/EIA	39
NO$_2^-$/NO$_3^-$ (µM)	20.2 (2.8)	16 (1.6)				No effect[0-1]	Not studied	G/F	39
NO$_3^-$ (µM)	9.6 (2.6–119.4)	62.5 (9.5–158)	24.1 (1.9–337)			551%↑[0-1] 151%↑[0-2]	Not studied	G/C	35

Note: The effect of disease or steroids is expressed as the comparison between, for example, control ([0]) and mild asthma ([1]) = [0-1]; Bud 400, 100, placebo = before and after treatment with 400 or 100 µg budesonide (Bud) or placebo. Data are mean ± (standard error of the mean), or [SD], or (95% confidence interval).

Abbreviations: COPD, chronic obstructive pulmonary disease; SNO, *S*-nitrosothiols; G, glass condenser; CA, colorimetric assay; SPh, spectrophotometry; EIA, specific enzyme immunoassay; F, fluorometric assay; G/C, gas chromatography.

Interestingly, the rate of protein nitration in lung tissue was directly related to iNOS expression and was associated with lower FEV_1 values.

In fact, treatment with steroids resulted in a significant reduction in both nitrotyrosine and iNOS immunoreactivity in sputum cells compared with pretreatment levels in COPD.[52] The reduction in nitrotyrosine and iNOS immunoreactivity also was correlated with the improvement in FEV_1. These results suggest that RNS may be involved in the reversible component of inflammation in COPD that is suppressed by steroids. Additional studies using specific inhibitors for RNS are needed to clarify their effects on the long-term progression of COPD.[52] This might also provide the rationale for simultaneous treatment of COPD and severe asthmatics with NO donors and iNOS-specific inhibitors.[2]

C. NO-DERIVED MARKERS IN LUNG DISEASE

1. Asthma

High levels of nitrite have been found in exhaled breath condensate[53] and sputum[54] of asthmatic patients, especially during acute exacerbations.[53] The ratio of airway wall thickness to lumen diameter measured by high-resolution computed tomography was significantly correlated with the sputum concentration of nitrite/nitrate.[54] We have shown that nitrotyrosine in EBC is increased in mild steroid-naïve asthma and is reduced in patients with severe asthma receiving steroid therapy[6] (Table 7.1). Additional increase of nitrotyrosine in EBC was associated with worsening of asthma symptoms and deterioration of lung function during inhaled steroid withdrawal in moderate asthma,[55] suggesting that nitrotyrosine not only might be a predictor of asthma deterioration, but might play a key role in the pathogenesis of airway remodeling.

Increased levels of NO_2^-/NO_3^- in the EBC of mild steroid-naïve asthmatics[56] might reflect airway inflammation and high NO production by iNOS, given that the levels NO_2^-/NO_3^- were significantly lower in stable steroid-treated asthmatics. This also might be a reflection of an increased oxidative stress in asthma, because of a significant positive correlation between NO_2^-/NO_3^- levels and H_2O_2 concentration in EBC, but not with airway obstruction and bronchial hyperreactivity as assessed by PC_{20} to histamine.

Children with asthma had significantly higher levels of nitrite compared to healthy subjects or subjects with cough,[57] suggesting that EBC collection and nitrite measurements are possible in children as young as 3 years of age, and might prove useful for the assessment of airway inflammation in a pediatric clinic.

A deficiency in S-nitrosothiols has been demonstrated in tracheal lining fluid in asthmatic children with respiratory failure,[29] suggesting that the levels of S-nitrosothiols, which are endogenous bronchodilators, might normally counteract increased airway tone in asthma. The levels of S-nitrosothiols in EBC were reduced after 3 weeks of treatment with a high (400 μg daily) but not a low dose (100 μg daily) of inhaled budesonide[58] (Figure 7.1). In contrast, there was a rapid and dose-dependent reduction in nitrite/nitrate in EBC in the same mild asthmatics, suggesting that nitrite/nitrate levels are more sensitive to anti-inflammatory treatment (Figures 7.2 and 7.3).

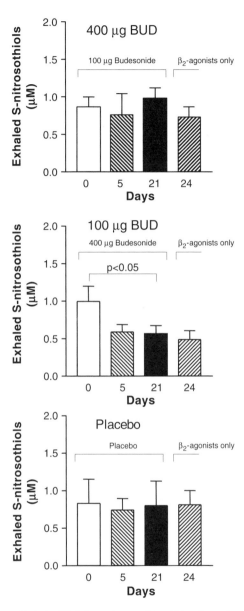

FIGURE 7.1 *S*-Nitrosothiols in EBC in patients with mild asthma during the onset (day 5), course of treatment (day 21), and cessation (day 24) of treatment with 100 or 400 µg of budesonide (BUD) or placebo. (From Chambers, D.C., Tunnicliffe, W.S., and Ayres, J.G., *Thorax*, 53, 677, 1998. With permission.)

2. Chronic Obstructive Pulmonary Disease

Habitual smokers have unusually high antioxidant concentrations in the epithelial lining fluid and higher resistance to oxidative pulmonary damage. NO can be trapped

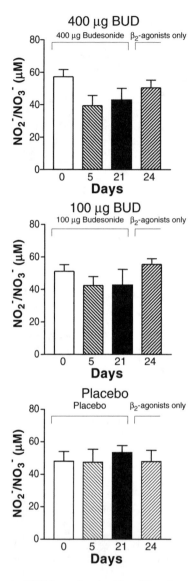

FIGURE 7.2 Nitrite/nitrate in EBC in patients with mild asthma during the onset (day 5), course of treatment (day 21), and cessation (day 24) of treatment with 100 or 400 μg of budesonide (BUD) or placebo. (From Chambers, D.C., Tunnicliffe, W.S., and Ayres, J.G., *Thorax*, 53, 677, 1998. With permission.)

in the epithelial lining fluid of the respiratory tract in the form of *S*-nitrosothiols or peroxynitrite and released thereafter, leading to transient elevation of exhaled NO after smoking of a cigarette.[59] Chronic oxidative stress presented to the lung by cigarette smoke might decrease the availability of thiol compounds and might

Onset of action

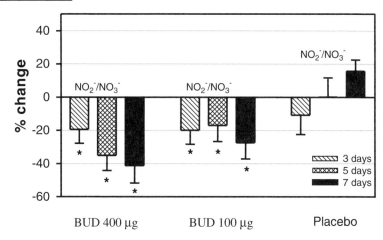

FIGURE 7.3 Dose-dependent effect of 100 or 400 μg of budesonide (BUD), or placebo on nitrite/nitrate in EBC of mild asthma during the onset (days 3, 5, and 7) of treatment with 100 or 400 μg of budesonide or placebo. (From Chambers, D.C., Tunnicliffe, W.S., and Ayres, J.G., *Thorax*, 53, 677, 1998. With permission.)

increase decomposition of nitrosothiols, explaining elevated levels of *S*-nitrosothiols in exhaled condensate in healthy smokers, which are related to smoking history, and increased EBC concentrations of NO_2^-/NO_3^- in COPD (Table 7.2).

Severe airway inflammation, prevalence of neutrophilic inflammation, oxidant/antioxidant imbalance, and high iNOS presence in sputum cells,[20] alveolar macrophages, alveolar walls, bronchial epithelium, and vascular smooth muscles of COPD patients[20,60] outweigh the effect of smoking on exhaled NO.[7] A significant negative correlation between FEV_1 and the amount of nitrotyrosine formation has been demonstrated in patients with COPD, but not in those with asthma and normal subjects,[20] suggesting that NO produced in the airways is consumed by its reaction with superoxide anion and/or peroxidase-dependent mechanisms and reactive nitrogen species play an important role in the pathobiology of the airway inflammatory and obstructive process in COPD. We have demonstrated that the peripheral airways/alveolar region is the predominant source of elevated exhaled NO in COPD. In contrast, increased exhaled NO levels in asthma are mainly from the larger airways/bronchial origin.[61] The prevalence of alveolar-derived NO in COPD is possibly related to the iNOS in macrophages, alveolar walls, and bronchial epithelium of COPD patients.[60]

Although the counts of nitrotyrosine-positive cells correlate with the severity of airway obstruction in COPD,[20] it is still unclear whether nitrotyrosine, including in EBC, is merely a biomarker of RNS or whether it actively contributes to cellular dysfunction and development of the airway inflammatory processes in COPD. In this respect, the recent discovery of apparent enzymatic nitrotyrosine dinitrase activity in rat spleen and lung homogenates[21] might suggest further the potential significance of nitration (and dinitration) as a signaling mechanism.

3. Primary Ciliary Dyskinesia

Despite the lower levels of exhaled NO in children with primary ciliary dyskinesia (PCD), no differences were found in the mean levels of NO_2^-, nitrite/nitrate (NO_2^-/NO_3^-), or S-nitrosothiol between children with PCD and healthy subjects.[62] These findings suggest that NO synthase activity might not be decreased as much as might be expected on the basis of low exhaled and nasal NO levels.

4. Cystic Fibrosis

Elevated levels of nitrite and nitrate[57,63,64] and nitrotyrosine[65] have been found in exhaled condensate and sputum[66] of patients with cystic fibrosis during both stable periods and exacerbations. This suggests that nitration of proteins by myeloperoxidase might be an additional source of nitrotyrosine in patients with cystic fibrosis who have a very low NO production. In fact, myeloperoxidase is elevated in cystic fibrosis sputum and correlates with nitrotyrosine concentrations,[66] suggesting that an absence of an increase in exhaled NO does not exclude the possibility of NO participating in airway inflammation, including cystic fibrosis.

In children with cystic fibrosis and normal lung function, however, the nitrite/nitrate concentrations in BAL are normal and concentrations of S-nitrosothiols are reduced.[67] In contrast, elevated levels of nitrite and S-nitrosothiols are found in exhaled breath condensate of adult patients with more severe cystic fibrosis.[68]

5. Mechanical Ventilation and Acute Respiratory Distress Syndrome

Mechanical ventilation may damage the lung, and nitrite concentration may increase with lung distension. Recently, it has been shown that measurements of NO_2^- in EBC correlated well with low tidal volume (VT) and expiratory minute volume but not with other ventilatory parameters or some inflammatory markers, such as interleukin (IL)-6 and IL-8, in both EBC and serum.[69] Interestingly, the ratio of NO_2^- in EBC and the size of the VT correlated directly with lung injury scores in these acute respiratory distress syndrome (ARDS) patients. An increase in this ratio might indicate a disproportional increase of NO_2^- production due to mechanical stress in acute respiratory distress syndrome (ARDS) lungs and might help to identify situations of critical mechanical stress.

6. Other Lung Diseases

Nitrite and nitrate concentrations are increased in EBC of patients with active pulmonary sarcoidosis.[70]

III. NOVEL TECHNIQUES TO DETECT NO-DERIVED MARKERS IN EXHALED BREATH CONDENSATE

A. REAL-TIME MEASUREMENT OF PEROXYNITRITE IN EXHALED BREATH CONDENSATE

Peroxynitrite ($ONOO^-$) detection is difficult due to a short half life (< 1 second) at 37°C and pH 7.4. Therefore, the measurement 3-nitrotyrosine as a footprint of $ONOO^-$ has been used in clinical samples.[6] We have developed a direct measurement of $ONOO^-$ using oxidation of 2′,7′-dichlorofluorescin (DCDHF) by $ONOO^-$ in EBC in normal subjects.[35] EBC was collected using an EcoScreen® condenser (Jaeger Toennies, Hoechberg, Germany). Levels of $ONOO^-$ were detectable (6.1 ± 2.5 nM) and reproducible. Inhalation of aminoguanidine, an iNOS inhibitor, significantly decreased exhaled NO and $ONOO^-$ in EBC,[36] suggesting that this noninvasive direct measurement of $ONOO^-$ in EBC might be very useful for monitoring airway inflammation and response to treatment in pulmonary diseases, such as asthma and COPD.

B. ELECTRON CAPTURE-NEGATIVE CHEMICAL IONIZATION-GAS CHROMATOGRAPHY/MASS SPECTROMETRY

A combination of mass spectrometric techniques allows the identification of nitrated proteins in complex protein mixtures from tissue samples,[30] and electron capture-negative chemical ionization-gas chromatography/mass spectrometry (EC-NCI GC/MS) is 100-fold more sensitive than liquid chromatography-electrospray ionization-tandem mass spectrometry (LC-MS/MS) for analyzing 3-chlorotyrosine, 3-bromotyrosine, and 3-nitrotyrosine *in vivo*.[71]

C. PROTEOMICS

Nitrotyrosine and tyrosine can be detected simultaneously by high-performance liquid chromatography (HPLC), which measures the specific ultraviolet absorbance of amino acids, the specific fluorescence of nitrotyrosine-fluorescence derivates, or the electrochemical properties of nitrotyrosine. None of these approaches, however, are capable of measuring nitrotyrosine in proteins or peptides.

Although an enzyme immunoassay (EIA) method combines sensitivity and specificity with the ability to process a large number of specimens to quantify nitrotyrosine, the proteomics approach might be preferential to enrich the samples, given that nitrotyrosine and protein content are very low in EBC.[6,65]

Specific antinitrotyrosine antibodies (immunoprecipitation) can be used to detect nitrotyrosine by immunohistochemistry (for example, in nasal mucosa of patients with allergic rhinits),[72] although Western blotting on a two-dimensional gel, followed by mass spectrometry[10] might offer higher sensitivity. Immunoprecipitation has certain limitations because it is limited to proteins for which specific antibodies are available and it cannot identify which specific tyrosine residue(s) has been nitrated.

Proteomics has the potential to identify novel targets of tyrosine nitration in cells and tissues to obtain a view of the nitro-[10] and phosphoproteome, or to identify proteins undergoing *S*-nitrosylation *in vivo*. Recently, a proteomic approach identified more than 40 nitrotyrosine-immunopositive proteins, including 30 not previously identified, which became modified as a consequence of the inflammatory response.[10] These targets include proteins involved in oxidative stress, apoptosis, adenosine triphosphate (ATP) production, and other metabolic functions.

We have identified low levels of proteins in EBC that are distinctive from saliva proteins (unpublished data). Proteomics allowed us to detect proteins that undergo endogenous nitration and, therefore, to eliminate artefacts that might arise when exposing breath condensate to exogenous NO or nitrating agents. Therefore, proteomics to detect exhaled breath proteins promises to be a sensitive means to initiate clinical studies in asthma and COPD on mechanisms, selectivity, and consequences of biological tyrosine nitration.

IV. CONCLUSION

Selective and more potent NOS inhibitors and NO donors, as well as noninvasive clinical methods such as EBC, to assess NO biochemistry will lead to a better understanding of its deleterious and beneficial effects and novel treatments in COPD and asthma patients.

FURTHER READING

1. Kharitonov, S.A. and Barnes, P.J., Exhaled markers of pulmonary disease, *Am. J. Respir. Crit. Care Med.*, 163, 1693, 2001.
2. Kharitonov, S.A. and Barnes, P.J., Nitric oxide, nitrotyrosine, and nitric oxide modulators in asthma and chronic obstructive pulmonary disease, *Curr. Allergy Asthma Rep.*, 3, 121, 2003.
3. Kharitonov, S.A. and Barnes, P.J., Biomarkers of some pulmonary diseases in exhaled breath, *Biomarkers*, 7, 1, 2002.
4. Kharitonov, S.A. and Barnes, P.J., Exhaled markers of inflammation, *Curr. Opin. Allergy Clin. Immunol.*, 1, 217, 2001.
5. Bartberger, M.D. et al., The reduction potential of nitric oxide (NO) and its importance to NO biochemistry, *Proc. Natl. Acad. Sci. U.S.A.*, 99, 10958, 2002.
6. Hanazawa, T., Kharitonov, S.A., and Barnes, P.J., Increased nitrotyrosine in exhaled breath condensate of patients with asthma, *Am. J. Respir. Crit. Care Med.*, 162, 1273, 2000.
7. Maziak, W. et al., Exhaled nitric oxide in chronic obstructive pulmonary disease, *Am. J. Respir. Crit. Care Med.*, 157, 998, 1998.
8. Gunther, M.R., Sturgeon, B.E., and Mason, R.P., Nitric oxide trapping of the tyrosyl radical-chemistry and biochemistry, *Toxicology*, 177, 1, 2002.
9. Kuo. W.N. and Kocis, J.M., Nitration/*S*-nitrosation of proteins by peroxynitrite-treatment and subsequent modification by glutathione *S*-transferase and glutathione peroxidase, *Mol. Cell. Biochem.*, 233, 57, 2002.
10. Aulak, K.S. et al., Proteomic method identifies proteins nitrated *in vivo* during inflammatory challenge, *Proc. Natl. Acad. Sci. U.S.A.*, 98, 12056, 2001.

11. Brown, G.C. and Borutaite, V., Nitric oxide, mitochondria, and cell death, *IUBMB Life*, 52, 189, 2001.
12. Bucchieri, F. et al., Asthmatic bronchial epithelium is more susceptible to oxidant-induced apoptosis, *Am. J. Respir. Cell Mol. Biol.*, 27, 179, 2002.
13. Tomita, K. et al., Increased p21(CIP1/WAF1) and B cell lymphoma leukemia-x(L) expression and reduced apoptosis in alveolar macrophages from smokers. *Am. J. Respir. Crit. Care Med.*, 166, 724, 2002.
14. Harju, T. et al., Diminished immunoreactivity of gamma-glutamylcysteine synthetase in the airways of smokers' lung, *Am. J. Respir. Crit. Care Med.*, 166, 754, 2002.
15. Yang, S. et al., Human surfactant protein a suppresses T cell-dependent inflammation and attenuates the manifestations of idiopathic pneumonia syndrome in mice, *Am. J. Respir. Cell. Mol. Biol.*, 24, 527, 2001.
16. Souza, J.M. et al., Proteolytic degradation of tyrosine nitrated proteins. *Arch. Biochem. Biophys.*, 380, 360, 2000.
17. Davis, K.L. et al., Novel effects of nitric oxide, *Annu. Rev. Pharmacol. Toxicol.*, 41, 203, 2001.
18. Eiserich, J.P. et al., Myeloperoxidase, a leukocyte-derived vascular NO oxidase, *Science*, 296, 2391, 2002.
19. Saleh, D. et al., Increased formation of the potent oxidant peroxynitrite in the airways of asthmatic patients is associated with induction of nitric oxide synthase: effect of inhaled glucocorticoid, *FASEB J.*, 12, 929, 1998.
20. Ichinose, M. et al., Increase in reactive nitrogen species production in chronic obstructive pulmonary disease airways, *Am. J. Respir. Crit. Care Med.*, 162, 701, 2000.
21. Kamisaki, Y. et al., An activity in rat tissues that modifies nitrotyrosine-containing proteins, *Proc. Natl. Acad. Sci. U.S.A.*, 95, 11584, 1998.
22. Cooke, C.L. and Davidge, S.T., Peroxynitrite increases iNOS through NF-kappaB and decreases prostacyclin synthase in endothelial cells, *Am. J. Physiol. Cell Physiol.*, 282, C395, 2002.
23. Ashutosh, K. et al., Use of nitric oxide inhalation in chronic obstructive pulmonary disease, *Thorax*, 55, 109, 2000.
24. Guo, X. et al., Surfactant protein gene A, B, and D marker alleles in chronic obstructive pulmonary disease of a Mexican population, *Eur. Respir. J.*, 18, 482, 2001.
25. Lawler, J.M. and Song, W., Specificity of antioxidant enzyme inhibition in skeletal muscle to reactive nitrogen species donors, *Biochem. Biophys. Res. Commun.*, 294, 1093, 2002.
26. Gow, A.J. et al., Basal and stimulated protein *S*-nitrosylation in multiple cell types and tissues, *J. Biol. Chem.*, 277, 9637, 2002.
27. Glare, E.M. et al., Beta-actin and GAPDH housekeeping gene expression in asthmatic airways is variable and not suitable for normalising mRNA levels *Thorax*, 57, 765, 2002.
28. Kasahara, Y. et al., Inhibition of VEGF receptors causes lung cell apoptosis and emphysema, *J. Clin. Invest.*, 106, 1311, 2000.
29. Gaston, B. et al., Bronchodilator *S*-nitrosothiol deficiency in asthmatic respiratory failure, *Lancet*, 351, 1317, 1998.
30. Haqqani, A.S., Kelly, J.F, and Birnboim, H.C., Selective nitration of histone tyrosine residues *in vivo* in mutatect tumors, *J. Biol. Chem.*, 277, 3614, 2002.
31. Ito, K. and Adcock, I.M., Histone acetylation and histone deacetylation, *Mol. Biotechnol.*, 20, 99, 2002.
32. Ito, K. et al., Expression and activity of histone deacetylases in human asthmatic airways, *Am. J. Respir. Crit. Care Med.*, 166, 392, 2002.

33. Kharitonov, S.A. and Barnes, P.J., Clinical aspects of exhaled nitric oxide, *Eur. Respir. J.*, 16, 781, 2000.
34. Corradi, M. et al., Nitrate in exhaled breath condensate of patients with different airway diseases, *Nitric Oxide*, 8, 26, 2003.
35. Ito, K. et al., Real-time measurement of peroxynitrite in exhaled breath condensate, *Eur. Respir. J.*, 22, Suppl. 45, 448s, 2003.
36. Kharitonov, S.A. et al., Acute and chronic effects of cigarette smoking on exhaled nitric oxide, *Am. J. Respir. Crit. Care Med.*, 152, 609, 1995.
37. Hoyt, J.C. et al., Cigarette smoke decreases inducible nitric oxide synthase in lung epithelial cells, *Exp. Lung Res.*, 29, 17, 2003.
38. Balint, B. et al., Increased nitric oxide metabolites in exhaled breath condensate after exposure to tobacco smoke, *Thorax*, 56, 456, 2001.
39. Olin, A.C. et al., Increased nitric oxide in exhaled air after intake of a nitrate-rich meal, *Respir. Med.*, 95, 153, 2001.
40. Sapienza, M.A. et al., Effect of inhaled L-arginine on exhaled nitric oxide in normal and asthmatic subjects, *Thorax*, 53, 172, 1998.
41. Kharitonov, S.A. et al., L-arginine increases exhaled nitric oxide in normal human subjects, *Clin. Sci. (Lond)*, 88, 135, 1995.
42. Kharitonov, S.A. et al., Increased nitric oxide in exhaled air of asthmatic patients, *Lancet*, 343, 133, 1994.
43. Yates, D.H. et al., Effect of a nitric oxide synthase inhibitor and a glucocorticosteroid on exhaled nitric oxide, *Am. J. Respir. Crit. Care Med.*, 152, 892, 1995.
44. Holden, W.E. et al., Temperature conditioning of nasal air: effects of vasoactive agents and involvement of nitric oxide, *J. Appl. Physiol.*, 87, 1260, 1999.
45. Sippel, J.M., Giraud, G.D., and Holden, W.E., Nasal administration of the nitric oxide synthase inhibitor L-NAME induces daytime somnolence, *Sleep*, 22, 786, 1999.
46. Hansel, T.T. et al., A selective inhibitor of inducible nitric oxide synthase inhibits exhaled breath nitric oxide in healthy volunteers and asthmatics, *FASEB J.*, 17, 1298, 2003.
47. Nightingale, J.A., Rogers, D.F., and Barnes, P.J., Effect of inhaled ozone on exhaled nitric oxide, pulmonary function, and induced sputum in normal and asthmatic subjects, *Thorax*, 54, 1061, 1999.
48. Latzin, P. and Griese, M., Exhaled hydrogen peroxide, nitrite and nitric oxide in healthy children: decrease of hydrogen peroxide by atmospheric nitric oxide, *Eur. J. Med. Res.*, 7, 353, 2002.
49. Stamler, J.S., *S*-nitrosothiols and the bioregulatory actions of nitrogen oxides through reactions with thiol groups, *Curr. Topics Microbiol. Immunol.*, 196, 19, 1995.
50. van der Vliet, A. et al., Reactive nitrogen species and tyrosine nitration in the respiratory tract. Epiphenomena or a pathobiologic mechanism of disease? *Am. J. Respir. Crit. Care Med.*, 160, 1, 1999.
51. Maestrelli, P. et al., Decreased haem oxygenase-1 and increased inducible nitric oxide synthase in the lung of severe COPD patients, *Eur. Respir. J.*, 21, 971, 2003.
52. Sugiura, H. et al., Correlation between change in pulmonary function and suppression of reactive nitrogen species production following steroid treatment in COPD, *Thorax*, 58, 299, 2003.
53. Hunt, J. et al., Condensed expirate nitrite as a home marker for acute asthma, *Lancet*, 346, 1235, 1995.
54. Gabazza, E.C. et al., Role of nitric oxide in airway remodelling, *Clin. Sci. (Colch)*, 98, 291, 2000.

55. Hanazawa, T. et al., Nitrotyrosine and cystenyl leukotrienes in breath condensates are increased after withdrawal of steroid treatment in patients with asthma, *Am. J. Respir. Crit. Care Med.*, 161, A919, 2000.

56. Ganas, K. et al., Total nitrite/nitrate in expired breath condensate of patients with asthma, *Respir. Med.*, 95, 649, 2001.

57. Formanek, W. et al., Elevated nitrite in breath condensates of children with respiratory disease, *Eur. Respir. J.*, 19, 487, 2002.

58. Kharitonov, S.A. et al., Dose-dependent onset and cessation of action of inhaled budesonide on exhaled nitric oxide and symptoms in mild asthma, *Thorax*, 57, 889, 2002.

59. Chambers, D.C., Tunnicliffe, W.S., and Ayres, J.G., Acute inhalation of cigarette smoke increases lower respiratory tract nitric oxide concentrations, *Thorax*, 53, 677, 1998.

60. Paska, C. et al., Increased expression of inducible NOS in peripheral lung of severe COPD patients, *Eur. Respir. J.*, 20, 95s, 2002.

61. Brindicci, C. et al., Extended exhaled NO measurements at different exhalation flows may differentiate between bronchial and alveolar inflammation in patients with asthma and COPD, *Eur. Respir. J.*, 20, 174s, 2002.

62. Csoma, Z. et al., Nitric oxide metabolites are not reduced in exhaled breath condensate of patients with primary ciliary dyskinesia, *Chest*, 124, 633, 2003.

63. Ho, L.P., Innes, J.A., and Greening, A.P., Nitrite levels in breath condensate of patients with cystic fibrosis is elevated in contrast to exhaled nitric oxide, *Thorax*, 53, 680, 1998.

64. Linnane, S.J. et al., Total sputum nitrate plus nitrite is raised during acute pulmonary infection in cystic fibrosis, *Am. J. Respir. Crit. Care Med.*, 158, 207, 1998.

65. Balint, B. et al., Increase nitrotyrosine in exhaled breath condensate in cystic fibrosis, *Eur. Respir. J.*, 17, 1201, 2001.

66. Jones, K.L. et al., Elevation of nitrotyrosine and nitrate concentrations in cystic fibrosis sputum, *Pediatr. Pulmonol.*, 30, 79, 2000.

67. Grasemann, H. et al., Decreased levels of nitrosothiols in the lower airways of patients with cystic fibrosis and normal pulmonary function, *J. Pediatr.*, 135, 770, 1999.

68. Corradi, M. et al., Nitrosothiols and nitrite in exhaled breath condensate of patients with cystic fibrosis, *Am. J. Respir. Crit. Care Med.*, 159, A682, 1999.

69. Gessner, C. et al., Exhaled breath condensate nitrite and its relation to tidal volume in acute lung injury, *Chest*, 124, 1046, 2003.

70. O'Donnell, D.M. et al., Exhaled nitric oxide and bronchoalveolar lavage nitrite/nitrate in active pulmonary sarcoidosis, *Am. J. Respir. Crit. Care Med.*, 156, 1892, 1997.

71. Gaut, J.P. et al., Artifact-free quantification of free 3-chlorotyrosine, 3-bromotyrosine, and 3-nitrotyrosine in human plasma by electron capture-negative chemical ionization gas chromatography mass spectrometry and liquid chromatography-electrospray ionization tandem mass spectrometry, *Anal. Biochem.*, 300, 252, 2002.

72. Hanazawa, T. et al., Intranasal administration of eotaxin increases nasal eosinophils and nitric oxide in patients with allergic rhinitis, *J. Allergy Clin. Immunol.*, 105, 58, 2000.

8 Analysis of Exhaled Breath Condensate in Children

Quirijn Jöbsis and Philippe P.R. Rosias

CONTENTS

I. INTRODUCTION

Airway inflammation plays an important role in various respiratory disorders of childhood, including recurrent wheezing, asthma, cystic fibrosis, bronchopulmonary dysplasia (BPD), and respiratory distress syndrome.[1-4] In daily clinical practice, indirect indices of airway inflammation such as symptoms and lung function measurements are used routinely for diagnosis and follow-up of inflammatory respiratory disorders. Especially in young children, these indirect indices of disease severity are less valuable than in adults; lung function studies in young children are often not possible because of lack of cooperation. Furthermore, reporting of symptoms by parents is very much dependent on perception of symptoms, with the potential risk for both under- and overperception. Therefore, in children, there is a strong need for objective and early criteria to detect and monitor airway inflammation to prevent or minimize the irreversible changes that are described in various chronic respiratory disorders including asthma, cystic fibrosis, and BPD.[1-5] The analysis of airway inflammatory cells and mediators traditionally has been performed by bronchoscopy on samples of bronchial mucosal biopsies or on bronchoalveolar lavage (BAL) fluid samples. In children both methods are limited in their applicability because of the invasive procedure of bronchoscopy. It is clear that in daily clinical practice, (serial) measurements of airway inflammation are not feasible using such invasive methods. A less invasive procedure to assess the presence and activity of airway inflammation would be of great benefit for early diagnosis and monitoring of inflammatory airway diseases in children.[6]

Inflammatory markers can be measured in blood or in urine.[6] The noninvasiveness of these methods is an advantage, but their indirect nature is a limitation. Measurements of certain inflammatory markers in blood and urine represent whole body production and do not necessarily reflect production of these inflammatory markers in the respiratory tract. It is reasonable to assume that the composition of respiratory tract secretions might more closely reflect airway inflammation than do substances in blood or urine. Sputum is one of the respiratory secretions that can be used in the assessment of airway inflammation.[7,8] Sputum can be obtained noninvasively, spontaneously, or during chest physiotherapy. Sputum examination has been limited by difficulties in obtaining adequate samples. When sputum cannot be produced spontaneously, it can be induced by inhalation of an aerosol of hypertonic saline. With this technique, sputum samples can be obtained in up to 75 to 100% of asthmatic and healthy adults.[8] In children, the success rate in obtaining adequate samples is definitely lower.[9] In general, sputum induction in children aged <6 years is not feasible. Other practical considerations of sputum induction include an inevitability of pretreatment with short-acting β_2-agonists to prevent an obstructive airway response provoked by inhalation of hypertonic saline, and the time-consuming procedure for inducing sputum and processing induced sputum samples. Furthermore, several studies have shown that repeated sputum induction in itself induces changes in airway inflammation within 8 to 24 hours after sputum induction, which limits the usefulness of this method for serial measurements .[10,11]

Exhaled breath condensate (EBC) is a recently rediscovered vehicle of substances from the respiratory tract, in which several potential markers of airway inflammation can be detected. In contrast with the other sampling methods mentioned above, EBC offers the advantage that it can be obtained completely noninvasively. Exhaled air carries components from the lower respiratory airways; it does not disturb the airways, in contrast to bronchial biopsies, BAL, and induced sputum; and it can be obtained with minimal risk and inconvenience from both adults and children.

II. COLLECTION OF EXHALED BREATH CONDENSATE IN CHILDREN

In children age 4 years and older, the EBC collection method(s) as used in adults can be applied in almost the same way. There are a variety of condenser systems to collect EBC, although they are fundamentally similar, based on condensation of exhaled air on a cold surface. In general, EBC is collected from adults and children from the age of 4 years by tidal breathing through a mouthpiece and a two-way nonrebreathing valve, which can also serve as a saliva trap, connected to a cooled condensing system. Minimal cooperation from the child is required for this technique of EBC collection. In children, the main issue for success of EBC sampling is if they are able to use a mouthpiece properly for approximately 10 to 15 minutes. Adequate instruction of the procedure and distraction of the child, for example by using video cartoons, increases the success rate of EBC collection in children.

Collecting EBC in children is not only a simple noninvasive procedure, but it is also a safe and feasible method of sampling substances from the respiratory tract. No adverse effects were seen in an EBC collection study in 93 healthy children aged 8 to 13 years, and all of the children were able to complete the EBC collection procedure successfully.[12] In a study of 91 children with asthma of varying severity, the EBC procedure proved to be safe even in children with an asthma exacerbation.[13] No significant changes in forced expiratory volume in 1 second (FEV_1) were found after the EBC collection. The success rate was 100% starting from 4 years of age. The volume of collected condensate depends on different variables, such as minute ventilation or total respired volume, condenser material and temperature, and turbulence characteristics.[14] Minute ventilation seems to be the most important determinant of the condensate volume over time. In children, it will take more time to collect the same amount of condensate as in adults. In general, a collection time of 15 to 20 minutes will yield 1 to 3 ml of EBC in children aged 4 years and older. It has been shown that the collected condensate volume significantly correlates with the age of children.[13]

In infants and young children, who are not able to use a mouthpiece properly, a face mask can be used. In a small number of infants, who are preferential nasal breathers, collection of EBC through a face mask was feasible.[15,16] In a sampling time of almost 30 minutes, a mean condensate volume of 101.6 µl was recoverd.[15] In the condensate of healthy infants and cystic fibrosis infants, nitrite and nitrate was detected. However, significant nasal contribution to the total nitrite/nitrate was found, suggesting that EBC analysis in infants should be limited to compounds not affected by nasal contribution, or EBC collection should be limited to sedated infants with induced oral breathing.[16]

Nasal collection of EBC is reported in minimal cooperative patients such as healthy infants from 4 weeks of age for the analysis of hydrogen peroxide.[17] Nasal prongs are serially connected to two polypropylene tubes, which are submerged in a cold trap, and in turn connected to an electric air suction pump. The condensate volume obtained increased significantly with age (up to 18 years) and was about 45% less in 1- to 6-year-old children. It averaged about 20 to 30% of the exhaled breath water vapor. However, contamination with nasal secretions might interfere with the actual concentration of inflammatory mediators in the lower respiratory tract.

III. INFLAMMATORY MEDIATORS DETECTED IN EXHALED BREATH CONDENSATE OF CHILDREN

EBC is presently an active research area. During recent years, an increasing number of EBC data are being presented. However, most data are obtained in adults. For the results of inflammatory mediators in EBC of children, we focus on data published in the international literature as peer-reviewed full articles.

A variety of inflammatory markers have been detected in EBC of children. In contrast to the condensate volume, the studied inflammatory marker levels in EBC are not age dependent.

The most commonly studied mediator is hydrogen peroxide (H_2O_2), a marker of oxidative stress. The concentration of H_2O_2 in EBC of stable asthmatic children is significantly increased compared with that in healthy children.[18] In stable asthmatic children the H_2O_2 concentrations were lower in those who used inhaled corticosteroids. In children with unstable asthma, higher concentrations have been reported than in stable asthmatic children.[19] Reference values of H_2O_2 have been described in a group of 93 healthy children with a mean age of 10 years.[20] H_2O_2 was not age dependent, nor was there a correlation with sex or lung function.[20] In children, it was demonstrated that atmospheric nitric oxide (NO) influenced exhaled H_2O_2 levels.[21] In addition to asthma, H_2O_2 concentration also has been detected in EBC of cystic fibrosis children with an acute infectious pulmonary exacerbation, and decreased significantly during intravenous antibiotic treatment.[22]

Another marker of oxidative stress that can be measured in the EBC of children is 8-isoprostane. Children with stable asthma had higher exhaled 8-isoprostane concentrations than healthy children.[23] In the asthmatic group, treatment with inhaled corticosteroids showed no difference in exhaled 8-isoprostane concentrations. The same study also showed, in contrast with the 8-isoprostane results, no significant difference in exhaled prostaglandin E_2 (PGE_2) concentrations between asthmatic and healthy children. In children with an asthma exacerbation, there is a significant reduction of exhaled 8-isoprostane after a 5-day course of oral prednisone.[24]

Leukotrienes also can be measured in EBC. In asthmatic children cysteinyl leukotrienes (cys-LTs) and leukotriene B_4 were significantly increased compared with healthy children.[25] After a course of oral corticosteroid therapy, cys-LTs were reduced in children with an asthma exacerbation.[24]

In children with asthma and cystic fibrosis, higher levels of nitrite in EBC have been found compared with children with nonasthmatic episodic cough and healthy children.[26] No significant differences were noted between the asthmatic and cystic fibrosis children, nor the episodic cough and healthy groups. In cystic fibrosis, there was no significant correlation between condensate nitrite levels and age, lung function (FEV_1, forced vital capacity [FVC]), or use of inhaled corticosteroids.[27] Children with primary ciliary dyskinesia (PCD) have been shown to have very low levels of exhaled oral and nasal NO.[28] However, no differences were found in the EBC levels of NO metabolites such as nitrite, nitrate, and S-nitrosothiol between children with PCD and healthy children, despite the marked decrease in exhaled NO levels in PCD patients.[29]

Cytokines reported in EBC of children include interleukin-8 (IL-8), IL-4, and interferon-γ (IFN-γ). In cystic fibrosis, IL-8 could only be detected in 33% of the condensate samples.[27] Although the IL-8 values were higher in cystic fibrosis children than in healthy controls, there was no statistically significant difference. Increased levels of IL-4 and decreased levels of IFN-γ were detected in EBC of stable asthmatic children.[30] The use of inhaled corticosteroids was associated with a significant change in IL-4 concentration, in contrast to IFN-γ concentration. IFN-γ was detectable in all EBC samples, whereas IL-4 was detectable in 92% of the samples.

Aldehydes and glutathione are biomarkers of oxidant-induced damage and antioxidant status, respectively. Malondialdehyde and glutathione are detectable in EBC

TABLE 8.1
Inflammatory Markers in EBC of Children with Asthma or Cystic Fibrosis

Marker	Asthma	Cystic Fibrosis	Reference
Hydrogen peroxide	⇑	⇑	18,19,22
8-Isoprostane	⇑	—	23,24
PGE$_2$	=	—	23
Cys-LTs	⇑	—	24,25
LTB$_4$	⇑	—	25
Nitrite	⇑	⇑	26,27
Interleukin-4	⇑	—	30
Interleukin-8	—	=	27
Interferon-γ	⇓	—	30
Aldehyde	⇑	—	31
Glutathione	⇓	—	31

Note: ⇑, Significantly increased compared with healthy children; ⇓, significantly decreased compared with healthy children; =, no significant difference compared with healthy children; —, no pediatric data.

of children.[31] In children with an asthma exacerbation, malondialdehyde levels were higher and glutathione levels were lower compared with healthy children.[31] After a 5-day course of oral prednisone, malondialdehyde decreased to values no longer different from those of the healthy control children, whereas glutathione levels increased. In healthy subjects as well as in asthmatic children, malondialdehyde and glutathione were negatively correlated. Malondialdehyde and glutathione concentrations were not dependent on exhaled flow rate (200, 150, 100, and 50 ml/s), and no correlation was found between spirometric values and these oxidant/antioxidant levels in EBC.

Table 8.1 summarizes pediatric results of inflammatory markers in EBC of children with asthma or cystic fibrosis.

IV. CONCLUSION

Assessment of inflammatory mediators in EBC is a challenging new technique for the diagnosis and management of various inflammatory lung diseases. Because of the noninvasive character of EBC and the general lack of other appropriate techniques to characterize airway inflammation in children, it is particularly interesting for pediatric respiratory medicine. EBC is not only a simple and noninvasive procedure, but it also is a safe and feasible method of sampling inflammatory mediators from the respiratory tract in children age 4 years and older. A variety of inflammatory markers have been detected in EBC of children. Potentially, this noninvasive method will allow early and appropriate anti-inflammatory treatment in children; it is hoped that this will prevent or at least limit the later development of chronic respiratory diseases in adults. However, the clinical relevance of exhaled inflammatory markers first needs to be established in longitudinal studies in various respiratory disorders, with repeated measurements in individual patients.

FURTHER READING

1. Tattersfield, A.E. et al., Asthma. *Lancet*, 360, 1313, 2002.
2. Dakin, C.J. et al., Inflammation, infection, and pulmonary function in infants and young children with cystic fibrosis. *Am. J. Respir. Crit. Care Med.*, 165, 904, 2002.
3. Özdemir, A., Brown, M.A., and Morgan, W.J., Markers and mediators of inflammation in neonatal lung disease, *Pediatr. Pulmonol.*, 23, 292, 1997.
4. Eber, E. and Zach, M.S., Long term sequellae of bronchopulmonary dysplasia (chronic lung disease of infancy), *Thorax*, 56, 317, 2001.
5. De Rose, V., Mechanisms and markers of airway inflammation in cystic fibrosis, *Eur. Respir. J.*, 19, 333, 2002.
6. Scheinmann, P. et al., Methods for assessment of airway inflammation: paediatrics, *Eur. Respir. J.*, 26, 53s, 1998.
7. Kim, J.S. et al., Sputum processing for evaluation of inflammatory mediators, *Pediatr. Pulmonol.*, 32, 152, 2001.
8. Kips, J.C. et al., Methods for sputum induction and analysis of induced sputum: a method for assessing airway inflammation in asthma, *Eur. Respir. J.*, 11, 9s, 1998.
9. Wilson, N.M. et al., Induced sputum in children: feasibility, repeatability, and relation of findings to asthma severity, *Thorax*, 55, 768, 2000.
10. Nightingale, J.A., Rogers, D.F., and Barnes, P.J., Effect of repeated sputum induction on cell counts in normal volunteers, *Thorax*, 53, 87, 1998.
11. Holz, O. et al., Changes in sputum composition between two inductions performed on consecutive days, *Thorax*, 53, 83, 1998.
12. Jöbsis, Q. et al., Hydrogen peroxide in exhaled air of healthy children: reference values, *Eur. Respir. J.*, 12, 483, 1998.
13. Baraldi, E. et al., Safety and success of exhaled breath condensate collection in asthma, *Arch. Dis. Child.*, 88, 358, 2003.
14. Hunt, J., Exhaled breath condensate: an evolving tool for noninvasive evaluating of lung disease, *J. Allergy Clin. Immuol.*, 110, 28, 2002.
15. Horak, F. et al., Measurement of nitrite in the breathing-condensate of healthy infants and infants with cystic fibrosis, *Am. J. Respir. Crit. Care Med.*, 165, A485, 2002.
16. Moeller, A. et al., Limitations of breath condensates in infants, *Am. J. Respir. Crit. Care Med.*, 167, A987, 2003.
17. Griese, M., Latzin, P., and Beck, J., A noninvasive method to collect nasally exhaled air condensate in humans of all ages, *Eur. J. Clin. Invest.*, 31, 915, 2001.
18. Jöbsis, Q. et al., Hydrogen peroxide in exhaled air is increased in stable asthmatic children, *Eur. Respir. J.*, 10, 519, 1997.
19. Dohlman, A.W., Black, H.R., and Royall, J.A., Expired breath hydrogen peroxide is a marker of acute airway inflammation in pediatric patients with asthma, *Am. Rev. Respir. Dis.*, 148, 955, 1993.
20. Jöbsis, Q. et al., Hydrogen peroxide in exhaled air of healthy children: reference values, *Eur. Respir. J.*, 12, 483, 1998.

21. Latzin, P. and Griese, M., Exhaled hydrogen peroxide, nitrite and nitric oxide in healthy children: decrease of hydrogen peroxide by atmospheric nitric oxide, *Eur. J. Med. Res.*, 30, 353, 2002.

22. Jöbsis, Q. et al., Hydrogen peroxide and nitric oxide in exhaled air of children with cystic fibrosis during antibiotic treatment, *Eur. Respir. J.*, 16, 95, 2000.

23. Baraldi, E. et al., Increased exhaled 8-isoprostane in childhood asthma, *Chest,* 124, 25, 2003

24. Baraldi, E. et al., Cysteinyl leukotrienes and 8-isoprostane in exhaled breath condensate of children with asthma exacerbations, *Thorax,* 58, 505, 2003.

25. Csoma, Z. et al., Increased leukotrienes in exhaled breath condensate in childhood asthma, *Am. J. Respir. Crit. Care. Med.*, 166, 1345, 2002.

26. Formanek, W. et al., Elevated nitrite in breath condensates of children with respiratory disease, *Eur. Respir. J.*, 19, 487, 2002.

27. Cunningham, S. et al., Measurement of inflammatory markers in the breath condensate of children with cystic fibrosis, *Eur. Respir. J.*, 15, 955, 2000.

28. Narang, I. et al., Nitric oxide in chronic airway inflammation in children: diagnostic use and pathophysiological significance, *Thorax,* 57, 586, 2002.

29. Csoma, Z. et al., Nitric oxide metabolites are not reduced in exhaled breath condensate of patients with primary ciliary dyskinesia, *Chest,* 124, 633, 2003.

30. Shahid, SK. et al., Increased interleukin-4 and decreased interferon-γ in exhaled breath condensate of children with asthma, *Am. J. Respir. Crit. Care Med.*, 165, 1290, 2002.

31. Corradi, M. et al., Aldehyde and glutathione in exhaled breath condensate of children with asthma exacerbation, *Am. J. Respir. Crit. Care Med.*, 167, 395 2003.

9 Exhaled Breath Condensate: Comparisons with Other Methods for Assessing Lung Inflammation

Christopher A. Bates and Philip E. Silkoff

CONTENTS

I. INTRODUCTION

It is important to have a thorough understanding of the inflammatory processes that occur in specific pulmonary diseases. With this understanding we are able to better identify and characterize the underlying phenotypes that are associated with syndromes. For example, in asthma it has been demonstrated that although a phenotype of inflammation involving eosinophils, their effector proteins (i.e., major basic protein),

113

and specific cytokines such as interleukin (IL)-5 is classically found, other phenotypes may exist, such as neutrophilic asthma. If we can identify patterns of lung
inflammation then an appropriate diagnosis can be made, and this might influence
the choice of therapy. In addition, these inflammatory markers can be observed over
time, allowing the clinician to follow the course of the disease and monitor the
response to therapy.

The field of exhaled breath condensate (EBC) offers a relatively new way of
evaluating lung inflammation and potentially can be applied to a wide array of pulmonary pathology. Multiple markers of inflammation can be measured, some of
which include hydrogen peroxide (H_2O_2), pH, nitric oxide metabolites, adenosine,
eicosanoids, leukotrienes, aldehydes, ammonia, and specific cytokines. EBC is one
of the newer methodologies available, and its evolving role in the assessment of
lung inflammation must be taken into context with what currently is available. Other
authors in this book discuss many aspects of EBC. This chapter compares EBC with
existing ways of assessing pulmonary inflammation.

II. WAYS TO ASSESS PULMONARY INFLAMMATION

Multiple methodologies are available to evaluate pulmonary inflammation. Each has
advantages and disadvantages. One must have an understanding of the limitations
of these methods to use them appropriately; there are costs and risks associated with
each method.

A. OPEN LUNG BIOPSY

Open lung biopsy (OLB) is routinely performed in clinical medicine for the diagnosis
of parenchymal lung disease.[1] The size of the lung sample often allows specific
diagnoses to be made when bronchoscopy has a low yield.[2] Although newer techniques such as video-assisted thorascopic biopsy have made the procedure safer,[3]
significant morbidity and mortality exist, especially in compromised patients, and
OLB is not performed in the research setting. Despite the fact that it would be
pertinent to compare less invasive methods with OLB where it is available, this has
been done only on rare occasions.

B. BRONCHOSCOPY

Bronchoscopy with endobronchial biopsy (EBBX), transbronchial biopsy (TBBX),
and bronchoalveolar lavage (BAL) have been the primary research and clinical tools
for assessing lung inflammation.[4–9] Aside from OLB, bronchoscopy allows the broad-
est perspective on pulmonary inflammation and pathology. It allows direct access
to inflammatory cells and mediators in the airways, samples for culture of microorganisms, and limited assessment of architecture, e.g., remodeling. For example,
bronchoscopy has been used to demonstrate eosinophil-positive versus eosinophil-
negative subpopulations in severe asthma,[10] and identification of these two groups
may have prognostic and therapeutic implications. Bronchoscopy yields small biopsies
compared with OLB and this reduces its ability to diagnose parenchymal lung
disease, e.g., idiopathic pulmonary fibrosis.[2] It is also difficult to obtain small airways

in transbronchial biopsies. BAL is limited by the dilutional effect of the instilled saline and a variable return of fluid, making quantitation problematic. Finally, there are inherent risks associated with bronchoscopy, such as oversedation, hemorrhage, bronchospasm, hypoxemia, and pneumothorax, with a small but significant risk of death. There is significant cost associated with this procedure as well. As a research tool, few protocols perform more than one or two bronchoscopies, given that the procedure is unsuitable for repeated application in both the research and clinical arenas.

C. BLOOD AND URINE

Peripheral blood markers have also been examined as a surrogate marker of pulmonary inflammation. There is minimal risk associated with venipuncture, but this is less acceptable for children on a repeated basis. Blood markers include cells and mediators. Eosinophilia, which is present in some asthmatics, has been shown to track reasonably well with atopic asthma and decreases in response to therapies aimed at treating this disease.[11] However, in many instances the inflammatory changes that are seen in the peripheral circulation do not correlate with the inflammatory changes seen in the lung. In addition, cytokine levels in the circulation can be at or below the level of detection with conventional methods of measurement.[12] Urinary markers of inflammation have been evaluated as well. An example is the measurement of urinary leukotrienes in asthma.[13] Although there is no risk, urine might not provide an accurate reflection of pulmonary inflammation, and not all asthmatics have elevated levels.

D. INDUCED SPUTUM

Blood and urine do not "go where the money is," but there are relatively noninvasive methods that more directly reflect inflammatory changes associated with the lung. Sputum that has been spontaneously expectorated or induced by inhalation of hypertonic saline (IS) has been employed extensively as a tool in the research arena. It can characterize inflammatory cells and mediators in the airway lumen, particularly in the large airways. Recently, Green et al.[14] showed that asthma control is improved by targeting induced sputum eosinophils as compared with standard monitoring. Its limitations include a lack of sensitivity and specificity, contamination by upper airway cells and organisms, and costly induction and processing of specimens. Induced sputum is suitable for repeated application but the cost might restrict its clinical applicability.

E. EXHALED NITRIC OXIDE

In more recent years, the development of exhaled nitric oxide (ENO) measurement has come to the forefront as a noninvasive means of assessing airway inflammation, particularly in asthma.[15] It has been standardized as a clinical tool through the American Thoracic Society,[16] and the U.S. Food and Drug Administration has recently approved an NO analyzer (NIOX®, Aerocrine AB, Stockholm, Sweden) for clinical use in asthma. ENO testing can be reproducibly performed in almost all age groups. It has been shown to be useful in establishing the diagnosis of asthma,[17] in the differential of chronic cough,[18] and has shown promise in being able to predict asthma exacerbations as well as follow responses to therapy.[19] The ENO result is immediate and the test is eminently suitable for repeated application. However, NO is just one marker/mediator of inflammation, and so ENO testing, although well established in asthma, cannot be applied to all forms of pulmonary inflammation. In addition, there is a high cost for NO analyzers, although the time investment and cost per test is low.

III. EXHALED BREATH CONDENSATE

Certain criteria must be met when a tool is used in the evaluation of a particular clinical process. These criteria include simplicity and practicality in its application. The cost associated with its use should not be so prohibitive in that it is impractical. The results should be reproducible in the individual being studied as well as between laboratories. It should be applicable in health and disease. The method also should provide a degree of specificity that allows a differentiation of one pathologic process from another. Finally, the method should be validated in multiple centers as being an accurate measuring device. Based on these criteria, where does EBC fit?

A. Collection Technique

OLB, bronchoscopy with BAL, induced sputum, and ENO measurement have been standardized, but EBC is new and not standardized as of yet.

EBC requires a collection technique, which is the most crucial step, followed by sample handling, storage, and analysis. As with spirometry, there is a need for standardization of collection procedures. A taskforce has been appointed by the European Respiratory and American Thoracic Societies, and there is a document in press. However, there are significant gaps in our knowledge that have made such standardization problematic. It also is possible that collection protocols will differ according to the mediator of interest.

The use of EBC currently is restricted to the research setting. Most methods for collecting EBC are based on cooling exhalate and have been developed by the investigators evaluating inflammatory mediators. A typical setup consists of a length of tubing that runs through a cooling device, which promotes condensation of expired air.[20] The study individual breathes through a one-way valve that prevents the mixture of ambient air with the exhaled condensate. The individual performs tidal breaths for 10 to 15 minutes until approximately 1 to 3 ml of condensate is collected. This condensate can then be analyzed for the inflammatory marker in question.

Two commercially available methods for obtaining EBC are available. One is the EcoScreen® (Jaeger Toennies, Hoechberg, Germany), which was modified from a cold air challenge device. It is a sizeable unit that makes it somewhat impractical for universal use. It uses a salivary trap to minimize oral contamination. Another device that has been developed is the RTube® (Respiratory Research, Inc., Charlottsville, VA). This consists of a mouthpiece and polypropylene collection tube that is portable. An aluminum cooling sleeve is kept in the freezer and then placed over the collection tube when needed for sample collection. The individual breathes through the one-way exhalation valve and gravity reduces salivary contamination. Once an adequate volume is collected, the tube can be sealed, stored, and shipped for further analysis.

The collected EBC can then be removed with a plunger. The commercial devices have been used in both children and adults. The RTube has the advantage in that it can be used easily at home.

The disadvantage of collection methods that rely on cooling is that the EBC sample is very dilute, as discussed in Chapter 3. In the future, it might be possible to trap nonvolatile particles in breath using other methods that do not use condensation, e.g., filters or other means.

B. Source of Exhaled Breath Condensate

The source of samples derived from lung biopsy, BAL, induced sputum, and ENO testing is clear. As of yet, it is difficult to determine exactly from where in the respiratory tract EBC originates. The alveolar region, airways, oral cavity, and nose might all contribute. For ENO, velum closure is essential to exclude nasal contamination, but the tidal breathing commonly used to collect EBC gives no assurance that nasal contamination is prevented. Initial studies of EBC would suggest that nasal contamination in healthy individuals does not matter much for specific mediators, but there is a significant impact when individuals with allergic rhinitis are included in the analysis for adenosine.[21] In tracheostomy samples, NH_4 levels were considerably lower than those taken via the oral route, suggesting that the oral cavity is the major source for this mediator.[22]

Opportunities for extraneous contamination exist in the handling of the samples. It is foreseeable that mishandling at this point could easily lead to contamination from ambient air or from the operator. This is especially true when measuring nitrite/nitrate, given that these are ubiquitous.[23] Samples also must be stored promptly and quickly, especially when reactive mediators such as H_2O_2 are involved.[24]

C. Simplicity and Invasiveness

Current methodology for EBC is the simplest of all the methods, both in concept and in performance. The collection devices available require minimal patient effort. EBC has been collected successfully in children as young as 2 years of age[25] who cannot perform single-breath online ENO measurement.[26] Once samples have been obtained, they can be stored and shipped by conventional methods that are similar to those used for blood samples.

In addition, EBC is entirely safe compared with bronchoscopy (which can result in bronchospasm, hemorrhage, infection, and pneumothorax) and compared with induced sputum (which has the possibility of causing bronchospasm and hypoxemia). Therefore, EBC facilitates repeated measurements in the same individual, which is a significant advantage over some of the other methodologies available for measuring inflammatory responses. ENO is also safe, simple, and suitable for repeated measurement.

D. Cost

Costs associated with EBC are uncertain. Capital costs for EBC collection devices vary from hundreds of U.S. dollars (homemade setups and RTube) to thousands of dollars (Jaeger ECoScreen), but the cost of the assays for various mediators add an extra expense and can vary widely, particularly if condensate requires special processing (e.g., concentration). Other methodologies for evaluating lung inflammation are no less expensive. Capital outlay for NO analyzers is currently very high but the per test cost is low. Induction of sputum requires 1 to 1.5 hours of technician time but processing costs of the specimens depends on which assays are performed. A cytospin takes 1 to 2 hours of laboratory technician time. Capital outlay for a bronchoscopy suite is high, although these facilities often are available. The procedure takes 4 to 6 hours of clinical care time or more, and the pathologic examination of tissue and processing of BAL for cells and mediators are associated with considerable cost.

E. REPRODUCIBILITY

Reproducibility with EBC is a problem at this point in its development, although for some mediators the data show reasonable short-term repeatability.[27,28] In disease in which airway inflammation can vary, longer term reproducibility might be low for biological reasons.

Technical factors also appear to be involved. Contamination of samples is one issue. A study in patients with cystic fibrosis required that more than 50% of the samples be discarded because of salivary contamination.[29] Attempts to overcome this issue include built-in salivary traps to minimize this problem, as incorporated in the RTube sampling system and the ECoScreen. Varying dilutional effects of collecting exhaled water vapor is another major factor, as discussed in Chapter 3 and other publications.[22,30] Attempts have been made to correct concentrations of mediators for solute content (such as sodium, potassium, or urea concentrations), similar to efforts described in the BAL literature. In cystic fibrosis patients, sodium content can be problematic as a correction factor, given the abnormalities associated with sodium transport. However, EBC concentrations have been shown to vary from sample to sample and from day to day. The heat expired by the subject (which can change by body size and temperature, hydration, breathing pattern, etc.) together with the efficiency of the collector are major factors that could result in variability. Flow dependence of mediator concentration also should be considered in reproducibility. This issue has been studied extensively in ENO measurements[31] and must be taken into consideration with EBC standardization. EBC levels of hydrogen peroxide have found to be flow dependent.[32] Finally, given that EBC is dilute, assays of many mediators are at the bottom or below the detection range of assays, and this is associated with poor reproducibility.

For other methods, ENO shows excellent short-term reproducibility,[33] as do induced sputum cell counts.[34] Few studies have examined reproducibility in bronchial biopsies, but short-term reproducibility in asthma is good.[35]

F. SENSITIVITY IN DISEASE

Sensitivity related to EBC measurements needs to be investigated further. Many mediators in EBC are detected at the lower levels of assay sensitivity (e.g., for nitrite measured in EBC in normal subjects versus individuals with asthma,[36] where the differences shown between health and disease were small). In contrast, EBC pH measurements show 2 to 3 log differences in asthma exacerbations when compared with normal controls.[37] At the other end of the spectrum are leukotriene measurements in stable asthma, in which levels are generally less than twice those of normal subjects.[25] In some cases, there are no differences between states of health and disease; e.g., H_2O_2 levels in healthy smokers versus patients with chronic obstructive pulmonary disease (COPD).[38] One would expect IL-8, a potent chemotactic factor for neutrophils, to be significantly elevated in cystic fibrosis, yet it was detected in only 30% of this population and there was no difference statistically compared with healthy controls.[29] Instability and volatility of some mediators might play a role in decreased sensitivity as well. This is particularly true with H_2O_2, which is reactive and should be measured directly or frozen immediately for future evaluation. As assays for mediators of interest become more sensitive, and collection techniques trap less water, EBC sensitivity might improve.

In comparison, ENO and induced sputum are sensitive for separating asthmatic from normal subjects.

G. SPECIFICITY

Perhaps one of the most difficult aspects thus far in evaluating EBC is the fact that most mediators studied lack specificity for particular disease processes. Multiple pulmonary diseases have been evaluated and include asthma, COPD, healthy smokers, bronchiectasis, cystic fibrosis, acute respiratory distress syndrome (ARDS), and sarcoidosis. Mediator levels, in general, typically are elevated when compared with those of normal controls. Studies involving pH, however, demonstrate a decrease in asthma and cystic fibrosis, but again this is nonspecific.[39] At present, established patterns of inflammation that correlate with definitive diseases have not been established. This lessens its clinical utility when compared with direct pathologic samples that can be obtained through biopsy. Although EBC lacks specificity with regard to diagnostic utility, it might ultimately be more useful in tracking disease course once the diagnosis has been established.

H. VALIDATION

Variability in reproducibility from one laboratory to the next remains the final hurdle. Being able to demonstrate that a method can be used consistently from institution to institution and can provide reproducible results in given research and clinical conditions is a necessity. Although studies have demonstrated a significant difference in leukotriene levels in diseases such as asthma,[40] confirmatory studies in many laboratories using methods soon to be recommended by the European Respiratory Society/American Thoracic Society (ERS/ATS) task force are required. Until that time, EBC will remain an experimental tool.

IV. CONCLUSION

Currently, EBC shows promise as a noninvasive tool in both the research and clinical setting for evaluating lung inflammation. Clearly, many issues remain regarding its further development as a useful methodology (Table 9.1). Standards remain to be

TABLE 9.1
Comparisons between Methods for Assessing Pulmonary Inflammation

Parameter	Bronchoscopy	BAL	Induced Sputum	Exhaled NO	EBC
Safety	Risk of oversedation, bleeding, hypoxemia, bronchospasm, pneumothorax, death	Risk of oversedation, hypoxemia, bronchospasm, death	Risk of bronchospasm, hypoxemia	No significant risk	No significant risk
Invasivity (0–5)	5	4	2	0	0
Suitability for repeated testing	Low	Low	Moderate	High	High
Procedure cost	High	High	Medium	Equipment cost currently high; low cost per test	Collection cost is low; processing cost depends on mediators of interest
Capital equipment	Bronchoscopy facility; equipment for biopsy processing, molecular biology, etc.	Bronchoscopy facility; equipment for BAL processing	Nebulizer; spirometer; equipment for cytospin preparation and mediator assays	NO analyzer; calibration gases; mouthpieces	EBC collector; equipment for mediator assays
Time investment	1–2 hours procedure time; 4–6 hours patient recovery time; 5–10 hours Biopsy processing	1–2 hours procedure time; 4–6 hours patient recovery time; 2 hours BAL cell differential; mediator assays: time varies	1 hour induction time; 2 hours to prepare cytospin and count differentials; mediator assays: time varies	Test is rapidly performed (10–15 minutes); online result is immediate	Collection time; mediator assays: time varies
Special skills required	Bronchoscopy; pathologic interpretation	Bronchoscopy; cytologic interpretation; specific mediator assays for BAL	Sputum preparation; cytologic interpretation; specific mediator assays for BAL	No special skills required	Specific mediator assays for EBC
Spectrum on inflammation (0–5)	5; Light microscopy with special stains; assessment of tissue architecture-remodeling; electron microscopy; molecular techniques, e.g., immunohistochemistry, Western, Northern blotting, RT-PCR, etc.; genetic processing	3; Characterize cells and mediators participating in inflammatory response	3; Characterize cells and mediators participating in inflammatory response	1; Measures only NO, a marker and mediator of the inflammatory response in asthma but not in all diseases	2; Measurement of wide range of mediators and chemicals
Validation	Gold standard	Well validated	Well validated	Well validated	Unvalidated

Abbreviation: RT-PCR, reverse transcriptase polymerase chain reaction.

determined pertaining to methods of collection, determining disease specificity, and distinguishing between health and disease. Once these have been clarified, EBC might move from bench to bedside and reduce the need for more invasive testing.

FURTHER READING

1. Allen, M.S. et al., Video-assisted thoracic surgical procedures: the Mayo experience, *Mayo Clin. Proc.*, 71, 351, 1996.
2. Chuang, M.T. et al., Bronchoscopy in diffuse lung disease: evaluation by open lung biopsy in nondiagnostic transbronchial lung biopsy, *Ann. Otol. Rhinol. Laryngol.*, 96, 654, 1987.
3. Kadokura, M. et al., Pathologic comparison of video-assisted thoracic surgical lung biopsy with traditional open lung biopsy, *J. Thorac. Cardiovasc. Surg.*, 109, 494, 1995.
4. Djukanovic, R. et al., Safety of biopsies and bronchoalveolar lavage, *Eur. Respir. J. Suppl.*, 26, 39S, 1998.
5. Jarjour, N.N. et al., Investigative use of bronchoscopy in asthma, *Am. J. Respir. Crit. Care Med.*, 157, 692, 1998.
6. Robinson, D.S. et al., Biopsies: bronchoscopic technique and sampling, *Eur. Respir. J. Suppl.*, 26, 16S, 1998.
7. Fabbri, L.M. et al., Assessment of airway inflammation: an overview, *Eur. Respir. J. Suppl.*, 26, 6S, 1998.
8. Saetta, M. et al., Biopsies: processing and assessment, *Eur. Respir. J. Suppl.*, 26, 20S, 1998.
9. Chanez, P. and Vignola, A.M., Bronchial brushing, *Eur. Respir. J. Suppl.*, 26, 26S, 1998.
10. Wenzel, S.E. et al., Evidence that severe asthma can be divided pathologically into two inflammatory subtypes with distinct physiologic and clinical characteristics, *Am. J. Respir. Crit. Care Med.*, 160, 1001, 1999.
11. Bousquet, J. et al., Eosinophilic inflammation in asthma, *N. Engl. J. Med.*, 323, 1033, 1990.
12. Stelmach, I., Jerzynska, J., and Kuna, P., Markers of allergic inflammation in peripheral blood of children with asthma after treatment with inhaled triamcinolone acetonide, *Ann. Allergy Asthma Immunol.*, 87, 319, 2001.
13. Westcott, J.Y. et al., Urinary leukotriene E_4 in patients with asthma. Effect of airways reactivity and sodium cromoglycate, *Am. Rev. Respir. Dis*, 143, 1322, 1991.
14. Green, R.H. et al., Asthma exacerbations and sputum eosinophil counts: a randomised controlled trial, *Lancet*, 360, 1715, 2002.
15. Bates, C.A. and Silkoff, P.E., Exhaled nitric oxide in asthma: from bench to bedside, *J. Allergy Clin. Immunol.*, 111, 256, 2003.
16. Recommendations for standardized procedures for the on-line and off-line measurement of exhaled lower respiratory nitric oxide and nasal nitric oxide in adults and children-1999. This official statement of the American Thoracic Society was adopted by the ATS Board of Directors, July 1999, *Am. J. Respir. Crit Care Med.*, 160, 2104, 1999.
17. Deykin, A. et al., Exhaled nitric oxide as a diagnostic test for asthma: online versus offline techniques and effect of flow rate, *Am. J. Respir. Crit. Care Med.*, 165, 1597, 2002.
18. Chatkin, J.M. et al., Exhaled nitric oxide as a noninvasive assessment of chronic cough, *Am. J. Respir. Crit. Care Med.*, 159, 1810, 1999.

19. Jones, S.L. et al., The predictive value of exhaled nitric oxide measurements in assessing changes in asthma control, *Am. J. Respir. Crit. Care Med.*, 164, 738, 2001.

20. Mutlu, G.M. et al., Collection and analysis of exhaled breath condensate in humans, *Am. J. Respir. Crit. Care Med.*, 164, 731, 2001.

21. Vass, G. et al., Comparison of nasal and oral inhalation during exhaled breath condensate collection, *Am. J. Respir. Crit. Care Med.*, 167, 850, 2003.

22. Effros, R.M. et al., Dilution of respiratory solutes in exhaled condensates, *Am. J. Respir. Crit. Care Med.*, 165, 663, 2002.

23. Hunt, J., Exhaled breath condensate: an evolving tool for noninvasive evaluation of lung disease, *J. Allergy Clin. Immunol.*, 110, 28, 2002.

24. van Beurden, W.J. et al., An efficient and reproducible method for measuring hydrogen peroxide in exhaled breath condensate, *Respir. Med.*, 96, 197, 2002.

25. Shahid, S.K. et al., Increased interleukin-4 and decreased interferon-gamma in exhaled breath condensate of children with asthma, *Am. J. Respir. Crit. Care Med.*, 165, 1290, 2002.

26. Canady, R.G. et al., Vital capacity reservoir and online measurement of childhood nitrosopnea are linearly related. Clinical implications, *Am. J. Respir. Crit. Care Med.*, 159, 311, 1999.

27. Huszar, E. et al., Adenosine in exhaled breath condensate in healthy volunteers and in patients with asthma, *Eur. Respir. J.*, 20, 1393, 2002.

28. Jöbsis, Q. et al., Hydrogen peroxide in exhaled air of healthy children: reference values, *Eur. Respir. J.*, 12, 483, 1998.

29. Cunningham, S. et al., Measurement of inflammatory markers in the breath condensate of children with cystic fibrosis, *Eur. Respir. J.*, 15, 955, 2000.

30. Mutti, A. et al., Reporting data on exhaled breath condensate, *Am. J. Respir. Crit. Care Med.*, 168, 719, 2003.

31. Silkoff, P.E. et al., Marked flow-dependence of exhaled nitric oxide using a new technique to exclude nasal nitric oxide, *Am. J. Respir. Crit. Care Med.*, 155, 260, 1997.

32. Schleiss, M.B. et al., The concentration of hydrogen peroxide in exhaled air depends on expiratory flow rate, *Eur. Respir. J.*, 16, 1115, 2000.

33. Silkoff, P.E. et al., Dose-response relationship and reproducibility of the fall in exhaled nitric oxide after inhaled beclomethasone dipropionate therapy in asthma patients, *Chest*, 119, 1322, 2001.

34. Fahy, J.V. et al., Safety and reproducibility of sputum induction in asthmatic subjects in a multicenter study, *Am. J. Respir. Crit. Care Med.*, 163, 1470, 2001.

35. Faul, J.L. et al., The reproducibility of repeat measures of airway inflammation in stable atopic asthma, *Am. J. Respir. Crit. Care Med.*, 160, 1457, 1999.

36. Ganas, K. et al., Total nitrite/nitrate in expired breath condensate of patients with asthma, *Respir. Med.*, 95, 649, 2001.

37. Hunt, J.F. et al., Endogenous airway acidification. Implications for asthma pathophysiology, *Am. J. Respir. Crit. Care Med.*, 161, 694, 2000.

38. Nowak, D. et al., Cigarette smoking does not increase hydrogen peroxide levels in expired breath condensate of patients with stable COPD, *Monaldi Arch. Chest Dis.*, 53, 268, 1998.

39. Tate, S. et al., Airways in cystic fibrosis are acidified: detection by exhaled breath condensate, *Thorax*, 57, 926, 2002.

40. Csoma, Z. et al., Increased leukotrienes in exhaled breath condensate in childhood asthma, *Am. J. Respir. Crit. Care Med.*, 166, 1345, 2002.

10 Analysis of Exhaled Breath Condensate: Potential Implications for Diagnosis and Therapy of Lung Diseases

Umur Hatipoğlu and Israel Rubinstein

CONTENTS

I. INTRODUCTION

Collection and analysis of nonvolatile compounds in exhaled breath condensate (EBC) provides a simple, nonintrusive, real-time, point-of-care clinical and research tool for evaluating lung pathobiology. Collection usually lasts 15 to 20 minutes and can be repeated in the same individual during a short time interval using, in some cases, portable devices. Hence, EBC represents a promising tool to address diagnostic and therapeutic challenges facing physicians caring for patients with pulmonary disorders.

TABLE 10.1

Inflammatory Mediators Detected in EBC in Various Pulmonary Diseases

Condition	Compound
Cigarette smoking	H_2O_2, 8-isoprostane, total protein, nitrite, cytokines (IL-1, TNF-α)
COPD	H_2O_2, 8-isoprostane, cytokines (IL-1, sIL-2R, TNF-α), aldehydes, LTB$_4$, PGE$_2$, nitrites, nitrosothiols
Asthma	H_2O_2, 8-isoprostane, nitrotyrosine, thiobarbituric acid reactive products, leukotrienes, pH, PGE$_2$, aldehydes, glutathione, adenosine, cytokines (IL-4, IFN-γ)
Bronchiectasis	H_2O_2
Cystic fibrosis	H_2O_2, 8-isoprostane, nitrite, nitrotyrosine, pH, IL-6, LTB$_4$
ALI/ARDS	H_2O_2, 8-isoprostane, PGE$_2$
Interstitial lung disease	H_2O_2, vitronectin, endothelin-1
Obstructive sleep apnea	IL-6, 8-isoprostane
Lung cancer	IL-6
Pneumonia	Hepatocyte growth factor
Common cold	H_2O_2

Abbreviations: ALI, acute lung injury; sIL-2R, soluble interleukin-2 receptor.

This chapter delineates current applications of EBC analysis in patients with certain pulmonary disorders (Table 10.1). It is based on a Medline search since 1966 to present for peer-reviewed articles published in English.

II. OBSTRUCTIVE LUNG DISEASES

A. Asthma

Asthma is a chronic inflammatory disease of the airway characterized by reversible airflow obstruction. Clinically, asthma severity is determined by measurement of expiratory flow rates and symptoms. Smoldering inflammation is present even in patients with mild to moderate asthma. Long-term presence of inflammation and repeated episodes of acute inflammation result in structural changes in the airway, collectively termed airway remodeling, which might cause chronic airflow obstruction. It is conceivable that detection of inflammatory biomarkers in the airway, before clinical symptoms develop, would allow optimal monitoring of inflammation and improve management of patients with asthma.

Various inflammatory markers present in EBC have been investigated as possible biomarkers of disease activity in asthma. Hydrogen peroxide (H_2O_2) is one of the best-studied markers. Activated cells in the airway including epithelial cells, mast cells, eosinophils, neutrophils, and macrophages are the likely source for H_2O_2 through conversion of superoxide anion by superoxide dismutase during respiratory burst. Antczak et al.[1] demonstrated increased concentrations of H_2O_2 and thiobarbituric acid-reactive (TBAR) substances (a marker of lipid peroxidation/oxidative damage) in patients with asthma compared with healthy volunteers. An increase in

H_2O_2 concentrations was associated with a decrease in forced expiratory volume at 1 second (FEV_1) in these patients. The same group of investigators subsequently showed a significant reduction in exhaled H_2O_2 concentrations in patients with asthma treated with inhaled corticosteroids compared with placebo in a double-blind study. Similar to their previous study, a negative correlation was noted between H_2O_2 concentration and FEV_1 after 1 month of treatment.[2] The decrease in H_2O_2 concentrations was maintained for 2 weeks after inhaled corticosteroids were discontinued.

In children with asthma, H_2O_2 concentrations are increased in EBC when compared with controls[3] and decrease with anti-inflammatory medications.[4] Other studies also have shown that exhaled H_2O_2 concentrations in asthmatic patients correlate with airway hyperresponsiveness,[5,6] sputum eosinophil count,[5] and serum eosinophil cationic protein.[6] Horváth et al.[5] studied 116 asthmatic patients and found that exhaled H_2O_2 was elevated in a subgroup of patients not well controlled with inhaled corticosteroids, although exhaled nitric oxide (ENO) was not. This finding suggested that exhaled H_2O_2 might be more useful than ENO in monitoring asthmatic patients. The enthusiasm for exhaled H_2O_2 monitoring is tempered by the observations that repeated measurements have high variability, measured concentrations are at the lower limits of detection of assays, concentrations are flow dependent, and up to 30% of patients with corticosteroid-naïve asthma might not have elevated concentrations.[5]

Exhaled nitric oxide (NO) is an established marker of airway inflammation and is increased in patients with asthma.[7] NO-related products such as nitrite, nitrate, nitrotyrosine, and nitrosothiols are nonvolatile and have been measured in EBC. Ganas et al.[8] measured total nitrite/nitrate in EBC of 50 patients with asthma and 10 normal nonatopic individuals. Concentrations of exhaled nitrite/nitrate were elevated in patients with asthma who were naïve to corticosteroids when compared to normals and inhaled corticosteroid-treated patients with asthma. Peroxynitrite is a highly unstable molecule that forms with the reaction of nitric oxide and superoxide anion; it is therefore an indicator of oxidative stress and inflammation in the lung. In contrast to peroxynitrite, nitrotyrosine is a stable compound produced when peroxynitrite reacts with tyrosine residues in proteins. Hanazawa et al.[9] compared concentrations of nitrotyrosine, NO, and leukotrienes in EBC of patients with asthma to those in normal nonsmoking controls. In patients with mild corticosteroid-naïve asthma, concentrations of nitrotyrosine were elevated when compared to patients with moderate and severe asthma who were taking corticosteroids and normal subjects. Leukotrienes (LTB_4 and cys-leukotrienes [cys-LTs] LTC_4, LTD_4, and LTE_4), on the other hand, were elevated in stepwise fashion, commensurating with asthma severity. In contrast to mild corticosteroid-naïve asthmatics, NO and nitrotyrosine concentrations were not elevated in patients with moderate and severe asthma who were taking corticosteroids, leading the authors to speculate that NO production played a critical role in nitrotyrosine production and that systemic corticosteroids inhibit oxidative stress.

Another group of stable NO metabolites, nitrosothiols (RS-NOs) are formed as a result of reaction between NO and glutathione, a marker of antioxidant response. RS-NOs in EBC were higher in patients with severe asthma when compared to patients with milder disease.[10]

Nonenzymatic peroxidation of membrane phospholipids (arachidonic acid) during oxidative stress leads to the formation of isoprostanes that have been investigated in EBC of patients with asthma.[11,12] Their stability and specificity for lipid peroxidation make them potentially reliable biomarkers of oxidative stress.[13] The concentration of 8-isoprostane in EBC is elevated in patients with asthma when compared with controls, and concentrations correlate with disease severity.[14]

Interestingly, concentrations of 8-isoprostane were not different between corticosteroid-naïve and corticosteroid-treated patients with asthma.[15] In the same study, in a subgroup of patients with aspirin-sensitive asthma, concentrations of 8-isoprostane were significantly lower in EBC in patients who have received corticosteroids, suggesting that there is a corticosteroid-dependent inhibitory mechanism of oxidative stress in aspirin-sensitive asthma that is not present in aspirin-tolerant asthma.

Such profiling of eicosanoids holds great promise in gaining further insight into asthma pathophysiology. Baraldi et al.[16] measured 8-isoprostane in EBC of children with asthma exacerbation before and after treatment with corticosteroids. Although 8-isoprostane concentrations decreased following a 5-day course of corticosteroids, they remained elevated when compared to control subjects, suggesting continued oxidative stress despite clinical improvement in children with asthma exacerbation. Prostaglandin E_2 (PGE$_2$), which is predominantly elaborated by epithelial and airway smooth muscle cells, relaxes airway smooth muscles and might have anti-inflammatory activity. Therefore, it has been hypothesized that deficiency of PGE$_2$ could lead to unchecked inflammation in asthma. In two studies measuring PGE$_2$ in EBC,[15,17] however, concentrations were not different between normal subjects and patients with asthma.

Leukotrienes, in particular cys-LTs (LTC$_4$, LTD$_4$, and LTE$_4$), have an important role in asthma pathophysiology. They induce airway smooth muscle contraction, increase vascular permeability, decrease mucociliary clearance, induce mucus hypersecretion, and recruit eosinophils to the lung. Concentrations of both cys-LTs and LTB$_4$, a potent neutrophil chemoattractant, were elevated in patients with asthma as compared to healthy controls.[9] Although there was no correlation between leukotrienes and FEV$_1$, concentrations of leukotrienes increased with asthma severity. In a study of 38 children with asthma of varying severity and 11 nonatopic children, Csoma et al.[18] found increased concentrations of cys-LTs and LTB$_4$ in EBC of patients with persistent asthma when compared to patients with mild intermittent asthma and nonatopic controls. Given that LTB$_4$ and cys-LTs were elevated particularly in children with severe asthma, the authors speculated that use of 5-lipoxygenase inhibitors could be more effective than leukotriene receptor antagonists because they inhibit synthesis of both LTB$_4$ and cys-LTs. A 5-day course of prednisone effectively lowers concentrations of cys-LTs in EBC of asthmatic children and brings their levels close to those of controls.[16]

Montuschi et al.[17] showed that concentrations of LTE$_4$ and LTB$_4$ were elevated in EBC of corticosteroid-naïve patients with mild asthma when compared to healthy nonsmoker control subjects. The concentrations of LTB$_4$ in EBC correlated with concentrations of ENO, suggesting interdependent roles in airway inflammation. The concentration of LTE$_4$, conversely, had no correlation with ENO, as reported by Csoma et al.[18]

Detection of elevated proinflammatory mediators in EBC of patients with relatively asymptomatic asthma and normal pulmonary function tests could offer a novel way to monitor lung inflammation and perhaps initiating treatment at an earlier time. In patients with corticosteroid-naïve aspirin-sensitive asthma, the concentrations of cys-LTs in EBC are significantly higher when compared to corticosteroid-naïve patients with aspirin-tolerant asthma,[15] indicating the importance of these eicosanoids in the pathogenesis of aspirin intolerance.

Aldehydes are produced from oxidation of cell membrane phospholipids. Concentrations of aldehydes and glutathione in biological fluids reflect lipid peroxidation and antioxidant status (i.e., oxidative stress). Aldehydes and glutathione were measured in EBC of children with asthma exacerbation, before and after treatment with prednisone, and in controls.[19] During exacerbation, malondialdehyde concentrations were higher in patients when compared to control subjects. After 5 days of treatment with prednisone, concentrations returned to values comparable to those in healthy individuals. Interestingly, glutathione concentrations were lower than those in controls and increased following therapy but not to normal concentrations. This study confirmed the presence of increased oxidative stress during asthma exacerbation.

Turbulent flow, such as would occur during an asthma exacerbation, theoretically can increase aerosolization of droplets and lead to a falsely elevated solute concentration in EBC.[20] The bidirectional changes in the biomarkers studied in the aforementioned study, in particular the increase in glutathione after treatment of asthma exacerbation, argued against this contention.

Low pH in EBC has been observed during acute asthma exacerbation and reverts to normal with corticosteroid therapy.[21] Kostikas et al.[22] studied pH in exhaled breath condensate of patients with various inflammatory airway diseases (asthma, chronic obstructive pulmonary disease [COPD], and bronchiectasis) and healthy subjects. The pH was lower in patients with asthma when compared to healthy subjects and correlated with sputum eosinophilia, FEV_1, H_2O_2, 8-isoprostane, and total nitrite and nitrate concentrations. A strong positive correlation between eosinophil count and EBC pH coupled with the observation that patients who had more severe asthma and were not taking corticosteroids had a lower pH suggested that eosinophilic inflammation could decrease pH.

Adenosine, a breakdown product of adenosine triphosphate (ATP), is a mediator of immediate bronchoconstriction and might have modulatory effect on inflammation. Huszár et al.[23] examined adenosine concentrations in EBC of 43 patients with asthma and 40 healthy volunteers. Adenosine concentrations were higher in corticosteroid-naïve patients compared with healthy controls and corticosteroid-treated patients. Adenosine concentration also increased with worsening symptoms of asthma. Because there was significant overlap of adenosine concentrations in healthy subjects and patients with asthma, adenosine did not appear to be a suitable diagnostic tool for bronchial asthma.

Interleukin-4 (IL-4) and interferon-γ (IFN-γ) are detected in EBC of normal children and children with asthma.[24] In asthma, there is an imbalance in lymphocyte subpopulations favoring Th2 cells, which produce IL-4, over Th1 cells, which elaborate IFN-γ. Indeed, the IL-4/IFN-γ ratio was elevated in children with asthma compared to healthy children. Inhaled corticosteroids brought the ratio close to that of healthy children.

Allergic rhinitis is present in more than half of patients with asthma. Sandrini et al.[25] demonstrated that nasal triamcinolone treatment of patients with allergic rhinitis with or without concomitant asthma resulted in lower levels of ENO (ENO) and H_2O_2 in EBC. Interestingly, patients who had allergic rhinitis without asthma displayed higher concentrations of H_2O_2 than patients with both conditions. ENO, on the other hand, was higher at baseline in patients with asthma, suggesting it could reflect lower airway inflammation better than H_2O_2 does. There were no changes in bronchial hyperresponsiveness, nasal and asthma symptoms, or peak expiratory flow with treatment, indicating that ENO and H_2O_2 are more sensitive than clinical parameters to assess airway inflammation.

B. Chronic Obstructive Pulmonary Disease

Persistent airway inflammation in COPD increases oxidative stress and might contribute to disease progression. Neutrophils appear to play a more central role in inflammation of COPD, in contrast to asthma, in which eosinophils predominate. The oxidative burden in COPD was assessed in EBC in a number of studies. Hydrogen peroxide concentration was increased in EBC of stable patients with COPD compared to healthy subjects, with further increases noted during acute exacerbation.[26] Notably, concentrations of H_2O_2 correlated with eosinophil count in induced sputum.

In a well-designed, randomized, placebo-controlled, crossover trial, administration of high-dose inhaled beclomethasone had no effect on EBC H_2O_2 concentrations in 20 patients with stable COPD.[27] ENO concentrations, however, were reduced while patients were on inhaled beclomethasone and increased while patients were on placebo. The lack of change in H_2O_2 concentrations was attributed, in part, to the ineffectiveness of corticosteroids in neutrophilic inflammation. In contrast, van Beurden et al.[28] found a significant reduction in the concentration of H_2O_2 in EBC after treatment with inhaled corticosteroids in a single-blinded, randomized, crossover study of stable COPD patients, suggesting that oxidative stress in COPD might be modified by inhaled corticosteroids. Of note, most patients in this study were current smokers and inhaled corticosteroids were administered for a relatively long period of time, two factors that may have accounted for the observed differences between the studies.

Kasielski and Nowak[29] showed in a double-blind, double-dummy study that long-term administration of N-acetylcysteine, a mucolytic drug that has antioxidant properties, reduced exhaled H_2O_2 concentrations in 22 patients with stable COPD when compared to placebo. It is noteworthy that changes occurred after 9 to 12 months of treatment. The clinical significance of this finding is unclear; however, administration of antioxidants holds promise in patients with inflammatory airway diseases such as COPD. Nonetheless, determination of H_2O_2 in EBC might allow appropriate patient selection for such intervention.

Montuschi et al.[30] demonstrated that 8-isoprostane concentrations were similar in COPD ex-smokers and COPD current smokers, and were increased 1.8-fold compared with healthy smokers. Current smokers with COPD had 2.2-fold higher 8-isoprostane concentrations than healthy nonsmokers. In addition, acute smoking increased 8-isoprostane concentrations by 50% within 15. Exacerbations of COPD also are associated with elevated 8-isoprostane concentrations in EBC that decrease after antibiotic treatment.[31]

Corradi et al.[32] showed that malondialdehyde, a marker of oxidative stress, is increased in EBC of patients with COPD. In a study of 20 patients with stable, moderate to severe COPD, concentrations of aldehydes (malondialdehyde, hexanal, heptanal, and nonanal) in EBC were elevated when compared with those in non-smoking control subjects. Only malondialdehyde, however, distinguished smoking control subjects from patients with COPD, with higher concentrations in the latter group. Moreover, malondialdehyde concentrations in EBC of COPD ex-smokers were higher than those in smoking control subjects, suggesting a mechanism other than smoking that accounted for the marked increase in lipid peroxidation in COPD.

The concentrations of certain eicosanoids in EBC have been determined by enzyme immunoassay in patients with COPD during clinically stable periods and exacerbations. In line with the neutrophilic nature of inflammation, LTB_4 concentrations in EBC were higher in patients with stable COPD (both in corticosteroid-naïve and corticosteroid-treated subjects) when compared to control subjects.[33] In contrast to patients with asthma, concentrations of LTE_4 in EBC of patients with COPD were not significantly elevated when compared to controls. Concentrations of PGE_2, an eicosanoid with anti-inflammatory effects, were elevated in EBC of patients with stable COPD, presumably counteracting the effects of LTB_4. In contrast, PGE_2 is not elevated in EBC of patients with asthma.[15,17]

Taken together, these findings suggest that the eicosanoid profiles in EBC are different in asthma and COPD. During an exacerbation, LTB_4 concentrations increase.[31] After a course of antibiotics but without systemic corticosteroids, concentrations decrease close to those of healthy subjects, albeit over a period of 2 months. Lastly, similar to asthma, patients with COPD have increased concentrations of nitrite and nitrosothiols compared to healthy subjects and healthy smokers.[10]

Cigarette smoking is clearly the greatest risk factor for developing of COPD. However, only 10 to 15% of habitual smokers develop COPD. Therefore, it is of great clinical interest to identify those smokers who are at higher risk of developing COPD. Nowak et al.[34] demonstrated a five-fold higher H_2O_2 concentration in EBC of cigarette smokers when compared to healthy nonsmokers. Male smokers appear to exhale more H_2O_2 than female subjects. In another study that correlated exhaled breath H_2O_2 with H_2O_2 generated from the alveolar lining fluid, exhaled H_2O_2 was 5×10^4 times lower than that produced in the alveolar lining fluid.[35] This difference was attributed to the presence of antioxidants in the lower respiratory tract epithelial lining fluid. Removal of H_2O_2 by the antioxidant system, which is also activated by smoking, might explain the lack of correlation between exposure to cigarette smoke and the concentration of H_2O_2 in EBC. To this end, H_2O_2 concentration in EBC of smokers is increased 30 minutes after combustion of one cigarette.[36] Nevertheless, cigarette smoking in patients with stable COPD does not appear to increase the concentration of exhaled H_2O_2 further.[37]

The concentrations of IL-6 and LTB$_4$ in EBC of smokers were also higher when compared to nonsmoking individuals.[38] The concentrations of IL-6 correlated with number of cigarettes smoked per day, exhaled carbon monoxide (CO), LTB$_4$, and lung function.

In a study of young healthy college students who smoked, Garey et al.[39] demonstrated higher concentrations of total protein, nitrite, and neutrophil chemotactic activity in comparison with nonsmoking controls. IL-1 and tumor necrosis factor alpha (TNF-α) concentrations were not different between the two groups. Although smoking one cigarette did not increase nitrite and nitrate concentrations in EBC of young healthy smokers in the latter study, Corradi et al.[40] showed that nitrate concentrations are increased more than six-fold in EBC of healthy smokers but not in patients with COPD, relative to nonsmoking healthy controls. Given that smokers reported by Garey et al. were younger, these seemingly discrepant results might indicate early and late effects of cigarette smoking on NO metabolites in the human airway. Whether EBC determination of NO metabolites, H$_2$O$_2$, and other inflammatory mediators in smokers could be helpful in predicting progression to COPD would be best addressed in a longitudinal study.

C. Bronchiectasis

Bronchiectasis is a suppurative lung disease characterized by recurrent chronic bacterial infections and consequent oxidant stress that has been quantitated using EBC H$_2$O$_2$. Loukides et al.[41] showed higher exhaled H$_2$O$_2$ concentrations in EBC of patients with bronchiectasis when compared to healthy controls. A negative correlation between H$_2$O$_2$ and FEV$_1$ was documented. In a follow-up study,[42] significant correlations were shown between H$_2$O$_2$ and percentage of neutrophils in induced sputum, severity of bronchiectasis on high-resolution computed tomography (CT) scan of the chest, and clinical symptoms scores. Long-term antibiotic therapy was associated with higher H$_2$O$_2$ concentrations, probably because persistently infected patients tended to receive long-term antibiotic therapy. Colonization with *Pseudomonas aeruginosa* was associated with higher H$_2$O$_2$ concentration in EBC of patients with bronchiectasis.[41,42]

However, both studies were cross-sectional and not powered to suggest causality between oxidant stress and bronchiectasis pathogenesis. Nonetheless, collection and analysis of EBC in patients with bronchiectasis could prove useful in early detection and treatment of heightened airway inflammation, thereby slowing further deterioration in lung function and improving quality of life.

D. Cystic Fibrosis

Cystic fibrosis is characterized by presence of copious and viscid secretions in the airways that lead to recurrent bacterial infections. Chronic bacterial infections, in particular *P. aeruginosa*, and subsequent oxidant stress lead to parenchymal scarring, bronchiectasis, and progressive loss of lung function. Preventing this vicious cycle of infection and lung damage is central to the management of cystic fibrosis. Given that inflammation is present even in asymptomatic patients with cystic fibrosis, there is a need to unravel biomarkers that could predict infective exacerbations before clinical symptoms develop. Several studies have sought to detect such markers in EBC.

The concentration of H_2O_2 in EBC of adult patients with clinically stable cystic fibrosis is not increased compared to that of healthy controls.[43] In a study of 16 children with cystic fibrosis exacerbation, however, H_2O_2 concentrations in EBC were elevated and decreased as patients improved clinically with antibiotic therapy.[44] There was no control group in this study. Although more longitudinal studies are needed, lack of elevated concentrations in EBC during clinically stable periods suggests that H_2O_2 might not be a suitable biomarker for smoldering inflammation in cystic fibrosis.

In contrast to H_2O_2, concentrations of nitrite in EBC are increased in adults[45] and children[46] with clinically stable cystic fibrosis when compared to controls. Interestingly, ENO concentrations were not elevated[44,45] (in fact, sometimes they are decreased[47,48]) in patients with cystic fibrosis. This discrepancy in the face of neutrophilic inflammation may be explained by release of superoxide anions during oxidative stress, which might result in formation of peroxynitrite (i.e., the scavenging effect of reactive oxygen species) or a defect in inducible NO synthase expression.[47] In addition to nitrite, elevation of nitrotyrosine[49] in EBC supports the notion that NO metabolism is increased in patients with cystic fibrosis.

The concentration of 8-isoprostane in EBC was elevated three-fold in clinically stable cystic fibrosis patients when compared to controls and correlated inversely with FEV_1.[48] A positive correlation was found between 8-isoprostane and exhaled CO concentrations, which could represent a physiological defense to counteract oxidative stress.

The pH of EBC in clinically stable cystic fibrosis patients is lower than in controls.[49] Values were further reduced during an exacerbation and increased significantly following antibiotic treatment. Low pH in cystic fibrosis airways is likely to be due to both neutrophilic inflammation and impaired epithelial cell bicarbonate secretion, which have been observed previously in cystic fibrosis.[50] Given that reduced pH may also have deleterious effects on lung defense, including increased mucus viscosity and reduced ciliary function, it is a clinically relevant parameter that could be monitored and be targeted for treatment in cystic fibrosis.

Carpagnano et al.[47] showed that the concentrations of LTB_4 and IL-6, two inflammatory mediators that are increased in chronic neutrophilic inflammation, are increased in EBC of patients with cystic fibrosis compared to age-matched healthy subjects. Concentrations of both mediators were elevated in EBC of cystic fibrosis patients when compared to controls. During an exacerbation, there were additional increases in LTB_4 and IL-6 concentration that reverted back to baseline with antibiotic therapy. Notably, higher concentrations of LTB_4 and IL-6 were present in patients with *P. aeruginosa* infection compared to other infectious agents. Two findings suggested that these mediators could be useful in monitoring disease activity in cystic fibrosis. First, normal values were clustered very tightly and there was virtually no overlap with stable cystic fibrosis patients. Second, the degree of reproducibility between two successive measurements was acceptable for both markers and with a coefficient of variation for LTB_4 measurements being 2%. In another study, IL-8 concentrations in EBC were found to be elevated in only one third of children with cystic fibrosis.[51]

III. PARENCHYMAL LUNG DISEASES

A. ACUTE LUNG INJURY/ACUTE RESPIRATORY DISTRESS SYNDROME

The concentration of H_2O_2 is increased in EBC collected from intubated and mechanically ventilated patients with acute respiratory distress syndrome (ARDS).[52,53] Although Baldwin et al.[52] reported higher concentrations of H_2O_2 compared with patients with other respiratory diseases, such a difference was not found by Sznajder et al.[53] In both studies, however, patients with pulmonary infiltrates tended to have higher concentrations of H_2O_2 compared to control subjects.

Interestingly, Sznajder et al.[53] showed higher concentrations of H_2O_2 in patients with sepsis independent of pulmonary infiltration. They proposed that monitoring and quantification of oxidant activity in EBC could be a useful tool in predicting risk of progression to ARDS. Kietzman et al.[54] also found elevated H_2O_2 in EBC of seven patients with ARDS compared to control subjects. However, the concentration of H_2O_2 in EBC did not correlate with prognosis over the study period of 9 days, an increase in H_2O_2 concentration did not herald the onset of ARDS, and a decrease in H_2O_2 concentration did not indicate improvement in lung injury.

Carpenter et al.[55] determined 8-isoprostane concentrations in EBC of patients with or at risk for acute lung injury/ARDS and in patients without lung disease who were intubated while undergoing minor surgical procedures. The concentration of 8-isoprostane in EBC of patients was more than 10 times that of control subjects. Given that PGE_2, which originates from monocytes and platelets, in EBC of patients was not elevated in comparison to control subjects, lipid peroxidation rather than cellular production appeared to be the predominant mechanism for 8-isoprostane formation in patients.

Collectively, these data support the hypothesis that oxidative stress is increased in ARDS. Reactive oxygen species formed during oxidative stress may cause lipid peroxidation and change membrane fluidity with consequent increased permeability. Although the finding of increased markers of oxidant stress is nonspecific, longitudinal measurement of such markers might help in monitoring effects of therapy and general management of patients with ARDS. Heard et al.[56] administered liposome-encapsulated PGE_1 intravenously to patients with ARDS. PGE_1 downregulates the CD11/CD18 receptor of the neutrophil, consequently limiting endothelial adhesion. The anticipated effect was reduction of neutrophil adhesion to the endothelium and thereby reduction of oxidative stress. However, H_2O_2 in EBC of patients who received therapy did not change over a period of 8 days when compared with patients who received placebo. Longitudinal studies could likely provide insight into the pathogenesis and management options in ARDS.

Mechanical ventilation may induce cytokine response that could be attenuated by minimizing overdistention and recruitment/derecruitment of the lung.[57] To this end, measurement of cytokines implicated in neutrophil recruitment (such as IL-6 and IL-8) in EBC of patients over time may assist in monitoring ventilator-associated lung injury in patients with ARDS.

B. INTERSTITIAL LUNG DISEASE

Interstitial lung diseases (ILDs) comprise a wide variety of conditions characterized by accumulation of mononuclear cells, fibroblasts with subsequent deposition of collagen, and fibrosis. The etiology of most ILDs is unknown. Because of the relative rarity of ILD, progress in "teasing out" cellular signaling and the biomarkers involved has been tedious. Examination of EBC for such mediators, especially in a longitudinal fashion, might be useful in identifying and using these biomarkers in monitoring disease process and ultimately tailoring therapies accordingly. In the seminal paper suggesting EBC as a diagnostic tool, Scheideler et al.[58] showed detectable concentrations of IL-1, soluble IL-2 receptor, and TNF-α in EBC of three patients with ILD.

Oxidative stress may be relevant to the pathophysiology of ILD.[59] In a study of 27 patients with systemic sclerosis, exhaled H_2O_2 was higher when compared to age- and sex-matched healthy controls.[60] The study was cross-sectional and there was significant overlap of exhaled H_2O_2 concentrations between patients and controls. All patients were treated with pentoxifylline and vitamin E, drugs with known antioxidant properties that might have affected results. Nevertheless, measurement of oxidative stress biomarkers may prove useful in monitoring disease activity in patients with systemic sclerosis.

Carpagnano et al.[61] measured the concentrations of vitronectin and endothelin-1, two established mediators of fibrosis, in EBC of patients with nonspecific interstitial pneumonia and fibrosing alveolitis caused by systemic sclerosis and compared them with those of normal subjects. Both were elevated in EBC of patients with fibrotic lung disease when compared to controls. Unstable patients and untreated patients tended to have higher concentrations of exhaled vitronectin. Similarly, patients who were treated with corticosteroids tended to have low concentrations of exhaled endothelin-1. The degree of reproducibility of endothelin-1 measurements appeared to be suboptimal, however.

The role of the T-helper cell subsets (Th1 and Th2) in the inflammatory response of the lung in idiopathic pulmonary fibrosis has been delineated and exploited therapeutically. A Th2 response leads to secretion of IL-4, IL-5, IL-10, and IL-13, the net effects of which are fibroblast activation and matrix deposition leading to fibrosis. As the counterpoint, Th1 response is characterized by secretion of IFN-γ, IL-2, IL-12, and IL-18, with the net effect of tissue restoration. A pilot study of patients with idiopathic pulmonary fibrosis showed that long-term treatment with IFN-1b probably benefits these patients by restoring the balance between Th1 and Th2 responses.[62] Measurement of cytokines involved in pulmonary repair in EBC of these patients could potentially be useful in identifying appropriate candidates for therapy as well as in developing new drugs.

IV. MISCELLANEOUS RESPIRATORY DISEASES

A. Obstructive Sleep Apnea Syndrome

Oxidative stress and systemic inflammation play important roles in the pathogenesis of obstructive sleep apnea syndrome (OSAS) and its cardiovascular complications.[63] In a study of patients with OSAS, obese subjects, and healthy age-matched subjects, IL-6 concentrations in EBC were higher in patients than those in obese subjects.[64] Both groups had higher concentrations in comparison with controls. These investigators found that 8-isoprostane concentrations were elevated only in patients with OSAS. These biomarkers might be useful in quantifying systemic inflammation and oxidative stress in OSAS, and in identifying obese individuals who might be at risk for developing OSAS. Given that EBC is simple and nonintrusive, it has the potential of being an important research tool in OSAS, particularly in nocturnal measurement of these substances.

B. Lung Cancer

Carpagnano et al.[65] determined IL-6 concentration in EBC of 20 patients with non-small-cell lung cancer and 15 healthy controls. They found that IL-6 concentration was increased compared to controls and that it correlated with the clinical stage of lung cancer. Although nonspecific for cancer, IL-6 and other cytokines might have potential for monitoring disease progression and prognostication.

C. Pulmonary Infections

EBC could also offer an efficient means of monitoring lung inflammation evoked by infectious agents. Hepatocyte growth factor (HGF), an epithelial growth factor produced in response to injury, was elevated in EBC of patients with pneumonia when compared to patients with nonrespiratory infections and healthy controls.[66] Serum concentrations of HGF decreased within a few days, whereas EBC levels remained elevated for weeks, suggesting local production of this compound. Thus, HGF might be a useful marker of lung injury and repair. Jöbsis et al.[67] demonstrated increased levels of H_2O_2 in EBC during common cold, with return to baseline after clinical recovery. These findings should be taken into account in studies using H_2O_2 as a marker of chronic lower airway inflammation.

V. SUMMARY AND FUTURE DIRECTIONS

There is a need for standardization of the exhaled breath condensate collection technique that is currently being addressed by an international task force. Further inquiry is necessary into diurnal variation, reproducibility of measurement, and origin of biomarkers measured in EBC. Correlating patient outcome data with concentrations of mediators is necessary to identify those related to distinct disease entities. It is desirable that finding new biomarkers also be correlated with more established methods such as bronchoalveolar lavage. In addition to markers for oxidative stress and cytokines, other proteins, lipids, and nucleic acids from mammalian cells and microorganisms as well as drugs might be present in exhaled breath. For instance, it is reasonable to assume that viral, bacterial, mycobacterial, and fungal proteins and/or RNA and DNA could be detected in EBC for early diagnosis and treatment of lung infections. However, the use of gene amplification test to detect *Mycobacterium tuberculosis* in EBC of patients being treated for active tuberculosis has been unsuccessful to date.[68]

Emphasis on patterns of inflammatory mediators rather than absolute concentrations of individual substances might provide more substantial clues about the pathophysiology of disease (e.g., low concentrations of cys-LTs in EBC of COPD patients compared to those in patients with asthma). It is also important to note that functional studies, such as neutrophil chemotaxis, are feasible as part of EBC analysis, and that the method is not necessarily restricted to identification of a single biomarker.[39] Surveillance for rejection after lung transplantation is an important potential area of EBC application. It is already established that ENO is a marker for clinical acute rejection in the EBC of lung transplant recipients distinguishable from infections or bronchiolitis obliterans.[69] Measurement of NO metabolites and other biomarkers in EBC of lung transplant recipients could afford closer monitoring for rejection and allow further insight into mechanisms of lung rejection. Monitoring of EBC might also be helpful in the postoperative setting. For instance, a prospective study of patients undergoing thoracotomy for lung resection revealed increased levels of H_2O_2 and malondialdehyde.[70] Measurement of oxidative stress in such patients could allow clinicians to monitor the degree of lung injury and repair process postoperatively.

Collection of EBC is a simple and convenient point-of-care intervention. It can be performed in virtually any clinical setting and with any patient group (including infants, children, and the elderly) and under virtually any conditions, such as mechanical ventilation. Collection can also be performed at home and its simplicity and acceptance by patients allows longitudinal sampling over time. Thus, EBC could represent a simple tool to monitor the natural history of pulmonary disorders and their responses to therapy.

ACKNOWLEDGMENTS

Supported, in part, by NIH grant HL72323 and VA Merit Review grant.

FURTHER READING

1. Antczak, A. et al., Increased hydrogen peroxide and thiobarbituric acid-reactive products in expired breath condensate of asthmatic patients, *Eur. Respir. J.*, 10, 1235, 1997.
2. Antczak, A. et al., Inhaled glucocorticosteroids decrease hydrogen peroxide level in expired air condensate in asthmatic patients, *Respir. Med.*, 94, 416, 2001.
3. Jöbsis, Q. et al., Hydrogen peroxide in exhaled air is increased in stable asthmatic children, *Eur. Respir. J.*, 10, 519, 1997.

4. Dohlman, A.W., Black, H.R., and Royall, J.A., Expired breath hydrogen peroxide is a marker of acute airway inflammation in pediatric patients with asthma, *Am. Rev. Respir. Dis.*, 148, 955, 1993.

5. Horváth, I. et al., Combined use of exhaled hydrogen peroxide and nitric oxide in monitoring asthma, *Am. J. Respir. Crit. Care Med.*, 158, 1042, 1998.

6. Emelyanov, A. et al., Elevated concentrations of exhaled hydrogen peroxide in asthmatic patients, *Chest*, 120,1136, 2001.

7. Kharitonov, S.A. and Barnes, P.J., Exhaled markers of pulmonary disease, *Am. J. Respir. Crit. Care Med.*, 163, 1693, 2001.

8. Ganas, K. et al., Total nitrites/nitrate in expired breath condensate of patients with asthma, *Respir. Med.*, 95, 649, 2001.

9. Hanazawa, T. et al., Increased nitrotyrosine in exhaled breath condensate of patients with asthma, *Am. J. Respir. Crit. Care Med.*, 162, 1273, 2000.

10. Corradi, M. et al., Increased nitrosothiols in exhaled breath condensate in inflammatory airway diseases, *Am. J. Respir. Crit. Care Med.*, 163, 854, 2001.

11. Roberts, L.J. and Morrow, J.D., The isoprostanes: novel markers of lipid peroxidation and potential mediators of oxidative injury, *Adv. Prostaglandin Thromboxane Leukotriene Res.*, 23, 219, 1995.

12. Morrow, J.D. et al., Non-cyclooxygenase derived prostanoids (F2-isoprostanes) are formed in situ on phospholipids, *Proc. Natl. Acad. Sci. U.S.A.*, 89, 10721, 1992.

13. Moore, K. and Roberts, L.J., Measurement of lipid peroxidation, *Free Radic. Res.*, 28, 659, 1998.

14. Montuschi, P., et al., Increased 8-isoprostane, a marker of oxidative stress, in exhaled condensate of asthma patients, *Am. J. Respir. Crit. Care Med.*, 160, 216, 1999.

15. Antczak, A. et al., Increased exhaled cysteinyl-leukotrienes and 8-isoprostane in aspirin induced asthma, *Am. J. Respir. Crit. Care Med.*, 166, 301, 2002.

16. Baraldi, E. et al., Cysteinyl leukotrienes and 8-isoprostane in exhaled breath condensate of children with asthma exacerbations, *Thorax*, 58, 505, 2003.

17. Montuschi, P. and Barnes, P.J., Exhaled leukotrienes and prostaglandins in asthma, *J. Allergy Clin. Immunol.*, 109,615, 2002.

18. Csoma, Z. et al., Increased leukotrienes in exhaled breath condensate in childhood asthma, *Am. J. Respir. Crit. Care Med.*, 166, 1345, 2002.

19. Corradi, M. et al., Aldehydes and glutathione in exhaled breath condensate of children with asthma exacerbation, *Am. J. Respir. Crit. Care Med.*, 167, 395, 2003.

20. Effros, R.M. et al., Dilution of respiratory solutes in exhaled condensate, *Am. J. Respir. Crit. Care Med.*, 165, 663, 2002.

21. Hunt, J.F. et al., Endogenous airway acidification: implications for asthma pathophysiology, *Am. J. Respir. Crit. Care Med.*, 161, 694, 2000.

22. Kostikas, K. et al., pH in expired breath condensate of patients with inflammatory airway diseases, *Am. J. Respir. Crit. Care Med.*, 165, 1364, 2002.

23. Huszár, É. Et al., Adenosine in exhaled breath condensate in healthy volunteers and in patients with asthma, *Eur. Respir. J.*, 20, 1393, 2002.

24. Shahid, S.K. et al., Increased interleukin-4 and decreased interferon-γ in exhaled breath condensate of children with asthma, *Am. J. Respir. Crit. Care Med.*, 165, 1290, 2002.

25. Sandrini, A. et al., Effect of nasal triamcinolone acetonide on lower airway inflammatory markers in patients with allergic rhinitis, *J. Allergy Clin. Immunol.*, 111, 313, 2003.

26. Dekhuijzen, P.N.R. et al., Increased exhalation of hydrogen peroxide in patients with stable and unstable chronic obstructive pulmonary disease, *Am. J. Respir. Crit. Care Med.*, 154, 813, 1996.

27. Ferreira Martens, I. et al., Exhaled nitric oxide and hydrogen peroxide in patients with chronic obstructive pulmonary disease, *Am. J. Respir. Crit. Care Med.*, 164, 1012, 2001.

28. Van Beurden, W.J.C. et al., Effects of inhaled corticosteroids with different lung deposition on exhaled hydrogen peroxide in stable COPD patients, *Respiration*, 70, 242, 2003.

29. Kasielski, M. and Nowak, D., Long-term administration of N-acetylcysteine decreases hydrogen peroxide exhalation in subjects with chronic obstructive pulmonary disease, *Respir. Med.*, 95, 448, 2001.

30. Montuschi, P. et al., Exhaled 8-isoprostane as an *in vivo* biomarker of lung oxidative stress in patients with COPD and healthy smokers, *Am. J. Respir. Crit. Care Med.*, 162, 1175, 2000.

31. Biernacki, W.A., Kharitonov, S.A., and Barnes, P.J., Increased leukotriene B4 and 8-isoprostane in exhaled breath condensate of patients with exacerbations of COPD, *Thorax*, 58, 294, 2003.

32. Corradi, M. et al., Aldehydes in exhaled breath condensate of patients with chronic obstructive pulmonary disease, *Am. J. Respir. Crit. Care Med.*, 167, 1380, 2003.

33. Montuschi, P. et al., Exhaled leukotrienes and prostaglandins in COPD. *Thorax*, 58, 585, 2003.

34. Nowak, D. et al., Increased content of hydrogen peroxide in the expired breath of cigarette smokers, *Eur. Respir. J.*, 9, 652, 1996.

35. Blue, M.L. and Janoff, A., Possible mechanisms of emphysema in cigarette smokers: release of elastase from human polymorphonuclear leukocytes by cigarette smoke condensate *in vitro*, *Am. Rev. Respir. Dis.*, 117,317, 1978.

36. Guatura, S.B. et al., Increased exhalation of hydrogen peroxide in healthy subjects following cigarette consumption, *Sao Paolo Med. J.*, 118, 93, 2000.

37. Nowak, D. et al., Cigarette smoking does not increase hydrogen peroxide levels in expired breath condensate of patients with stable COPD, *Monaldi Arch. Chest Dis.*, 53, 268, 1998.

38. Carpagnano, G.E. et al., Increased inflammatory markers in the exhaled breath condensate of cigarette smokers, *Eur. Respir. J.*, 21, 589, 2003.

39. Garey, K.W. et al., Markers of inflammation in exhaled breath condensate of young healthy smokers, *Chest*, 125, 22, 2004.

40. Corradi, M., Pesci, A., and Casana, R., Nitrates in exhaled breath condensate of patients with different airway diseases, *Nitric Oxide*, 8, 26, 2003.

41. Loukides, S. et al., Elevated levels of expired breath hydrogen peroxide in bronchiectasis, *Am. J. Respir. Crit. Care Med.*, 158, 991, 1998.

42. Loukides, S. et al., Exhaled H_2O_2 in steady-state bronchiectasis: relationship with cellular composition in induced sputum, spirometry, and extent and severity of disease, *Chest*, 121, 81, 2002.

43. Ho, L.P. et al., Expired hydrogen peroxide in breath condensate of cystic fibrosis patients, *Eur. Respir. J.*, 13, 103, 1999.

44. Jöbsis, Q. et al., Hydrogen peroxide and nitric oxide in exhaled air of children with cystic fibrosis during antibiotic treatment, *Eur. Respir. J.*, 16, 95, 2000.

45. Ho, L.P., Innes, J.A., and Greening, A.P., Nitrite levels in breath condensate of patients with cystic fibrosis is elevated in contrast exhaled nitric oxide, *Thorax*, 53, 680, 1998.

46. Cunningham, S. et al., Measurement of inflammatory markers in the breath condensate of children with cystic fibrosis, *Eur. Respir. J.*, 15, 955, 2000.

47. Carpagnano, G.E. et al., Increased leukotriene B_4 and interleukin-6 in exhaled breath condensate in cystic fibrosis, *Am. J. Respir. Crit. Care Med.*, 167, 1109, 2003.

48. Montuschi, P. et al., Exhaled 8-isoprostane as new non-invasive biomarker of oxidative stress in cystic fibrosis, *Thorax*, 55, 205, 2000.

49. Balint, B. et al., Increased nitrotyrosine in exhaled breath condensate in cystic fibrosis, *Eur. Respir. J.*, 17, 1201, 2001.

50. Tate, S. et al., Airways in cystic fibrosis are acidified: detection by exhaled condensate, *Thorax*, 57, 926, 2002.

51. Smith, J.J. and Welsh, M.J., cAMP stimulates bicarbonate secretion across normal, but not cystic fibrosis airway epithelia, *J. Clin. Invest.*, 89, 1148, 1992.

52. Baldwin, S.R. et al., Oxidant activity in expired breath of patients with adult respiratory distress syndrome, *Lancet*, 1, 11, 1986.

53. Sznajder, J.I. et al., Increased hydrogen peroxide in the expired breath of patients with acute hypoxemia respiratory failure, *Chest*, 96, 606, 1989.

54. Kietzman, D. et al., Hydrogen peroxide in expired breath condensate of patients with acute respiratory failure and with ARDS, *Intensive Care Med.*, 19, 78, 1993.

55. Carpenter, C.T., Price, P.V., and Christman, B.W., Exhaled breath condensate isoprostanes are elevated in patients with acute lung injury or ARDS, *Chest*, 114, 1653, 1998.

56. Heard, S.O. et al., The influence of liposome-encapsulated prostaglandin E_1 on hydrogen peroxide concentrations in the exhaled breath of patients with the acute respiratory distress syndrome, *Anesth. Analg.*, 89, 353, 1999.

57. Ranieri, V.M. et al., Effect of mechanical ventilation on inflammatory mediators in patients with acute respiratory distress syndrome: a randomized controlled trial, *JAMA*, 1282, 54, 1999.

58. Scheideler, L. et al., Detection of nonvolatile macromolecules in breath, *Am. Rev. Respir. Dis.*, 148, 774, 1993.

59. Montuschi, P. et al., 8-isoprostane as a biomarker of oxidative stress in interstitial lung diseases, *Am. J. Respir. Crit. Care Med.*, 158, 1524, 1998.

60. Łuczyňska, M. et al., Elevated exhalation of hydrogen peroxide in patients with systemic sclerosis, *Eur. J. Clin. Invest.*, 33, 274, 2003.

61. Carpagnano, G.E. et al., Increased vitronectin and endothelin-1 in the breath condensate of patients with fibrosing lung disease, *Respiration*, 70, 154, 2003.

62. Ziesche, R. et al., A preliminary study of long-term treatment with interferon gamma-1b and low-dose prednisone in patients with idiopathic pulmonary fibrosis, *N. Engl. J. Med.*, 341, 1264, 1999.

63. Hatipoğlu, U. and Rubinstein, I., Inflammation and obstructive sleep apnea syndrome pathogenesis: a working hypothesis, *Respiration*, 70, 665, 2003.

64. Carpagnano, G.E. et al., Increased 8-isoprostane and interleukin-6 in breath condensate of obstructive sleep apnea patients, *Chest*, 122, 1162, 2002.

65. Carpagnano, G.E. et al., Interleukin-6 is increased in breath condensate of patients with non small cell lung cancer, *Int. J. Biol. Markers*, 17, 141, 2002.

66. Nayeri, F. et al., Exhaled breath condensate and serum levels of hepatocyte growth factor in pneumonia, *Respir. Med.*, 96,115. 2002.

67. Jöbsis, R.Q. et al., Hydrogen peroxide in breath condensate during a common cold, *Mediators Inflamm.*, 10, 351, 2001.

68. Schreiber, J. et al., Mycobacterium tuberculosis gene amplification in breath condensate of patients with lung tuberculosis, *Eur. J. Med. Res.*, 7, 290, 2002.

69. Silkoff, P.E., et al., Exhaled nitric oxide in human lung transplantation, *Am. J. Crit. Care Med.*, 157, 1822, 1998.

70. Lases, E.C. et al., Oxidative stress after lung resection therapy: A pilot study, *Chest*, 117, 999, 2000.

11 Future of Exhaled Breath Condensate

Jon L. Freels and Richard A. Robbins

CONTENTS

I. INTRODUCTION

The exact future of exhaled breath condensate (EBC) is unclear, and how it will impact research and the practice of medicine is equally vague, yet promising. Sidorenko et al.[1] published the pilot article on EBC, entitled "Surface-active properties of the exhaled air condensate" in 1980. Since then there have been more than 200 articles published on EBC and thousands of subjects studied; published studies are growing exponentially. The method of collecting EBC and measuring different volatile and nonvolatile particles in normal and disease-state subjects encompass the present research objectives. An international task force composed of several investigators throughout the world has been organized to further guide and broaden the scope of research in EBC. The task force also hopes to stimulate new investigators to get involved in the process of tackling the problematic issues, to find new uses for EBC, and to solidify the future. EBC is in its infancy and has great potential for use in the research and subsequently the clinical communities.

Lung disease research *in vitro* is extensive, yet studies *in vivo* are limited in part by the invasive nature of obtaining samples from within the lung, as in bronchoalveolar lavage (BAL), radiographic guidance needle biopsies, or open lung sampling. Sputum collection, although a widely used and noninvasive sampling method, requires experience and training to obtain proper and reliable results, and is limited to evaluating either infectious or malignant etiologies of disease states at best.[2] EBC is simple, noninvasive, and contains many volatile and nonvolatile substances, thus providing researchers with a method to study the lung *in vivo*.[3] New potential uses for EBC in the laboratory are being explored. Polymerase chain reaction (PCR) is being used to measure potential DNA fragments for infectious etiologies, with investigators finding mixed results.[4,5] Other fields being applied to EBC include metabonomics and proteonomics. Metabonomics is the measurement of many metabolites in biological fluid using high-resolution nuclear magnetic resonance spectrometry or liquid chromatography/mass spectrometry.[6,7] Proteonomics applies high-resolution gel electrophoresis or mass spectrometry to detect multiple proteins in biological samples. These methods might enable the investigator to evaluate multiple products at once; however, it is unclear if the current methodology of collection provides adequate material for usable results.

The clinical field also might benefit from this simple noninvasive method driven by the findings from research protocols. Categorizing variations of disease (such as in asthma), longitudinally studying different diseases, and diagnostically evaluating infectious etiologies are just a few areas that could evolve. In addition, development of in-line real-time measurements using nanotechnology will further benefit both the research and clinical fields. These advancements could lead to the use of EBC in asthma clinics, pulmonary offices, and even intensive care units by providing the clinician with a simple noninvasive tool to investigate, follow, and/or diagnose their patients. The potential of EBC in research and the clinical setting is yet to be fully realized. Some of the limiting factors hindering these advancements include the collection device, method of collection, and assay sensitivity.

II. EQUIPMENT

The collection device for EBC at its basic level is composed of a mouthpiece, salivary trap, and a condenser surrounded by a cooling apparatus. Variations on this theme seen in laboratories throughout the world include one-way valves, noseclips, and filters. Commercially available and homemade systems are being used. However, it is unclear whether standardizing these systems would decrease intraobserver variability between research sites. A major obstacle limiting a single standard setup is that substrates might react differently within the same environment. One substrate stabilized with freezing during condensing differs from another that is broken down during the same process. Therefore, the setup and equipment used might need to be individualized for each substance desired to be measured. This situation would prohibit the use of a test battery on a single sample. Therefore, serial sampling with differing setups would be required in an effort to obtain material to measure. Not only does this take time but it also likely introduces potential confounding variables. EBC is simple and noninvasive, and there have been no reported adverse events to date even during serial sampling,[8] but the time needed between sample acquisition and how many serial samples can be processed is not completely clear.

A. SALIVARY TRAP

A salivary trap composed of either a chamber or tubing is placed lower than the subject's mouth and the condenser to limit the potential contamination from the upper airway, primarily the oral contents. Amylase measured in the EBC has been used to determine the amount of oral contamination. Several studies using the trap have shown that minimal amounts of amylase have contaminated the sample.[3] However, it is unclear whether amylase is a good marker of oral contamination. Evidence could be interpreted to indicate that amylase is not a good marker. NH_4^+ has been found to be lower when collected through a tracheostomy tube than through the mouth, suggesting that there is some input from the upper airway during oral collection.[9,10] This could indicate that oral contamination might occur in EBC that is not detected by amylase. The major component of EBC is water vapor that has trapped mainly volatile solutes. This water vapor is then condensed by cooling as it passes through the condenser. Multiple factors alter the collection of these volatile substances into the condensing chamber. Air velocity, temperature, and adhesion and releasing properties of the desired particles might all play a role. This leads to the assumption that for each measured substance one might need to change and control how it is collected. To date, the mechanisms or importance have not been determined.

The salivary trap is proximal to the condenser, which leads to the potential that some substances might be trapped there instead of continuing to be delivered to the condenser. This leads to a decrease in concentration of the substance collected. This might not be problematic if the same collection device is used during a longitudinal study because the equipment would decrease the concentration equally between subjects. The limitation is when multiple sites are used with different collection systems or comparison between studies is being attempted. The adhesion properties of the equipment used for the salivary trap and even the condenser might alter the concentration outcome, and individual substances need to be evaluated for this potential alteration in outcome.

B. CONDENSER

1. Temperature

The adhesion properties of the condenser also need to be considered. The condenser is tubing surrounded by a cooling apparatus. Cooled water is not the only possible cooling apparatus; other methods include a metal sleeve precooled to various temperatures or a refrigeration unit that can sustain a preset temperature. The variation in cooling temperature causes the condensed air to be liquefied, frozen, or a combination of the two. Substances collected vary in their stability and possible trapping capability by the condenser under various temperature conditions, thus limiting specific substances from being in the same batter. Substances that have similar collection modalities could be processed in batches, but which substances should be processed together is yet unknown. Further studies are needed to determine the optimal temperature needed for the individual substance to be measured.

2. Flow Dynamics

The internal diameter and wall thickness of the condenser also must be evaluated. Flow dynamics through a tube with laminar flow occurs at the innermost aspect of the tube and this area is larger in larger diameter tubes. The most turbulent flow is found at the interface between the moving air and the condenser wall. It is thought that this interface is where the water vapor is condensed. This has led some investigators to add internal surface area to increase the turbulence and thus increase the amount of condensate. Turbulence also is altered by the flow rate of the air in the tube, formation of ice particles, and the ambient temperature inside the condensing unit. This varied turbulence and its effect on the stability and collection ability of individually measured substances is not known at present. The wall thickness of the condenser also might be important. Varying the wall thickness alters the temperature conductance from the cooling unit into the air space of the condenser, further changing the internal ambient temperature of the condenser. The difference might be negligible but is not reported and might provide further confounded variables. If this difference is found to alter outcomes, then comparison between investigations will be hindered.

3. Length and Resistance

The length of the condenser might alter the concentration of the measured substances. If the tube is too short, the potential of the water vapor to be condensed is limited. If the tube is too long, resistance and possible contamination from the outside ambient air might be a factor.[11] Different substances might have a propensity to be condensed at different parts of the condenser, potentially because of the speed of the exhaled air, weight of the water vapor, and exposure time to the cooled air. Therefore, temperature of ambient air inside the condenser, internal diameter, wall thickness, and length of the tube all need to be considered when measuring individual substances.

C. ONE-WAY VALVE

One-way valves have been used by some investigators to limit the potential contamination of the condensed material by outside ambient air particles entering the system without being mixed within the airway. Depending on the substance being measured, this might be of some significance. Cells have not been found in EBC but some investigators have performed PCR on collected fluid to find DNA fragments, particularly in the field of infectious disease. The results of these investigations have been varied, but if DNA fragments are exhaled, then the potential for ambient air to contain such particles is possible. Ambient air might also contain substances that could alter the adhesion potential, condenser air environment, and even the chemical properties of the desired substance to be measured. This information would seem to favor using a one-way valve all the time. Unfortunately, the alteration in flow dynamics and in breathing patterns of subjects has not been evaluated and thus might change the measured outcome. Using a one-way valve also requires nasal inhalation on the part of the subject. Air movement through the nose and upper pharyngeal passages could add volatile substances to the exhaled breath that do not originate from the lower airways. Depending on the physiologic state of this upper airway subset in a specific subject, this addition could alter the measured results significantly, as has been found with adenosine. These data suggest that there might be a significant influence of the upper airway in the concentration of certain samples, especially in subjects with upper airway pathology.

III. COLLECTION PROTOCOL

The collection apparatus might alter the end result but the method of collection also can introduce variability. Duration of collection, subject breathing pattern, and circumstances surrounding the subject have the potential to alter outcomes. Traditionally, EBC has been collected in an individual subject for a predetermined length of time.[12-14] However, the amount of water vapor presented to the condenser over a preset time is variable, depending on the breathing pattern and physiology of the subject. Taller subjects have larger tidal volumes compared with those of shorter subjects; therefore, over a given time, taller subjects present more water vapor to the condenser. Given that the majority of the breath condensate is water, higher dilutions potentially occur in taller subjects without adding a significant amount of the desired material to be measured. This might not be true, but only if one makes the presupposition that each water vapor molecule contains equal parts of water and the measured substance. The complexity of the airway system makes the supposition unlikely. In addition, variation in respiratory rate dose alters minute ventilation. Higher respiratory rates have the potential of drying out the airway, thus decreasing the amount of water vapor and allowing a higher concentration of volatile substances in the water vapor. Lower respiratory rates, conversely, could increase the amount of water in the water vapor and further dilute the desired particles to be measured. These factors have yet to be evaluated to determine their importance in the final results.

A. BREATHING PATTERN

In addition to issues surrounding sample collection, subjects react differently under testing conditions. Tidal breathing and respiratory rate have inter- and intrasubject variability, both of which have a multitude of causes. Subjects might have underlying disease states, such as emphysema, that could alter the amount of EBC and possibly the location from which the EBC comes. This alteration in the ratio of dead space to tidal volume further determines how much of the substances would come from the lower respiratory tract. Diurnal variation has been found in some substances, thus indicating that time of day at which the EBC is collected might be of some importance.[15-17] Subject medications and proximity of smoking, eating, or drinking to the collection time might all vary among different measured substances.[18-26] Unpublished data suggest that regardless of the subject's breathing pattern, a consistent amount of condensate is collected if preset minute ventilation is used in contrast to a preset time. This consistent volume of collection might decrease some of the intra- and intersubject variability and variability between different research sites.

B. HUMIDITY

Location of and the season during which exhaled breath is collected might alter results. A general assumption is made that the breath is fully saturated with water vapor, yet this has not been published. The amount of exhaled air saturation might be related to the ambient air humidity and temperature, which may vary considerably (for example from the arid southwest to the snowy Appalachian Mountains in the United States).[27,28] Studies are needed to evaluate the variables involved that would maximally extract the water vapor from the exhaled breath and yet not compromise the integrity of the substance to be measured and studied. A first step in doing this is to investigate the humidity of the exhaled breath and to determine if variables such as breathing pattern alter humidity. Then one would need to establish the humidity found after the condenser, and that ratio would need to be maximized by altering all the variables thought to be involved in EBC.

IV. ORIGIN OF CONDENSATE

Where does the exhaled breath water vapor come from and how is it generated? Studies attempting to ascertain where the water vapor comes from have determined that EBC comes from the lower and the upper airways, but it is unclear what percentage of EBC comes from each. To answer this question, researchers have sought markers found specifically at the aforementioned sites with little success. Other researchers believe that to determine the contribution of EBC from the said sites, one needs first to find a marker to determine a solubility constant.[10] This solubility standard would not only aid in determining the contributing location of EBC but would also allow researchers to more accurately compare studies by gaining a corrected concentration of the studied substances. This is not a new question and has been a problem with BAL. One knows the location from which BAL is obtained but the dilution and the corrected concentration are still unknown. Dilution has been estimated with a variety of techniques, including the ratio of the measured substance to albumin or total protein, or an estimate of the dilution of the epithelial lining fluid with methylene blue or urea.[10,13,29] The answer to this question might or might not be vital to the future of EBC. Despite not knowing the exact extent of epithelial lining fluid dilution, BAL is a useful tool in respiratory medicine in the clinical and research arena. Likewise, EBC might prove to have similar benefits regardless of whether the exact amount of dilution of epithelial lining fluid can be determined.

V. ASSAYS

The concentrations of substances found in EBC generally have been lower compared with BAL or, in some instances, induced sputum. Many of the concentrations are measured at or below the range of sensitivity of the currently available assays. This variability decreases the reproducibility of the tests and subsequently the validity. Good reproducibility has been found for adenosine, aldehydes, glutathione, 8-isoprostane, leukotrienes, prostaglandin E_2, and pH.[17,19,30,31] As the collection devices, method of collection, and surrounding confounded variables are evaluated and controlled for, maximization of concentration of measured substances will occur. However, more sensitive assays will need to be created to enhance the reproducibility and validity of experiments.

To achieve the objective of optimizing the concentration of measured substances without their being altered by determining the variables involved for each individual substance, research with particular attention to details is mandatory. Publishing this material that meticulously describes the parts, assembly, method, and circumstances surrounding the collection is vital to this future endeavor.

To speculate, EBC in the future might not be EBC at all, but real-time, in-line, nanotechnological measurement of the volatile and nonvolatile substances that make up one's exhaled breath. The optimistic futurist might conjecture that an EBC battery of test results might be found next to those for temperature and blood pressure, along with the other vital signs. Perhaps EBC is a method that will give a result of an individual blueprint, much like a thumbprint. In this age in which novel methods of personal identification are being proposed, it might be possible in the future to access your bank account by just breathing. This might lend a new meaning to the phrase "take your breath away," especially if it is accompanied by a drop in your bank balance!

The clinical relevance of EBC measurement of these volatile and nonvolatile substances is unclear and is an essential question to address. Bronchoscopy gives the investigator and clinician the ability to visualize the lower respiratory tract, obtain lung tissue for pathological examination, and sample the lower respiratory tract by BAL. However, biopsy and BAL both depend on cellular sampling. EBC has the disadvantage of not visualizing the lower respiratory tract and has no ability to sample tissue. This might dramatically reduce its utility compared with BAL. In addition, BAL might not be an appropriate gold standard with which to compare EBC. The advantage of EBC is the noninvasiveness and apparent safety in a wide range of ages and disease states. This suggests that it might have utility in patients with exacerbation of obstructive lung disease or other similar situations in which BAL is generally thought to carry unacceptable increased risk. If a correlation is found between the inflammatory markers found in EBC to the actual inflammatory cells found in BAL, and if lung infections could be evaluated with EBC, then the future will be very bright indeed.

Understanding of the medical implications of these substances has yet to be ascertained. Further evaluation of the correlation between EBC, sputum collection, and BAL is a critical step in determining the future of EBC. First, we need to find what we can measure. Second, we must optimize and be able to replicate these findings in a controlled manner. Third, we must evaluate and understand the implications of these substances with regard to health and the disease state.

This chapter is meant to provide some background to stimulate the investigator and clinician to go further and look beyond what we know or do not know. The future of medicine is directly dependent on the enthusiasm, imagination, and support of those investigators who are willing to step out and grasp new ideas without letting what is not known hinder their drive. We hope that this book helps readers take that step.

FURTHER READING

1. Sidorenko, G.I., Zborovskii, E.I., and Levina, D.I., Surface-active properties of the exhaled air condensate (a new method of studying lung function), *Ter. Arkh.*, 52, 65, 1980.

2. Hargreave, F.E., Pizzichini, M.M., and Pizzichini, E., Assessment of airway inflammation, in *Asthma*, Barnes, P.J., Grunstein, M.M., Leff, A.R., and Woolcock, A.J., Eds., Lippincott-Raven, Philadelphia, 1997, pp. 1433–1450.

3. Hunt, J., Exhaled breath condensate: an evolving tool for noninvasive evaluation of lung disease, *J. Allergy Clin. Immunol.* 110, 28, 2002.

4. Vogelberg, C. et al., *Pseudomonas aeruginosa* and *Burkholderia cepacia* cannot be detected by PCR in the breath condensate of patients with cystic fibrosis, *Pediatr. Pulmonol.*, 36, 348, 2003.

5. Scheideler, L. et al., Detection of nonvolatile macromolecules in breath. A possible diagnostic tool? *Am. Rev. Respir. Dis.*, 148, 778, 1993.

6. Nicholson, J.K. et al., Metabonomics: a platform for studying drug toxicity and gene function, *Nat. Rev. Drug Discov.*, 1, 153, 2002.

7. Brindle, et al., Rapid and no-invasive diagnosis of the presence and severity of coronary heart diseases using 1H-NMR based metabonomics, *Nat. Med.*, 8, 1439, 2002.

8. Kharitonov, S.A. and Barnes, P.J., Biomarkers of some pulmonary diseases in exhaled breath, *Biomarkers*, 7, 1, 2002.

9. Vass, G. et al., Comparison of nasal and oral inhalation during exhaled breath condensate collection, *Am. J. Respir. Crit. Care Med.*, 167, 850, 2003.

10. Effros, R.M. et al., Dilution of respiratory solutes in exhaled condensates, *Am. J. Respir. Crit. Care Med.*, 65, 663, 2002.

11. Latzin, P. and Griese, M., Exhaled hydrogen peroxide, nitrite and nitric oxide in healthy children: decrease of hydrogen peroxide by atmospheric nitric oxide, *Eur. J. Med. Res.*, 7, 353, 2002.

12. Sznajder, J.I. et al., Increased hydrogen peroxide in the expired breath of patients with acute hypoxemic respiratory failure, *Chest*, 96, 606, 1989.

13. Gessner, C. et al., Factors influencing breath condensate volume, *Pneumologie*, 55, 414, 2001.

14. Schleiss, M.B. et al., The concentration of hydrogen peroxide in exhaled air depends on expiratory flow rate, *Eur. Respir. J.*, 16, 1115, 2000.

15. Van Beurden, W.C.J. et al., Variability of exhaled hydrogen peroxide in stable COPD and matched healthy controls, *Respiration*, 69, 211, 2002.

16. Nowak, D. et al., Exhalation of H_2O_2 and thiobarbituric acid reactive substances (TBARS) by healthy subjects, *Free Rad. Biol. Med.*, 30, 178, 2001.

17. Vaughan, J. et al., Exhaled breath condensate pH is a robust and reproducible assay of airway acidity, *Eur. Respir. J.*, 22, 889, 2003.

18. Shahid, S.K. et al., Increased interleukin-4 and decreased interferon-γ in exhaled breath condensate of children with asthma, *Am. J. Respir. Crit. Care Med.*, 165, 1290, 2002.

19. Corradi, M. et al., Aldehydes and glutathione in exhaled breath condensate of children with asthma exacerbation, *Am. J. Respir. Crit. Care Med.*, 167, 395, 2003.

20. Nowak, D. et al., Increased content of hydrogen peroxide in the expired breath of cigarette smokers, *Eur. Respir. J.*, 9, 652, 1996.

21. Balint, B. et al., Increased nitric oxide metabolites in exhaled breath condensate after exposure to tobacco smoke, *Thorax*, 56, 456, 2001.

22. Montuschi, P. et al., Exhaled 8-isoprostane as an *in vivo* biomarker of lung oxidative stress in patients with COPD and healthy smokers, *Am. J. Respir. Crit. Care Med.*, 162, 1175, 2001.

23. Nowak, D. et al., Increased content of thiobarbituric acid-reactive substances and hydrogen peroxide in the expired breath condensate of patients with stable chronic obstructive pulmonary disease: no significant effect of cigarette smoking, *Respir. Med.*, 93, 389, 1999.

24. Dekhuijzen, P.N.R. et al., Increased exhalation of hydrogen peroxide in patients with stable and unstable chronic obstructive pulmonary diseases, *Am. J. Respir. Crit. Care Med.*, 154, 813, 1996.

25. Nowak, D. et al., Cigarette smoking does not increase hydrogen peroxide levels in expired breath condensate of patients with stable COPD, *Monaldi Arch. Chest Dis.*, 53, 268, 1998.

26. Kasielski, M. and Nowak, D., Long-term administration of N-acetylcysteine decreases hydrogen peroxide exhalation in subjects with chronic obstructive pulmonary disease, *Respir. Med.* 95, 448, 2001.

27. McFadden, E.R., Jr., Respiratory heat and water exchange: physiological and clinical implications, *J. Appl. Physiol.*, 54, 331, 1983.

28. Baile, E.M. et al., Role of tracheal and bronchial circulation in respiratory heat exchange, *J. Appl. Physiol.*, 58, 217, 1985.

29. Haslam, P.L. and Baughman, R.P., Report of ERS Task Force: guidelines for measurement of acellular components and standardization of BAL, *Eur. Respir. J.*, 14, 245, 1999.

30. Huszar, E. et al., Adenosine in exhaled breath condensate in healthy volunteers and in patients with asthma, *Eur. Respir. J.*, 20, 1393, 2002.

31. Montuschi, P. et al., Validation of 8-isoprostane and prostaglandin E_2 measurements in exhaled breath condensate, *Inflamm. Res.*, 2003 (in press).

12 The Role of Leukotrienes and Prostanoids in Airway Inflammation

Ryszard Dworski, R. Stokes Peebles, Jr., and James R. Sheller

CONTENTS

I. BIOCHEMISTRY AND FUNCTION OF PROSTANOIDS AND LEUKOTRIENES

Prostanoids and leukotrienes belong to a large family of metabolites of arachidonic acid (AA) collectively known as eicosanoids. AA is a 20-carbon polyunsaturated fatty acid esterified in cell membrane phospholipids that is hydrolyzed upon cell activation by the phospholipases.[1] Free AA may serve itself as a signaling molecule.[2] However, the majority of liberated AA is metabolized through different enzymatic or nonenzymatic pathways. The two major cascades of AA metabolism depend on the cyclooxygenase (COX) and 5-lipoxygenase (5-LO) enzymes (Figure 12.1). Other classes of eicosanoids (e.g., lipoxins, cytochrome P450 metabolites, and isoprostanes) will not be discussed in this chapter.

A. CYCLOOXYGENASE PATHWAY

Prostaglandin endoperoxide H synthase, frequently designated as COX, is the enzyme regulating the conversion of AA released by various stimuli to prostaglandin

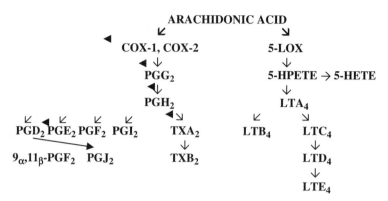

FIGURE 12.1 Cyclooxygenase (COX) and 5-lipoxygenase (5-LO) cascades of arachidonic acid metabolism.

H_2 (PGH_2), the common precursor to all prostaglandins (PG) and thromboxane A_2 (TXA_2). There are at least two distinct isozymes for COX: COX-1 (PGHS-1), which is constitutively expressed in most cell types and tissues, and is encoded by a 2.8-kb transcript, and a 4.4-kb transcript designated COX-2 (PGHS-2). In most cells COX-2 is present in very low amounts at baseline; however, the expression of the enzyme can be stimulated by lipopolysaccharide, phorbol ester, cytokines (e.g., interleukin [IL]-1α), growth factors (e.g., transforming growth factor-α), and hormones.[3,4] Conversely, corticosteroids, IL-4, IL-10, and IL-13 are potent inhibitors of COX-2 expression. The major differences between the COX-1 and COX-2 isoforms are the two termini. At the N-terminus, only COX-1 contains a 17-amino acid stretch within the signal peptide. In contrast, there is a unique 18-amino acid region at the carboxy terminus of the COX-2 enzyme.[5] Recently, an alternative splice variant of COX has been described; the biological role of this enzyme has not yet been defined.[6]

Although COX-1 and COX-2 share many catalytic and kinetic properties, a growing body of evidence suggests that the enzymes function independently. For example, it has been suggested that coupling to signaling pathways,[7] use of arachidonate pools,[8,9] compartmentalization with specific prostaglandin synthases,[10] and exhibition of affinity toward some fatty acid substrates and nonsteroidal anti-inflammatory drugs[11] differ between COX-1 and COX-2. The distinctive physiological roles of COX-1 and COX-2 isozymes have been demonstrated in mice in which the genes coding for the enzymes have been selectively deleted.[12–15]

The synthesis of the major prostanoids PGD_2, PGE_2, $PGF_{2\alpha}$, prostacyclin (PGI_2), and TXA_2 results from cell-specific isomerization or reduction of PGH_2 by unique synthases (isomerases) or reductases. The primary prostanoids can be further metabolized to either inactive products or biologically active mediators. For example, $9_\alpha,11$-PGF_2 is a biologically active metabolite of PGD_2 generated by a stereospecific metabolism of PGD_2 by 11-ketoreductase.[16] Prostaglandins of the J_2 and A series are formed from PGD_2 and PGE_2, respectively, spontaneously and catalytically in aqueous solution in the presence of albumins. These chemicals, also known as

TABLE 12.1
Proinflammatory Actions of Prostanoids

Prostanoid	Effect
PGD$_2$[33-37]	Airway constriction and hyperresponsiveness
	Recruitment and activation of eosinophils
	Recruitment of basophils and Th2 cells
	Inhibition of IL-12 in APC
	Promotion of allergic inflammation
	Augmentation of capillary permeability
	Increased mucus production
PGE$_2$[38-40]	Bronchoconstriction (in some subjects)
	Cough
	Enhanced capillary permeability
	Inhibition of IL-12 production and IL-12 receptor on APC
PGF$_{2\alpha}$	Bronchoconstriction
PGI$_2$[41]	Cough and airway irritation
TXA$_2$[42-43]	Bronchoconstriction
	Induction of extracellular matrix proteins synthesis
	Enhancement of proinflammatory cytokine synthesis
PGJ$_2$ series	Mobilization and priming of eosinophils

cyclopentenone prostaglandins (PGJ$_2$, Δ^{12}-PGJ$_2$, 15-deoxy-Δ12,14-PGD$_2$, 15-deoxy-Δ12,14-PGJ$_2$, PGA$_1$, and PGA$_2$) are of increasing interest because they have been shown to possess both pro- and anti-inflammatory actions.[17,18] The expression of the terminal enzymes in the COX cascade can be regulated by environmental factors. For instance, IL-1 is capable of inducing the glutathione-dependent isoform of PGE synthase.[19] Moreover, a compartmentalization of these enzymes with COX-1 or COX-2, and differences in a substrate affinity and kinetics, have been demonstrated.[10,20]

The biological activities of prostanoids are mediated through (1) distinct cell surface receptors that have been identified and cloned, each with unique signal transduction mechanisms as a result of coupling to different G proteins, (2) G protein-independent nuclear receptors, and (3) direct molecular interactions.[21] PGD$_2$, PGE$_2$, PGF$_{2\alpha}$, PGI$_2$, and TXA$_2$ couple to their own receptors (delineated DP, EP, FP, etc.;[22] Table 12.1). Some prostaglandins act through multiple receptors and therefore can trigger opposite actions and physiological responses. There are four distinctly encoded receptors for PGE$_2$ (EP1-EP4). PGD$_2$ accomplishes its actions through the DP1 and DP2/chemoattractant receptor-homologous molecule (CRTH2), which was found on Th2 lymphocytes, basophils, and eosinophils.[23,24] Activation of DP, EP2, EP4, one isoform of the EP3, and IP receptors coupled to G$_s$ results in increased activity of adenylyl cyclase, thereby increasing intracellular cyclic adenosine mono-phosphate (cAMP). Stimulation of the EP1, some EP3 isoforms, FP, IP, and TP coupled to G$_q$ receptors provokes a boost in intracellular calcium. Activation of the CRTH2, TP, and EP3 isoform receptors coupled to G$_i$ causes a simultaneous decrease in cAMP and an increase in intracellular calcium. Cyclopentenone prostaglandins

---

TABLE 12.2
Potential Salutary Actions of Prostanoids

Prostanoid	Effect
PGE$_2$[44-52]	Bronchodilation
	Attenuation of allergen-induced airway responses and inflammation
	Lessening of exercise-induced bronchoconstriction
	Attenuation of aspirin-induced asthmatic reaction
	Downregulation of 5-LO, FLAP, and leukotrienes synthesis
	Inhibition of mast cell degranulation
	Suppression of proinflammatory cytokines
	Inhibition of eosinophils chemotaxis and survival
	Inhibition of dendritic cell function
	Limitation of fibroproliferation
PGI$_2$[53]	Bronchodilation
	Limitation of the Th2 immune response
PGJ$_2$ series	Inhibition of expression of cytokines and growth factors

---

have been shown to exert anti-inflammatory activity through peroxisome proliferator-activated receptor- (PPAR-),[25,26] although a PPAR-independent mechanism has also been suggested. For example, a receptor-independent inhibition of IB kinase by 15-deoxy-Δ12,14-PGD2 through a direct molecular interaction has been reported.[27-30] CRTH2 on eosinophils can also be activated by Δ12-PGJ$_2$, resulting in eosinophil mobilization from bone marrow and priming for chemotaxis.[31] The presence of prostanoid receptors in the cell nucleus suggests that these chemicals might also act as autocrine mediators and regulators of gene expression.[32]

The pattern of the expression of prostanoid receptors on immune effector cells, resident airway, or lung parenchymal cells and neurons dictates the final biological effects of prostanoids. Because this receptor expression might differ depending on the pathophysiological state, the effect of prostaglandins might also vary. The role and coordination of these multiple signals in an individual cell is unclear. Several polymorphisms of the prostanoid receptors have been reported; however, the physiological role of these variants remains unknown. The major biological activities of prostanoids that might be relevant to airway biology are shown in Tables 12.2 and 12.3.[33-53]

B. LIPOXYGENASE PATHWAY

The three major enzymes of lipoxygenation are designated 5-, 12-, and 15-lipoxygenase, for the number of the carbon atom of AA at which one molecule of oxygen is introduced. The conversion of AA to leukotrienes, a group of potent inflammatory mediators, is initiated by the enzyme 5-LO. In resting cells, 5-LO is located in the euchromatin of the nucleus but it translocates to the nuclear envelope upon cell activation.[54] The initiation of leukotriene biosynthesis is a complex process that requires (1) stimulation by an agonist (e.g., allergen crosslinking of IgE on the mast

TABLE 12.3
Activities of Leukotrienes

Leukotriene	Effect
LTB$_4$	Neutrophil chemotaxis
	Leukocyte secretion
	Promotion of IgE synthesis
	Nuclear transcription
Cys-LTs	Bronchoconstriction
	Airway hyperresponsiveness
	Plasma exudation
	Promotion of Th-2 responses
	Inhibition of Th-1 cytokines
	Eosinophil infiltration and degranulation
	Mucus gland hyperplasia
	Mucus hypersecretion
	Inhibition of respiratory cilia
	Smooth muscle hyperplasia
	Epithelial cell proliferation
	Collagen deposition
	Vasodilation or vasoconstriction

cell membrane); (2) hydrolysis of AA from membrane phospholipids by cytosolic phospholipase A$_2$; and (3) interaction of 5-LO with a membrane-bound protein, designated 5-LO-activating protein (FLAP). 5-LO catalyzes the conversion of AA first to 5-hydroperoxyeicosatetraenoic acid (HPETE), which might be reduced to 5-hydroeicosatetraenoic (5-HETE) by the action of peroxidases, or converted by the dehydrase activity of 5-LO to form the labile epoxide, leukotriene A$_4$ (LTA$_4$). In alveolar macrophages, monocytes, and neutrophils, LTA$_4$ is converted by LTA$_4$ hydrolase to form leukotriene B$_4$ (LTB$_4$). Mast cells, eosinophils, and basophils, the predominant cells of allergic inflammation, transform LTA$_4$ to the initial cysteine-containing leukotriene C$_4$ (LTC$_4$), through LTC$_4$ synthase.[55,56] Transcellular metabolism of AA products leading to leukotriene synthesis has been described in cells that do not express 5-LO (e.g., platelets express LTC$_4$ synthase and may generate LTC$_4$ from LTA$_4$ donated by neutrophils); however, the importance of this mechanism *in vivo* is unclear.[57] LTC$_4$ and its extracellular metabolites LTD$_4$ and LTE$_4$ are collectively known as the cysteinyl-leukotrienes (cys-LTs) or peptidoleukotrienes, previously known as slow reacting substance of anaphylaxis (SRSA). Effects of leukotrienes are mediated via the G protein-coupled receptors BLT for LTB$_4$, and CysLT$_1$ and CysLT$_2$ for the cysteinyl-LT. Most actions of the cys-LTs in human airways are mediated by the CysLT$_1$ receptor. All cys-LTs bind to CysLT$_1$, although LTE$_4$ has a greatly reduced binding capacity. CysLT$_2$ appears to mediate mainly pulmonary vein constriction.[58,59] Genetic variations in the human 5-LO gene promoter have been reported but the functional role of these variants is unclear.[60] Table 12.4 shows different activities of LTB$_4$ and cys-LTs.[61]

TABLE 12.4
Prostanoid and Leukotriene Receptors

Prostanoids

PGD_2	DP1, CRTH2 (DP2)
PGE_2	EP1, EP2, EP3, EP4
$PGF_{2\alpha}$	FP
PGI_2	IP
TXA_2	TP
PGJ_2 series	PPAR-, CRTH2

Leukotrienes

LTB_4	BLT
Cys-LTs	CysLT1, CysLT2

II. THE ROLE OF PROSTANOIDS AND LEUKOTRIENES IN AIRWAY DISEASES

A. EICOSANOIDS AND ASTHMA

Bronchoalveolar lavage (BAL) fluid,[62–66] sputum,[67,68] and exhaled breath condensates (EBCs)[69,70] from atopic asthmatics contain detectable levels of prostanoids and leukotrienes at baseline, indicating that ongoing chronic airway inflammation is present even in the airways of subjects with mild asthma, and that these chemicals are the biochemical markers of that inflammation. After instillation of allergen or inhaled allergen challenge to which the individual is sensitive, the levels of phospholipase A_2, arachidonate,[71] and eicosanoids increase still further. PGD_2 is the principal COX product, and LTC_4 is the main 5-LO product released following allergen stimulation, but other prostanoids, including $9_\alpha,11_\beta$-PGF_2, $PGF_{2\alpha}$, TXB_2, and 6-keto-$PGF_{1\alpha}$ as well as LO products, LTB_4, and 5-, 12-, and 15-HETE, are also augmented.[62,63,65,66] Twenty-four hours after segmental allergen challenge in human atopics, the levels of LTE_4 in BAL fluid remain elevated, whereas the COX products are only slightly increased compared with baseline.[72] Likewise, sputum cys-LTs increase 24 hours after allergen inhalation in atopic asthmatics.[73] In addition to local increases in the airways, elevated eicosanoid levels have been detected in urine of asthmatics undergoing specific inhalation challenges,[74,77] in exercise-induced bronchoconstriction,[78] and during acute asthma.[74,79,80] Augmented synthesis of cys-LTs also has been demonstrated in aspirin-intolerant asthmatics after inhaled or local aspirin challenge,[81,82] in patients with nocturnal asthma[83] and occupational asthma (e.g., during plicatic acid-induced bronchoconstriction),[84] and following exposure to ozone.[85] Increased formation of LTB_4 has been found in subjects with acute asthma,[80] nocturnal asthma,[83] severe persistent asthma,[80] and following exposure to toluene diisocyanate.[86] Patients with chronic hyperplastic sinusitis, nasal polyposis, and tissue eosinophilia have an augmented expression of LTC_4 synthase and local production of cys-LTs.[87] LTB_4 appears to be involved predominantly in asthmatic airway inflammation characterized by infiltration of neutrophils.[88]

Several types of cells can contribute to the spectrum of lipid mediators present in asthmatic airways. Prostanoids can be generated by mast cells, eosinophils, basophils, alveolar macrophages, antigen-presenting cells, epithelial cells, lymphocytes, fibroblasts, and airway smooth muscle cells. Mast cells predominantly generate PGD_2 (although macrophages, antigen-presenting cells, and human helper T-cell subsets also release PGD_2), whereas macrophages generate PGE_2 and TXA_2.

The data on the expression of COX-1 and COX-2 in the asthmatic airway are conflicting. Some studies reported no difference in the expression of COX-1 and COX-2 in alveolar macrophages and blood monocytes,[89] and in epithelial cells[90] between asthmatic and normal subjects at baseline, and during natural exposure to an offending antigen.[91] Likewise, PGD_2 synthase was unchanged in bronchial biopsies of seasonal atopic asthmatics during the pollen season.[91] A decreased expression of COX-2 was reported in polyps from aspirin-intolerant asthmatics compared with polyps from aspirin-tolerant asthmatics.[92] Conversely, other investigators found increased amounts of COX-2 in the epithelium and submucosa as well as sputum cells of asthmatics compared with controls.[93–95] Mast cells and eosinophils from aspirin-intolerant asthmatics were particularly rich in the COX-2 isozyme in one study,[93] although disturbances in COX expression in these patient have not been reported uniformly.[96]

The 5-LO has a narrow cellular distribution, and the predominant cells with the full enzymatic pathway capable of producing cys-LTs are mast cells, eosinophils, and basophils. A significant increase in an immunostaining for 5-LO, FLAP, LTA_4 hydrolase, and LTC_4 synthase that correlated with the deterioration of lung performance was found in airway eosinophils and macrophages obtained from seasonal asthmatics during the pollen season.[91] Patients with aspirin-intolerant asthma had overexpressed LTC_4 synthase in bronchial biopsies compared with subjects with aspirin-tolerant asthma and normal subjects.[96] Other investigators found an increased expression of $cysLT_1$ on nasal inflammatory cells, which was downregulated after local aspirin desensitization.[97] These findings suggest that cys-LTs might indeed play a central role in aspirin-intolerant asthma, but the pathomechanism of this syndrome is complex and does not result simply from shifting of AA metabolism from COX pathways to 5-LO cascade. In addition, macrophages, lymphocytes, and neutrophils have been suggested as sources of 5-HETE. 15-HETE is produced in the lung predominantly by epithelial cells and eosinophils, but macrophages and monocytes are also capable of expressing 15-LO and synthesize 15-HETE when stimulated with IL-4 or IL-13.[98] Both epithelial cells and platelets are sources of 12-HETE.[99]

B. EICOSANOIDS AND OTHER INFLAMMATORY AIRWAY DISORDERS

In patients with acute exacerbation of chronic obstructive lung disease (COPD), levels of LTB_4 in sputum[100] and exhaled breath concentrate[101] are elevated, suggesting a contribution of LTB_4 in neutrophil recruitment into the airways. Increased immunoreactivity for COX-1 and COX-2 has been found on induced sputum cells in patients with COPD.[94]

Enhanced levels of LTB$_4$ and cys-LTs, as well as prostanoids, have been demonstrated in sputum,[102,103] BAL fluid,[104] EBC,[105] and nasal secretions[106] from patients with cystic fibrosis. Given that LTB$_4$ and IL-6 were particularly increased in subjects with acute exacerbation of the disease, it has been suggested that these chemicals could be used to monitor neutrophilic airway inflammation typically seen in patients with cystic fibrosis.[105] A correlation between total cys-LTs in sputum and the overall severity of cystic fibrosis based on chest radiograph score was found.[103] However, another study demonstrated that the elevation in urinary cys-LTs, which correlated with the degree of bronchoconstriction and responsiveness to bronchodilators, occurred predominantly in atopic children with cystic fibrosis.[107]

Patients with eosinophilic bronchitis associated with chronic cough but not airway obstruction or increased airway hyperresponsiveness had elevated levels of cys-LT and PGD$_2$ in induced sputum.[108] Increased levels of LTB$_4$ and LTE$_4$ in BAL fluid have been reported recently in scleroderma lung disease.[109]

C. ROLE OF PROSTANOIDS IN AIRWAY DISORDERS

The COXs and prostanoids should be viewed as both promoters and inhibitors of airway tone, inflammation, and remodeling. Pharmacologic studies in animals *in vivo,* and experiments in mice with targeted mutations of genes encoding enzymes and receptors are invaluable in creating hypotheses regarding the functions of prostanoids in airway pathologies. A new intriguing paradigm has been proposed, suggesting that the major role of prostaglandins, particularly COX-2-derived PGE$_2$ during the acute phase of inflammation, is not simply to amplify inflammatory responses (although such actions might certainly occur) but rather to inhibit inflammation by reprogramming the metabolism of AA from inflammatory pathways, e.g., 5-LO and LTB$_4$, to anti-inflammatory and antifibrotic cascades such as 15-LO and lipoxin A$_4$.[110,111] Although there are some data supporting the concept of the dual role of prostanoids in human subjects, more extensive research in this area is necessary. Examples of intriguing questions illustrating uncertainties regarding the role of prostanoids in airway disorders are listed below.

What is the role of PGE$_2$ in the regulation of airway tone? PGE$_2$ can provoke both bronchoconstriction through EP1 and EP3, and bronchodilation upon stimulation of EP2.[112,113] Indeed, human studies have demonstrated inconsistent effects of inhaled PGE$_2$ on bronchial tone, with most asthmatics showing a bronchodilator action but some developing profound bronchoconstriction.[38,114]

How does PGE$_2$ affect allergic inflammation? Both selective and nonselective inhibition of the COX isozymes during allergen sensitization in ovalbumin-sensitized mice caused an increased airway reactivity, lung tissue eosinophilia, enhanced mRNA expression for the chemokine receptors CCR1 through CCR5 (expressed on eosinophils, basophils, lymphocytes, and dendritic cells), and promotion of Th2 responses (a finding contradictory to some *in vitro* studies).[115,116] Conversely, in genetically manipulated ovalbumin-sensitized mice, only COX-1- but not COX-2-deficient animals developed increased numbers of CD4+ and CD8+ T cells; enhanced levels of IL-4, IL-5, IL-13; eotaxin in BAL fluid; and a greater airway responsiveness to antigen exposure compared with the wild type.[15] Collectively, these findings suggest that at least some COX products modulate allergic responses in the lung. Indeed, many animal and human experiments support the notion that PGE_2, and possibly PGI_2,[53] might inhibit different stages of immune and inflammatory responses such as mast cell degranulation, eosinophil chemotaxis and activation, release of proinflammatory cytokines, and synthesis of leukotrienes, and also might promote resolution of allergic inflammation. Some studies suggest a unique role of COX-2-derived PGE_2 in these processes.[117,118]

Does PGE_2 promote neutrophilic inflammation in the airways? PGE_2 generated by COX-2 might have some deleterious effects in neutrophilic inflammation associated with COPD and some asthma fenotypes.[88,119,120] Therefore, the role of COX-2 and prostanoids in these disorders requires clarification.

Does PGE_2 inhibit airway remodeling? PGE_2 might inhibit the airway remodeling process through inhibition of fibroblast chemotaxis, fibroblast proliferation, collagen synthesis, proliferation of smooth muscle cells, and reduction in airway smooth muscle growth.[121–126] In one study, severe inflammatory responses and pulmonary fibrosis to vanadium pentoxide exposure developed only in COX-2-deficient mice but not in COX-1 or wild-type mice. Although PGE_2 levels in BAL fluid under experimental conditions were significantly upregulated in wild-type and COX-1 mice, this effect was not observed in COX-2-deficient animals, suggesting that the COX-2-derived PGE_2 could be an important factor in resolving inflammation and protecting against lung fibrogenesis.[127] A special role in this process could be played by COX-2-derived prostanoids generated by epithelial cells.[122] Interestingly, patients with pulmonary fibrosis might have an impaired expression of COX-2 compared with that in normal lung.[128]

How is prostanoid receptor expression regulated in different airway inflammatory disorders? Understanding the mechanisms of the expression and distribution of prostanoid receptors on airway residential and inflammatory cells is critical for defining the role of prostanoids in human airway inflammatory diseases.

Are prostanoids involved in development of lung cancer? Although this subject is beyond the scope of this chapter, it is worth mentioning that several experimental studies suggest tumor-promoting roles of COX-2-derived prostanoids in the lung and other organs.[129]

In general, employing nonspecific COX inhibitors to study functions of COX isozymes and prostanoids in airway disorders might lead to erroneous conclusions. These drugs simply remove all prostanoids (good and bad) from the scene of the inflammation. Specific COX-1 (not available for human research) or COX-2 inhibitors provide more advanced probes in this regard. For example, tolerance of specific anti-COX-2 agents by subjects with aspirin-intolerant asthma strongly suggests an unequal role of COX-1- and COX-2-derived prostanoids in this syndrome.[130] Clinically relevant doses of corticosteroids have been reported to upregulate the expression of COX-2 in alveolar macrophages and peripheral-blood monocytes from atopic nonasthmatics and atopic asthmatics,[131] but decrease the immunoreactivity of the enzyme in the epithelial cells.[95]

Drugs specifically targeting individual prostanoid syntheses or prostanoid receptors would be of great importance to identify the role of these chemicals in airway inflammatory conditions. For example, a specific inhibition of DP receptor resulted in a significant inhibition of allergic responses in a guinea pig model.[132] Nevertheless, with few exceptions these inhibitors have not been approved for human studies. For example, specific inhibition of thromboxane synthetase or thromboxane receptor in human asthmatics demonstrated mild protection from bronchoconstriction and airway inflammation.[133–135] Recently, some new antithromboxane drugs have been evaluated in human asthmatics.[43]

Regulation of immune and inflammatory responses by prostanoids distally from the lung (e.g., in the thymus or bone marrow) that might have important consequences on the airways in normal and pathologic states will not be discussed in this chapter.

D. ROLE OF LEUKOTRIENES IN INFLAMMATORY AIRWAY DISORDERS

The involvement of leukotrienes in airway inflammation, particularly in asthma and atopy, is undeniable. Antileukotriene drugs have been found to improve clinical control of atopic asthma, nocturnal asthma, aspirin-intolerant asthma, occupational asthma, exercise-induced asthma, and acute asthma exacerbation.[136,137] These are remarkable facts because other attempts to control asthma by eliminating a single inflammatory mediator (e.g., histamine, IL-5, lymphocyte function antigen [LFA-1]) were unsuccessful. Both bronchodilatory and anti-inflammatory properties are likely to have an important role in the mechanism of the protection offered by leukotriene antagonists.[138] It is unclear, however, what factors determine the heterogeneity of patient responses to these drugs.[139] Growing evidence points to a possible role of leukotrienes in the lung remodeling processes by promoting proliferation of fibroblasts, smooth muscle cells, and collagen synthesis. In a model of bleomycin-stimulated pulmonary fibrosis, 5-LO-deficient mice were protected substantially from developing lung fibrotic changes.[140] This is an important area to investigate because corticosteroids, which offer the most effective treatment for asthma, have an inconsistent inhibitory effect on leukotriene synthesis and might actually stimulate their production in certain types of cells.[141]

III. CONCLUSIONS

A growing body of evidence strongly suggests that prostanoids and leukotrienes are involved in various airway inflammatory disorders. The profile of generated eicosanoids depends on the expression of the enzymes involved in AA cascades that can be regulated by many environmental factors. Likewise, the expression of prostanoid and leukotriene receptors is influenced by coexisting inflammatory mediators. Consequently, the same mediators might have diverse functions under different inflammatory conditions. Therefore, eicosanoids, especially some prostanoids, should be viewed as both pro- and anti-inflammatory mediators. A better understanding of the role of eicosanoids in distinct physiological and pathophysiological conditions might result in development of new valuable pharmacologic agents.

FURTHER READING

1. Dennis, E.A., Phospholipase A_2 in eicosanoid generation, *Am. J. Respir. Crit. Care Med.*, 161, S32, 2000.
2. Kuebler, W. et al., A novel signaling mechanism between gas and blood compartments of the lung, *J. Clin. Invest.* 105, 905, 2000.
3. Xie, W. et al., Expression of a mitogen-responsive gene encoding prostaglandin synthase is regulated by mRNA splicing, *Proc. Natl. Acad. Sci. U.S.A.*, 88, 2692, 1991.
4. Kujubu, D.A. et al., TIS10, a phorbol ester tumor promoter-inducible mRNA from Swiss 3T3 cells, encodes a novel prostaglandin synthase-cyclooxygenase homologue, *J. Biol. Chem.* 266, 12866, 1991.
5. Smith, W.L. and DeWitt, D.L., Biochemistry of prostaglandin endoperoxide H synthase-1 and synthase-2 and their differential susceptibility to nonsteroidal antiinflammatory drugs, *Sem. Nephrol.* 15, 179, 1995.
6. Chandrasekharan, N.V. et al., COX-3, a cyclooxygenase-1 variant inhibited by acetaminophen and other analgesic/antipyretic drugs: cloning, structure, and expression, *Proc. Natl. Acad. Sci. U.S.A.*, 99, 13926, 2002.
7. Murakami, M. et al., Prostaglandin endoperoxide synthase-1 and -2 couple to different transmembrane stimuli to generate prostaglandin D_2 in mouse bone marrow-derived mast cells, *J. Biol. Chem.* 269, 22269, 1994.
8. Brock, T.G., McNish, R.W., and Peters-Golden, M., Arachidonic acid is preferentially metabolized by cyclooxygenase-2 to prostacyclin and prostaglandin E_2, *J. Biol. Chem.*, 274, 11660, 1999.
9. Reddy, S.T. and Herschman, H.R., Prostaglandin synthase-1 and prostaglandin synthase-2 are coupled to distinct phospholipases for the generation of prostaglandin D_2 in activated mast cells, *J. Biol. Chem.*, 272, 3231, 1997.
10. Naraba, H. et al., Segregated coupling of phospholipases A_2, cyclooxygenases and terminal prostanoid synthases in different phases of prostanoid biosynthesis in rat peritoneal macrophages, *J. Immunol.*, 160, 2974, 1998.
11. Meade, E.A., Smith, W.L., and DeWitt, D.L., Differential inhibition of prostaglandin endoperoxide synthase (cyclooxygenase) isozymes by aspirin and other non-steroidal anti-inflammatory drugs, *J. Biol. Chem.*, 268, 6610, 1993.
12. Dinchuk, J.E. et al., Renal abnormalities and an altered inflammatory response in mice lacking cyclooxygenase II, *Nature*, 378, 406, 1995.
13. Langenbach, R. et al., Prostaglandin synthase 1 gene disruption in mice reduces arachidonic acid-induced inflammation and indomethacin-induced gastric ulceration, *Cell*, 83, 483, 1995.
14. Gavett, S.H. et al., Allergic lung responses are increased in prostaglandin H synthase-deficient mice, *J. Clin. Invest.*, 104, 721, 1999.
15. Carey, M.A., et al., Accentuated T helper type 2 airway response after allergen challenge in cyclooxygenase-1-/- but not cyclooxygenase-2-/- mice, *Am. J. Respir. Crit. Care Med.*, 167, 1509, 2003.
16. Liston, T.E. and Roberts, L.J., Transformation of prostaglandin D_2 to 9a,11b-(15S)-trihydroxy-prosta-(5Z,13E)-dien-1-oic acid (9a,11b-PGF_2): a unique biologically active prostaglandin produced enzymatically *in vivo* in humans, *Proc. Natl. Acad. Sci. U.S.A.*, 82, 6030, 1985.
17. Fitzpatrick, F.A. and Wynalda, M.A., Albumin-catalyzed metabolism of prostaglandin D_2, *J. Biol. Chem.*, 258, 11713, 1983.

18. Fukushima, M., Prostaglandin J_2: antitumor and antiviral activities and the mechanisms involved, *Eicosanoids*, 3,189, 1990.

19. Jakobsson, P.-J. et al., Identification of human prostaglandin E synthase: a microsomal, glutathione-dependent, inducible enzyme, constituting a potential novel drug target, *Proc. Natl. Acad. Sci. U.S.A.*, 96, 7220, 1999.

20. Penglis, P.S. et al., Differential regulation of prostaglandin E_2 and thromboxane A_2 production in human monocytes: implications for the use of cyclooxygenase inhibitors, *J. Immunol.*, 165, 1605, 2000.

21. Tilley, S.L., Coffman, T.M., and Koller, B.H., Mixed messages: modulation of inflammation and immune responses by prostaglandins and thromboxanes, *J. Clin. Invest.*, 108, 15, 2001.

22. Narumiya, S., Sugimoto, Y., and Ushikubi, F., Prostanoid receptors: structures, properties, and functions, *Physiol. Rev.*, 79, 1193, 1999.

23. Hirai, H. et al., Prostaglandin D_2 selectively induces chemotaxis in T helper type 2 cells, eosinophils, and basophils via seven-transmembrane receptor CRTH2, *J. Exp. Med.*, 193, 255, 2001.

24. Monneret, G. et al., Prostaglandin D_2 is a potent chemoattractant for human eosinophils that acts via a novel DP receptor, *Blood*, 98, 1942, 2001.

25. Jiang, C., Ting, A.T., and Seed, B., PPAR-agonists inhibit production of monocyte inflammatory cytokines, *Nature*, 391, 82, 1998.

26. Gilroy, D.W. et al., Inducible cyclooxygenase may have anti-inflammatory properties, *Nat. Med.*, 5, 698, 1999.

27. Tsubouchi, Y. et al., Feedback control of the arachidonate cascade in rheumatoid synoviocytes by 15-deoxy-delta(12,14)-prostaglandin J_2, *Biochem. Biophys. Res. Commun.*, 283, 750, 2001.

28. Rossi, P. et al., Anti-inflammatory cyclopentenone prostaglandins are direct inhibitors of IκB kinase, *Nature*, 403, 103, 2000.

29. Straus, D.S., 15-deoxy-Δ12,14-prostaglandin J_2 inhibits multiple steps in the NK-B signaling pathway, *Proc. Natl. Acad. Sci. U.S.A.*, 97, 4844, 2000.

30. Hinz, B., Brune, K., and Pahl, A., 15-deoxy-delta(12,14)-prostaglandin J_2 inhibits the expression of proinflammatory genes in human blood monocytes via a PPAR-gamma independent mechanism, *Biochem. Biophys. Res. Commun.*, 302, 415, 2003.

31. Heinemann, R. et al., Δ12-Prostaglandin J_2, a plasma metabolite of prostaglandin D_2, causes eosinophil mobilization from bone marrow and primes eosinophils for chemotaxis, *J. Immunol.*, 170, 4752, 2003.

32. Bhattacharya, M. et al., Nuclear localization of prostaglandin E_2 receptors, *Proc. Natl. Acad. Sci. U.S.A.*, 95, 15792, 1998.

33. Hardy, C.C. et al., The bronchoconstrictor effect of inhaled prostaglandin D_2 in normal and asthmatic men, *N. Engl. J. Med.*, 311, 209, 1984.

34. Matsuoka, T. et al., Prostaglandin D_2 as a mediator of allergic asthma, *Science*, 287, 2013, 2000.

35. Fujitani, Y. et al., Pronounced eosinophilic lung inflammation and Th2 cytokine release in human lipocalin-type prostaglandin D synthase transgenic mice, *J. Immunol.*, 168, 443, 2002.

36. Faveeuw, C. et al., Prostaglandin D_2 inhibits the production of interleukin-12 in murine dendritic cells through multiple signaling pathways, *Eur. J. Immunol.*, 33, 889, 2003.

37. Wright, D.H. et al., A novel biological role for prostaglandin D_2 is suggested by distribution studies of the rat DP prostanoid receptor, *Eur. J. Pharmacol.*, 377, 101, 1999.

38. Mathe, A.A. and Hedqvist, P., Effect of prostaglandin $F_{2\alpha}$ and E_2 on airway conductance in healthy subjects and asthmatic patients, *Am. Rev. Respir. Dis.*, 111, 313, 1975.

39. van der Pouw Kraan, T.C.T.M. et al., Prostaglandin E_2 is a potent inhibitor of human interleukin 12 production, *J. Exp. Med.*, 181, 775, 1995.

40. Wu, C.Y. et al., Prostaglandin E_2 and dexamethasone inhibit IL-12 receptor expression and IL-12 responsiveness, *J. Immunol.*, 161, 2723, 1998.

41. Hardy, C. et al., Airway and cardiovascular responses to inhaled prostacyclin in normal and asthmatic subjects, *Am. Rev. Respir. Dis.*, 131, 18, 1985.

42. Bruggeman, L.A. et al., Thromboxane stimulates synthesis of extracellular matrix proteins *in vitro*, *Am. J. Physiol.*, 261, F488, 1991.

43. Dogne, J.M. et al., Therapeutic potential of thromboxane inhibitors in asthma, *Expert Opin. Investig. Drugs*, 11, 275, 2002.

44. Kambayashi, T., Wallin, R., and Ljunggren, H-G., cAMP-elevating agents suppress dendritic cell function, *J. Leukoc. Biol.*, 70, 903, 2001.

45. Hartert, T.V. et al., Prostaglandin E_2 decreases allergen-stimulated release of prostaglandin D_2 in airways of subjects with asthma, *Am. J. Respir. Crit. Care Med.*, 162, 637, 2000.

46. Harizi, H. et al., Prostaglandins inhibit 5-lipoxygenase-activating protein expression and leukotriene B_4 production from dendritic cells via an IL-10 dependent mechanism, *J. Immunol.*, 170, 139, 2003.

47. Charbeneau, R.P. et al., Impaired synthesis of prostaglandin E_2 by lung fibroblasts and alveolar epithelial cells from GM-CSF -/- mice: implications for fibroproliferation, *Am. J. Physiol.*, 284, L1103, 2003.

48. Christman, B.W., Prostaglandin E_2 limits arachidonic acid availability and inhibits leukotriene B_4 synthesis in rat alveolar macrophages by a nonphospholipase A_2 mechanism, *J. Immunol.*, 151, 2096, 1993.

49. Fadok, V.A. et al., Macrophages that have ingested apoptotic cells *in vitro* inhibit proinflammatory cytokine production through autocrine/paracrine mechanisms involving TGF-β, PGE_2, and PAF, *J. Clin. Invest.*, 101, 890, 1998.

50. Pavord, I.D. et al., Effect of inhaled prostaglandin E_2 on allergen-induced asthma, *Am. Rev. Respir. Dis.*, 148, 87, 1993.

51. Pavord, I.D. and Tattersfield, A.E., Bronchoprotective role of endogenous prostaglandin E_2, *Lancet*, 344, 436, 1994.

52. Gauvreau, G.M., Watson, R.M., and O'Byrne, P.M., Protective effects of inhaled PGE_2 on allergen-induced airway responses and airway inflammation, *Am. J. Respir. Crit. Care Med.*, 159, 31, 1999.

53. Jaffar, Z., Wan, K-S., and Roberts, K. A key role for prostaglandin I_2 in limiting lung mucosal Th2, but not Th1, responses to inhaled allergen, *J. Immunol.*, 169, 5997, 2002.

54. Woods, J.E. et al., 5-lipoxygenase is located in the euchromatin of the nucleus in resting human alveolar macrophages and translocates to the nuclear envelope upon cell activation, *J. Clin. Invest.*, 95, 2035, 1995.

55. Samuelsson, B., The discovery of the leukotrienes, *Am. J. Respir. Crit. Care Med.*, 161, S2, 2000.

56. Lewis, R.A., Austen, K.F., and Soberman, R.J., Leukotrienes and other products of the 5-lipoxygenase pathway, *N. Engl. J. Med.*, 323, 645, 1990.

57. Chavis, C. et al., 5(S),15(S)-dihydroeicosatetraenoic acid and lipoxin generation in human polymorphonuclear cells: dual specificity of 5-lipoxygenases towards endogenous precursors, *J. Exp. Med.*, 183, 1633, 1996.

58. Barnes, N.C., and Smith, L.J., The role of leukotrienes in asthma and allergic rhinitis, *Clin. Rev. Allergy Immunol.*, 17, 27, 1999.

59. Izumi, T. et al., Leukotriene receptors: classification, gene expression, and signal transduction, *J. Biochem.*, 132, 1, 2002.
60. Silverman, E.S. and Drazen, J.M., Genetic variations in the 5-lipoxygenase core promoter. Description and functional implications, *Am. J. Respir. Crit. Care Med.*, 161, S77, 2000.
61. Leff, A., Role of leukotrienes in bronchial hyperresponsiveness and cellular responses in airways, *Am. J. Respir. Crit. Care Med.*, 161, S125, 2001.
62. Murray, J.J. et al., Release of prostaglandin D_2 into human airways during acute antigen challenge, *N. Engl. J. Med.*, 315, 800, 1986.
63. Wenzel, S.E., et al., Spectrum of prostanoid release after bronchoalveolar lavage allergen challenge in atopic asthmatics and control groups, *Am. Rev. Respir. Dis.*, 139, 450, 1989.
64. Liu, M.C., et al., Evidence for elevated levels of histamine, prostaglandin D_2, and other bronchoconstricting prostaglandins in the airways of subjects with mild asthma, *Am. Rev. Respir. Dis.*, 142, 126, 1990.
65. Wenzel, S.E., Westcott, J.Y., and Larsen, G.L., Bronchoalveolar lavage fluid mediator levels 5 minutes after allergen challenge in atopic subjects with asthma: relationship to the development of late asthmatic responses, *J. Allergy Clin. Immunol.*, 87, 540, 1991.
66. Dworski, R. et al., Effect of oral prednisone on airway inflammatory mediators in atopic asthma, *Am. Rev. Respir. Dis.*, 149, 953, 1994.
67. Pavord, I.D. et al., Induced sputum eicosanoid concentrations in asthma, *Am. J. Respir. Crit. Care Med.*, 160, 1905, 1999.
68. Higashi, N. et al., A comparative study of eicosanoid concentrations in sputum and urine in patients with aspirin-intolerant asthma, *Clin. Exp. Allergy*, 32, 1484, 2002.
69. Montuschi, P. and Barnes, P.J. Exhaled leukotrienes and prostaglandins in asthma, *J. Allergy. Clin. Immunol.*, 109, 615, 2002.
70. Csoma, Z. et al., Increased leukotrienes in exhaled breath condensate in childhood asthma, *Am. J. Respir. Crit. Care Med.*, 166, 1345, 2002.
71. Bowton, D.L. et al., Phospholipase A_2 and arachidonate increase in bronchoalveolar lavage fluid after inhaled antigen challenge in asthmatics, *Am. J. Respir. Crit. Care Med.*, 155, 421, 1997.
72. Kane, G.C. et al., Insights into IgE-mediated lung inflammation derived from a study employing a 5-lipoxygenase inhibitor, *Prostaglandins*, 50, 1, 1995.
73. Macfarlane, A.J., Sputum cysteinyl leukotrienes increase 24 hours after allergen inhalation in atopic asthmatics, *Am. J. Respir. Crit. Care Med.*, 161, 1553, 2000.
74. Taylor, G.W. et al., Urinary leukotriene E_4 after antigen challenge and in acute asthma and allergic rhinitis, *Lancet*, 1, 584, 1989.
75. Sladek, K., Allergen-stimulated release of thromboxane A_2 and leukotriene E_4 in humans, *Am. Rev. Respir. Dis.*, 141, 1441, 1990.
76. Sladek, K. et al., Formation of PGD_2 after allergen inhalation in atopic asthmatics, *Adv. Prostagl. Thromb. Leuk. Res.*, 21A, 433, 1990.
77. Knapp, H.R., Sladek, K., and FitzGerald, G.A., Increased excretion of leukotriene E_4 during aspirin-induced asthma, *J. Lab. Clin. Med.*, 119, 48, 1992.
78. Reiss, T.F. et al., Increased urinary excretion of LTE_4 after exercise and attenuation of exercise-induced bronchospasm by montelukast, a cysteinyl leukotriene antagonist, *Thorax*, 52, 1030, 1997.
79. Taylor, I.K. et al., Thromboxane A_2 biosynthesis in acute asthma and after antigen challenge, *Am. Rev. Respir. Dis.*, 143, 119, 1991.
80. Sampson, A.P. et al., Persistent increase in plasma and urinary leukotrienes after acute asthma, *Arch. Dis. Child.*, 73, 221, 1995.

81. Sladek, K. et al., Eicosanoids in bronchoalveolar lavage fluid of aspirin-intolerant patients with asthma after aspirin challenge, *Am. J. Respir. Crit. Care Med.*, 149, 940, 1994.

82. Szczeklik, K. et al., Bronchial aspirin challenge causes specific eicosanoid response in aspirin-sensitive asthmatics, *Am. J. Respir. Crit. Care Med.*, 154, 1608, 1996.

83. Wenzel, S.E. et al., Effect of 5-lipoxygenase inhibition on bronchoconstriction and airway inflammation in nocturnal asthma, *Am. J. Respir. Crit. Care Med.*, 152, 897, 1995.

84. Chan-Yeung, M. et al., Histamine and leukotrienes release in bronchoalveolar fluid during plicatic acid-induced bronchoconstriction, *J. Allergy. Clin. Immunol.*, 84, 762, 1989.

85. Coffey, M.J. et al., Increased 5-lipoxygenase metabolism in the lungs of human subjects exposed to ozone, *Toxicology*, 114, 118, 1996.

86. Zocca, E. et al., Leukotriene B$_4$ and late asthmatic reactions induced by toluene diisocyanate, *J. Appl. Physiol.*, 68, 1576, 1990.

87. Steinke, J.W. et al., Cysteinyl leukotriene expression in chronic hyperplastic sinusitis-nasal polyposis: importance to eosinophilia and asthma, *J. Allergy. Clin. Immunol.*, 111, 342, 2003.

88. Sampson, A.P., The role of eosinophils and neutrophils in inflammation, *Clin. Exp. Allergy*, 30, S22, 2000.

89. Dworski, R. et al., Prednisone increases PGH-synthase 2 in human atopics *in vivo*, *Am. J. Respir. Crit. Care Med.*, 155, 351, 1997.

90. Demoly, P. et al., Prostaglandin H synthase 1 and 2 immunoreactivities in the bronchial mucosa of asthmatics, *Am. J. Respir. Crit. Care Med.*, 155, 670, 1997.

91. Seymour, M.L. et al., Leukotriene and prostanoid pathway enzymes in bronchial biopsies of seasonal allergic asthmatics, *Am. J. Respir. Crit. Care Med.*, 164, 2051, 2001.

92. Picado, C. et al., Cyclooxygenase-2 mRNA is downexpressed in nasal polyps from aspirin-sensitive asthmatics, *Am. J. Respir. Crit. Care Med.*, 160, 291, 1999.

93. Sousa, A.R. et al., Enhanced expression of cyclooxygenase isoenzyme 2 (COX-2) in asthmatic airways and its cellular distribution in aspirin sensitive asthma, *Thorax*, 52, 940, 1997.

94. Taha, R. et al., Prostaglandin H synthase 2 expression in airways cells from patients with asthma and chronic obstructive pulmonary disease, *Am. J. Respir. Crit. Care Med.*, 161, 636, 2000.

95. Redington, A.E. et al., Increased expression of inducible nitric oxide synthase and cyclooxygenase 2 in the airway epithelium of asthmatic subjects and regulation by corticosteroid treatment, *Thorax*, 56, 351, 2001.

96. Cowburn, A.S. et al., Overexpression of leukotriene C$_4$ synthase in bronchial biopsies from patients with aspirin-intolerant asthma, *J. Clin. Invest.*, 101, 834, 1998.

97. Sousa, A.R., et al., Leukotriene-receptor expression on nasal inflammatory cells in aspirin-sensitive rhinosinusitis, *N. Engl. J. Med.*, 347, 1493, 2002.

98. Kuhn, H., Walther, M., and Kuban, R.J., Mammalian arachidonate 15-lipoxygenases structure, and biological implications, *Prostaglandins Other Lipid Mediat.*, 68–69, 263, 2002.

99. Spector, A.A., Gordon, J.A., and Moore, S.A. Hydroxyeicosatetraenoic acids (HETEs). *Prog. Lipid Res.*, 27, 271, 1988.

100. Hill A.T. et al., Evidence for excessive bronchial inflammation during an acute exacerbation of chronic obstructive pulmonary disease in patients with α_1-antitrypsin deficiency, *Am. J. Respir. Crit. Care Med.*, 160, 1968, 1999.

101. Biernacki, W.A., Kharitonov, S.A., and Barnes, P.J. Increased leukotriene B_4 and 8-isoprostane in exhaled breath condensate of patients with exacerbations of COPD, *Thorax*, 58, 294, 2003.

102. Zakrzewski, J.T. et al., Lipid mediators in cystic fibrosis and chronic obstructive pulmonary disease, *Am. Rev. Respir. Dis.*, 136, 779, 1987.

103. Spencer, D.A. et al., Sputum cysteinyl-leukotriene levels correlate with the severity of pulmonary disease in children with cystic fibrosis, *Pediatr. Pulmonol.*, 12, 90, 1992.

104. Konstan, M.W. et al., Leukotriene B_4 markedly elevated in the epithelial lining fluid of patients with cystic fibrosis, *Am. Rev. Respir. Dis.*, 148, 896, 1993.

105. Carpagnano, G.E. et al., Increased leukotriene B_4 and interleukin-6 in exhaled breath condensate in cystic fibrosis, *Am. J. Respir. Crit. Care Med.*, 167, 1109, 2003.

106. Wang, D. et al., Clement. Inflammatory cells and mediator concentrations in nasal secretions of patients with cystic fibrosis, *Acta Otolaryngol.*, 116, 472, 1996.

107. Greally, P. et al., Atopic children with cystic fibrosis have increased urinary leukotriene E_4 concentrations and more severe pulmonary disease, *J. Allergy Clin. Immunol.*, 93, 100, 1994.

108. Brighling, C.E. et al., Induced sputum inflammatory mediator concentrations in eosinophilic bronchitis and asthma, *Am. J. Respir. Crit. Care Med.*, 162, 878, 2000

109. Kowal-Bielecka, O. et al., Elevated levels of leukotriene B_4 and leukotriene E_4 in bronchoalveolar lavage fluid from patients with scleroderma lung disease, *Arthritis Rheum.*, 48, 1639, 2003.

110. Gilroy, D.W. et al., Inducible cyclooxygenase may have anti-inflammatory properties, *Nat. Med.*, 5, 698, 1999.

111. Levy, D. et al., Lipid mediator class switching during acute inflammation: signals in resolution, *Nat. Immunol.*, 2, 612, 2001.

112. Sheller, J.R. et al., EP2 receptor mediates bronchodilation by PGE_2 in mice, *J. Appl. Physiol.*, 88, 2214, 2000.

113. Tilley, S.L. et al., Receptors and pathways mediating the effects of prostaglandin E_2 on airway tone, *Am. J. Physiol.*, 284, L599, 2003.

114. Cuthbert, M.F., Effect on airways resistance of prostaglandin E_1 given by aerosol to healthy and asthmatic volunteers, *BMJ*, 4, 723, 1969.

115. Peebles, R.S., Jr. et al., Cyclooxygenase inhibition increases interleukin 5 and interleukin 13 production and airway hyperresponsiveness in allergic mice, *Am. J. Respir. Crit. Care Med.*, 162, 676, 2000.

116. Peebles, R.S., Jr. et al., Selective cyclooxygenase-1 and -2 inhibitors each increase allergic inflammation and airway hyperresponsiveness in mice, *Am. J. Respir. Crit. Care Med.*, 165, 1154, 2002.

117. Raud, J. et al., Enhancement of acute allergic inflammation by indomethacin is reversed by prostaglandin E_2: apparent correlation with *in vivo* modulation of mediator release, *Proc. Natl. Acad. Sci. U.S.A.*, 85, 2315, 1988.

118. Melo-Bandeira, C. et al., Cyclooxygenase-2-derived prostaglandin E_2 and lipoxin A4 accelerate resolution of allergic edema in *Angiostrongylus costaricensis*-infected rats: relationship with concurrent eosinophilia, *J. Immunol.*, 164, 1029, 2000.

119. Rodgers, H.C. et al., Bradykinin increases IL-8 generation in airway epithelial cells via COX-2 derived prostanoids. *Am. J. Physiol.*, 283, L612, 2002.

120. Smith, R.S. et al., The *Pseudomonas* autoinducer N-(3-oxododecanoyl) homoserine lactone induces cyclooxygenase-2 and prostaglandin E_2 production in human lung fibroblasts: implications for inflammation, *J. Immunol.*, 169, 2636, 2002.

121. Kohyama, T. et al., Prostaglandin E_2 inhibits fibroblast chemotaxis, *Am. J. Physiol.*, 281, L257, 2001.

122. Lama, V. et al., Prostaglandin E_2 synthesis and suppression of fibroblast proliferation by alveolar epithelial cells is cyclooxygenase-2 dependent, *Am. J. Respir. Cell Mol. Biol.*, 27, 2002, 752.

123. Moore, B.B. et al., GM-CSF regulates bleomycin-induced pulmonary fibrosis via a prostaglandin-depended mechanism, *J. Immunol.*, 165, 4032, 2000.

124. Moore, B.B. et al., Alveolar epithelial cell inhibition of fibroblast proliferation is regulated by MCP-1/CCR2 and mediated by PGE_2, *Am. J. Physiol.*, 284, L342, 2003.

125. Yang, X. et al., Hypoxic induction of COX-2 regulates proliferation of human pulmonary artery smooth muscle cells, *Am. J. Respir. Cell Mol. Biol.*, 27, 688, 2002.

126. Belvisi, M.G. et al., Expression of cyclo-oxygenase in human airway smooth muscle is associated with profound reductions in cell growth, *Brit. J. Pharmacol.*, 125, 1102, 1998.

127. Bonner, J.C. et al., Susceptibility of cyclooxygenase-2-deficient mice to pulmonary fibrosis, *Am. J. Pathol.*, 161, 459, 2002.

128. Wilborn, J. et al., Cultured lung fibroblasts isolated from patients with idiopathic pulmonary fibrosis have a diminished capacity to synthesize prostaglandin E_2 and to express cyclooxygenase-2, *J. Clin. Invest.*, 95, 1861, 1995.

129. Gridelli, C. et al., Selective cyclooxygenase-2 inhibitors and non-small cell lung cancer, *Curr. Med. Chem.*, 9, 1851, 2002.

130. Gyllfors, P. et al., Biochemical and clinical evidence that aspirin-intolerant asthmatic subjects tolerate the cyclooxygenase 2-selective analgesic drug celecoxib, *J. Allergy Clin. Immunol.*, 111, 1116, 2003.

131. Dworski, R.T. et al., Prednisone increases PGH-synthase 2 in atopic humans *in vivo*, *Am. J. Respir. Crit. Care Med.*, 155, 351, 1997.

132. Arimura, K. et al., Prevention of allergic inflammation by a novel prostaglandin receptor antagonist, S-5751, *J. Pharmacol. Exp. Ther.*, 298, 411, 2001.

133. Fujimura, M. et al., Effects of aerosol administration of a thromboxane synthetase inhibitor (OKY-046) on bronchial responsiveness to acetylcholine in asthmatic subjects, *Chest*, 98, 276, 1990.

134. Finnerty, J.P., Effect of GR32191, a potent thromboxane receptor antagonist, on exercise induced bronchoconstriction in asthma, *Thorax*, 46, 190, 1991.

135. Hoshino, M. et al., Effect of AA-2414, a thromboxane A_2 receptor antagonist, on airway inflammation in subjects with asthma, *J. Allergy Clin. Immunol.*, 103, 1054, 1999.

136. Drazen, M., Israel, E., and O'Byrne, P.M., Treatment of asthma with drugs modifying the leukotriene pathway, *N. Engl. J. Med.*, 340, 197, 1999.

137. Camargo, C.A., Jr. et al., A randomized controlled trial of intravenous montelukast in acute asthma, *Am. J. Respir. Crit. Care Med.*, 167, 528, 2003.

138. Holgate, S.T. et al., Roles of leukotrienes in airway inflammation, smooth muscle function, and remodeling, *J. Allergy Clin. Immunol.*, 111, S18, 2003.

139. Peters, S.P., Leukotriene receptor antagonists in asthma therapy, *J. Allergy Clin. Immunol.*, 111, S62, 2003.

140. Peters-Golden, M. et al., Protection from pulmonary fibrosis in leukotriene-deficient mice, *Am. J. Respir. Crit. Care Med.*, 165, 229, 2002.

141. Dworski, R., Eicosanoid regulation by glucocorticoids in asthma, in *Eicosanoids, Aspirin and Asthma*, Szczeklik, A., Gryglewski, R.J., and Vane, J.R., Eds., Marcel Dekker, Inc., New York, 1998, pp. 283–298.

13 Neurogenic Inflammation in the Airways: Role of Tachykinins

Guy F. Joos, Katelijne O. De Swert, and Romain A. Pauwels

CONTENTS

I. INTRODUCTION

The inflammation that results from the release of substances from primary sensory nerve terminals is called neurogenic inflammation. More than one century ago, the first observations were made that activation of dorsal root ganglia neurons results in vasodilation. Since then, abundant evidence has been accumulated to suggest that activation of peripheral terminals of sensory neurons by local depolarization, axonal reflexes, or dorsal root reflexes releases bioactive substances. These substances act on target cells in the periphery, such as mast cells, immune cells, and vascular smooth muscle cells, to produce inflammation (redness and warmth, swelling, and hypersensitivity).[1]

Small-diameter sensory neurons that are sensitive to capsaicin are of major importance in the generation of neurogenic inflammation. The neuropeptides substance P (SP) and calcitonin gene-related peptide (CGRP) are considered to be the major initiators of neurogenic inflammation.[2,3] SP and neurokinin A (NKA) are members of the tachykinin peptide family and are potent vasodilators and contractors of smooth muscle.[4] In studies on rodent airways, SP and NKA have been implicated as the neurotransmitters mediating the excitatory part of the nonadrenergic noncholinergic (NANC) nervous system. These noncholinergic excitatory nerves can be activated by mechanical and chemical stimuli, generating antidromic impulses and a local axon reflex that leads to noncholinergic bronchoconstriction and neurogenic inflammation.[5,6]

SP and NKA have various effects that could contribute to the changes observed in airways of patients with asthma or chronic obstructive pulmonary diseases (COPD). These include smooth muscle contraction, submucosal gland secretion, vasodilation, increase in vascular permeability, stimulation of cholinergic nerves, stimulation of mast cells, stimulation of B and T lymphocytes, stimulation of macrophages, chemoattraction of eosinophils and neutrophils, and the vascular adhesion of neutrophils. SP and NKA interact with the different targets in the airways by stimulation of tachykinin NK_1, NK_2, and NK_3 receptors.[7,8] The physiological activity of both exogenously administered and endogenously released neuropeptides is modulated through enzymatic cleavage and inactivation by peptidases.[9] This chapter describes the role of tachykinins and their receptors in airway inflammation.

II. THE NONADRENERGIC NONCHOLINERGIC AIRWAY INNERVATION

In the 1970s and 1980s, the classical view that cholinergic excitatory and adrenergic inhibitory nerves regulate airways was considerably changed by the demonstration of the NANC system. The NANC system can be either inhibitory or excitatory. Various purines and peptides have been suggested as candidate neurotransmitters for the NANC system. Some of these coexist with acetylcholine or noradrenaline in the classical nerves, for example, vasoactive intestinal peptide (VIP) in cholinergic nerves and neuropeptide Y (NPY) in noradrenergic nerves.[10] Both afferent sensory and efferent motor nerves are present within the lung (Figure 13.1).[11]

A nonadrenergic inhibitory airway innervation was first demonstrated in the guinea pig trachea[12]: electrical field stimulation produced a biphasic response, an initial contraction that was blocked by atropine, followed by a relaxation that was only partially inhibited by propranolol. This propranolol-resistant relaxation was abolished after pretreatment with the neurotoxin, tetrodotoxin (TTX), indicating a nerve-mediated response. The nonadrenergic bronchodilation has been demonstrated in several animal species, both *in vivo* and *in vitro*, with the exception of the rat and the dog. It is also present in human airways; *in vitro* studies have indicated that the inhibitory response to electrical stimulation is not influenced practically by β-adrenergic blockade.[13,14]

The nonadrenergic inhibitory nervous pathway can be reflex activated. In feline airways mechanical stimulation of the laryngeal mucosa elicited a transient bronchoconstriction, abolished by atropine, and a prolonged bronchodilation, which was resistant to β-adrenergic blockade with propranolol.[15] Reflex activation of nonadrenergic inhibitory nerves is also present within human airways.[16,17]

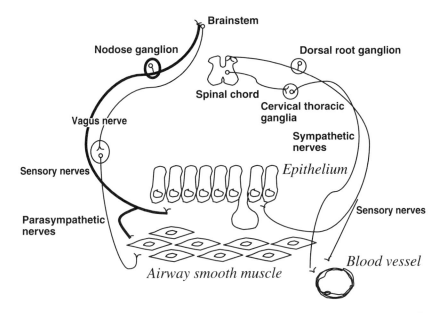

FIGURE 13.1 Schematic view of the lung innervation. The afferent (sensory) part allows the transmission of stimuli to the central nervous system. The efferent (parasympathetic, sympathetic, local reflex) part transmits the response to the target(s), which include the airway smooth muscle and the mucus secreting cells. The vagus nerve contains the parasympathetic part as well as most of the sensory nerves. A small part of the sensory innervation is dependent on the dorsal root ganglia; these nerve fibers are running along with the efferent spinal sympathetic nerve fibers.

Noncholinergic excitatory nerves have been demonstrated in guinea pig airways, *in vivo* and *in vitro*.[18–20] In the presence of atropine and propranolol, the hilus and main bronchi of the guinea pig contract slowly in response to electrical field stimulation. This atropine-resistant contraction comprises about 60% of the contractions that can be induced by electrical field stimulation. It is absent in animals that were pretreated with capsaicin, a neurotoxin that damages unmyelinated C fibers. These nerves can also be demonstrated, by bilateral electrical stimulation of the cervical vagal nerves, which induces a bronchoconstriction that is only reduced by approximately 60% after pretreatment with atropine.[20] These noncholinergic excitatory nerves also can be stimulated by mechanical irritation and chemical irritants such as ether, formalin, capsaicin, and cigarette smoke.[6]

A noncholinergic bronchoconstriction has not been consistently demonstrated in human airways.[21] Nevertheless, the existence of noncholinergic excitatory nerves in human airways has been claimed by the finding that capsaicin induces contractions of isolated bronchi.[21] Capsaicin degranulates C fiber endings and releases different neuropeptides from them. Inhalation of capsaicin caused a dose-dependent coughing in normal volunteers and subjects with mild asthma.[22] It also caused a dose-dependent decrease in specific airway conductance (SG_{aw}) in normal and asthmatic subjects, an effect that was significantly reduced after pretreatment with ipratropium bromide. The time course of this bronchoconstriction (maximal decrease in SG_{aw} within 20 seconds of exposure and lasting less than 60 seconds) and its reduction by an anticholinergic agent have been taken as indication that the bronchoconstrictor response to capsaicin inhalation is due mainly to a vagally mediated cholinergic reflex and not to a local axon reflex with release of neuropeptides.[23]

NANC nerves also can control mucus secretion. Adrenergic- and cholinergic-blocking drugs inhibited only partially the mucus secretion that occurred in the trachea of the cat after stimulation of the vagus nerves.[24]

III. NEUROGENIC AIRWAY INFLAMMATION

Antidromic stimulation of sensory nerves C-fiber afferents produces vasodilation in skin, dental pulp, and nasal mucosa, and local edema due to an increase in vascular permeability to plasma proteins in skin and respiratory tract. These responses are known as neurogenic inflammation.[5,7,25] In 1901, Bayliss described vasodilator fibers in peripheral sensory nerves that, when stimulated antidromically, dilated blood vessels in the skin. Langley proposed the concept of an axon-reflex, suggesting that sensory nerves can have a peripheral effector function. Stimulation of sensory nerves not only initiates orthodromic impulses that travel upward to the spinal cord but also induces antidromic impulses that spread through the terminal arborizations (axon collaterals) of the sensory nerves. The concept of the axon reflex was further developed in the skin by Lewis in 1927, who showed that the flare response or vasodilation, which spreads for several centimeters beyond the point of injury, is mediated by axon reflexes in sensory nerve terminals.

Neurogenic inflammation has been described in the airways of rodents. A wide array of stimuli can induce neurogenic inflammation in rodent airways. Lundberg et al.[26] were the first to describe neurogenic inflammation in the respiratory tract. They found that in rats and guinea pigs topical application of capsaicin, inhalation of cigarette smoke, or electrical stimulation of the vagus nerve induced an increase in the plasma protein extravasation in the airways. This neurogenic plasma extravasation occurred both in the upper airways nasal mucosa, epiglottis, and vocal cords, and in the lower airways from the trachea down to the bronchioles. The increase in vascular permeability was abolished by capsaicin pretreatment and inhibited by an antagonist for SP. Administration of exogenous SP mimicked the plasma leakage induced by either capsaicin or electrical nerve stimulation. Furthermore, the effect of SP was not affected by depletion of sensory nerves with capsaicin. Consequently, they postulated that SP released from capsaicin-sensitive nerve fibers mediates the neurogenic inflammation in the airways.[26,27]

Subsequent studies have shown that the plasma extravasation induced by cold air, hypertonic saline, or isocapnic hyperpnea depends on capsaicin-sensitive sensory nerves and is inhibited by tachykinin receptor antagonists. Furthermore, part of the increase in vascular permeability produced by histamine, bradykinin, acetylcholine, or antigen challenge involves tachykinins released from capsaicin-sensitive nerves.[6]

IV. NEURONAL AND NONNEURONAL SOURCES OF TACHYKININS IN HUMAN AIRWAYS

SP and NKA are contained in a distinct subpopulation of primary afferent nerves that are characterized by sensitivity to capsaicin. In man, SP and NKA are present in nerve profiles, found beneath and within the epithelium, around blood vessels and submucosal glands, and within the bronchial smooth muscle layer.[28,29] Using confocal laser scanning microscopy and immunohistochemistry for the protein gene product 9.5 (PGP-IR), Lamb and Sparrow[30] demonstrated an arrangement of epithelial nerves in human bronchi, which was very similar to that of porcine nerves containing sensory neuropeptides. An apical layer of varicose processes terminated in enlarged varicosities, and these fibers encircled goblet cells. These processes arose from fibers that had crossed the epithelium from a basal plexus that was supplied by nerve bundles in the lamina propria. As in other studies, SP-immunoreactive nerves were faintly stained in human bronchi.

Tachykinins have been measured in bronchoalveolar lavage (BAL), induced sputum, and plasma. Various studies have shown that tachykinins can be released into the airways after exposure to allergen, ozone, or hypertonic saline. Nieber et al.[31] found a significantly larger amount of SP in BAL fluid of atopic compared with nonallergic subjects. After intrasegmental provocation with allergen, a significant increase in BAL SP levels was observed. Heaney et al.[32] also recovered NKA from BAL fluid from normal and asthmatic patients. NKA was increased in the asthmatic patients 4 hours after inhalation challenge with house dust mite. Exposure of healthy individuals to ozone increased the concentration of SP in BAL fluid[33] and decreased the immunoreactivity for SP, assessed on bronchial biopsies.[34] Nasal application of hypertonic saline also induced release of SP.[35]

Although increased amounts of tachykinins have been recovered from the airways, there has been debate about a possible upregulation of SP-containing nerves in patients with asthma or COPD. Ollerenshaw et al.[37] reported that in tissue obtained at autopsy, after lobectomy and at bronchoscopy, both the number and the length of SP-immunoreactive nerve fibers was increased in airways of subjects with asthma, when compared with airways from subjects without asthma [36]. However, Howarth et al.[37] could not identify any SP-containing nerves in endobronchial biopsies from patients with mild asthma. In a study on 49 asthmatic patients, including 16 patients with severe asthma, Chanez et al.[38] did not find evidence for an upregulation of SP-containing nerves in asthma. Nerves were present in most of the endobronchial biopsies, as demonstrated by the neural marker PGP 9.5, and were found within and below the epithelium and adjacent to smooth muscle, glands, and blood vessels. However, nerves positive for SP and CGRP were rarely found in the biopsy specimens. Moreover no increase in patients with asthma was observed. Conversely, SP-like immunoreactivity was decreased in tracheal tissue of asthmatic subjects studied at autopsy. This might reflect augmented release of SP, followed by degradation.[39] Lucchini et al.[40] studied lung tissue obtained at thoracotomy from patients with chronic bronchitis. The lung tissue in chronic bronchitis did not contain more nerves, and did not show a change in the amount of SP- or CGRP-containing nerves.

In contrast, the density of VIP-containing nerves was significantly higher in the glands of patients with chronic bronchitis compared with control subjects.

In recent years, it has become clear from both animal and human studies that immune cells might form an additional source of tachykinins.[8,41] Evidence for the production of SP by eosinophils (mouse, man), monocytes and macrophages (rat, man), lymphocytes (man), and dendritic cells (mice) has been reported. Inflammatory stimuli such as lipopolysaccharide (LPS) can upregulate the concentration of tachykinins in these cells.[42,43] These findings can help to explain the paradox between the relatively few SP- and NKA-containing nerves observed in human airways and the recovery of SP and NKA from sputum and BAL. Thus, increased amounts of immune cells attracted to the inflamed airways might be responsible for an increased content of SP and NKA in patients with asthma or COPD. Moreover, the release of tachykinins from these inflammatory cells might further stimulate and activate these cells in an autocrine or paracrine fashion. Indeed, these inflammatory cells produce and secrete SP and possess tachykinin NK_1 receptors on their membranes.[42]

Epithelial or endothelial cells might be an additional nonneuronal source of SP.[8] Chu et al.[44] reported staining for SP in the epithelium on human biopsy specimens. In comparison with control subjects, patients with asthma showed a significantly higher expression of SP in the epithelium but not in the submucosa. It is of interest to note that in their study the epithelial expression of SP was correlated with the epithelial mucus content.

V. AIRWAY TACHYKININ RECEPTORS

Most of the biological actions of tachykinins are mediated via activation of one of three tachykinin receptors, denoted NK_1, NK_2, and NK_3. The NK_1, NK_2, and NK_3 tachykinin receptors have the highest affinity for SP, NKA, and neurokinin B, respectively. There is, however, a wide cross-talk between natural tachykinin peptides and their receptors: for instance it is presently accepted that NKA is a high-affinity and effective endogenous ligand for NK_1 receptors at many synapses and/or neuro-effector junctions.[45]

The tachykinins SP and NKA interact with the targets on the airways by specific tachykinin receptors. The tachykinin NK_1 and NK_2 receptors have been characterized in human airways, both pharmacologically and by cloning. In in vitro studies on isolated human bronchi and bronchioli, tachykinin NK_2 receptors were found to be present on smooth muscle of both large and small airways, and to mediate part of the bronchoconstrictor effect of the tachykinins [46]. Tachykinin NK_1 receptors are localized on smooth muscle of small airways and are responsible for a transient, low-intensity contraction.[47] Most of the proinflammatory effects of SP are mediated by the tachykinin NK_1 receptor (reviewed by Advenier et al.[48]). The tachykinin NK_3 receptor has been demonstrated in guinea pig airways, where it mediates citric acid-induced cough and changes in airway responsiveness induced by SP and citric acid.[49,50] Moreover, the tachykinin NK_3 receptor mediates the neurokinin-induced facilitation of synaptic neurotransmission in parasympathetic ganglia.[51]

Various studies have explored possible changes in the expression of airway tachykinin receptors as a consequence of inflammatory changes in the airways.

Smoking increases the tachykinin NK_1 receptor mRNA.[52] In asthmatics, the expression of the tachykinin NK_2 receptor mRNA is increased.[53] Glucocorticoids can reduce the level of tachykinin receptor mRNA.[54] Using antibodies to the tachykinin NK_1 and NK_2 receptors, Mapp et al.[55] found expression of both tachykinin receptors in bronchial glands, bronchial vessels, and bronchial smooth muscle. Receptors were occasionally found in nerves (NK_1) and in inflammatory cells (NK_2) such as T lymphocytes, macrophages, and mast cells. The distribution of both tachykinin NK_1 and NK_2 receptors was similar in the tissues examined from nonsmokers, asymptomatic smokers, symptomatic smokers with normal lung function, and symptomatic smokers with chronic airflow limitation. In a study on endobronchial biopsies by Chu et al.,[44] immunoreactivity for the tachykinin NK_1 receptor was found in the epithelium and submucosa. The NK_1 receptor expression was mainly seen on cell surfaces of the upper half of the epithelial layer. Goblet cells appeared to be the cells with the strongest staining. In the submucosa, the tachykinin NK_1 receptor was primarily localized on the endothelial cells of the blood vessels, the surfaces of inflammatory cells, and some smooth muscle cells. In this study the expression of SP as well as the tachykinin NK_1 receptor was significantly higher in the epithelium of asthmatic subjects.[44]

VI. BRONCHOCONSTRICTOR EFFECTS OF TACHYKININS

Tachykinins are potent contractors of airways. The *in vitro* contractile effect of SP and NKA has been studied extensively. SP contracts human bronchi and bronchioli[56,57] but is less potent than histamine or acetylcholine.[58] NKA is a more potent constrictor of human bronchi than SP and was reported to be, on a molar basis, 2 to 3 orders of magnitude more potent than histamine or acetylcholine.

It has long been thought that only tachykinin NK_2 receptors are involved in contraction of isolated human airways.[59] However, in small-diameter bronchi (~1 mm in diameter) tachykinins also cause contraction via NK_1 tachykinin receptor stimulation. The NK_1-mediated contraction of small bronchi appears to be mediated by prostanoids.[47] In a study of medium-sized human isolated bronchi (2 to 5 mm in diameter) the specific NK_1 receptor agonist $[Sar^9,Met(O_2)^{11}]SP$ was found to induce contraction in about 60% of the preparations — an effect that was not mediated by prostanoids, but from a direct activation of smooth muscle receptors and release of inositol phosphate.[60] Thus, part of the airway contraction induced by tachykinins in man is mediated by tachykinin NK_1 receptors.

Several groups have studied the *in vivo* bronchoconstrictor effect of SP and NKA, administered via inhalation or intravenous infusion. NKA was found to be a more potent bronchoconstrictor than SP. Patients with asthma are hyperresponsive to SP and NKA (reviewed by Joos et al.[61]). The bronchoconstrictor effect of inhaled SP and NKA in asthmatics can be prevented by pretreatment with sodium cromoglycate and nedocromil sodium.[62,63] This has led us to postulate that SP and NKA are indirect bronchoconstrictors in man. This indirect bronchoconstrictor effect could arise from an effect on inflammatory cells (e.g., mast cells) and/or nerves.[64,65] In experimental animals, tachykinins are able to cause acetylcholine release from postganglionic cholinergic airway nerve endings,[66–68] and to activate mast cells.[69–72] The exact mechanism of tachykinin-induced bronchoconstriction in man, however, is not yet known. In some patients cholinergic mechanisms do play a role.[73,74] Histamine, however, does not seem to be involved because pretreatment with different H_1 receptor antagonists (astemizole and terfenadine) did not inhibit NKA-induced bronchoconstriction.[73,75] It was demonstrated recently that leukotrienes mediate part of the bronchoconstrictor effect of NKA: the cys-LT1 receptor antagonists zafirlukast and montelukast partially inhibited bronchoconstriction induced by inhaled NKA in patients with asthma.[76,77] Thus, NKA causes bronchoconstriction in patients with asthma by indirect mechanisms, involving mast cells, leukotrienes, and cholinergic nerves.[78]

VII. TACHYKININS AND AIRWAY PLASMA EXTRAVASATION

Ablation of sensory nerves by capsaicin pretreatment abolishes airways plasma extravasation induced by a variety of mediators and stimuli, including histamine, serotonin, and cigarette smoke.[27,79] Tachykinin NK_1 receptors that mediate neurogenic plasma extravasation have been visualized on postcapillary endothelial cells.[80] Once plasma extravasation occurs, leukocytes initiate a process that results in slowing down their velocity, and rolling on and adhering to the venular endothelium. The involvement of tachykinin NK_1 receptors in the neurogenic plasma extravasation in the central airways of rats and guinea pigs has been demonstrated by the use of selective tachykinin receptor agonists and antagonists. The tachykinin NK_1 receptors are also implicated in the extravasation caused by hypertonic saline, bradykinin, antigen challenge, or acetylcholine. Tachykinin NK_2 receptors mediate part of the neurogenic plasma extravasation in the secondary bronchi and intraparenchymal airways of the guinea pig.[81,82]

Bowden et al.[80] have demonstrated that in the rat trachea, tachykinin NK_1 receptors are present on the endothelial cells of the postcapillary venules. These receptors are internalized in endosomes upon binding with SP. They also observed an increase in the number of tachykinin NK_1 receptor immunoreactive endosomes when the vagus nerve is electrically stimulated, indicating that SP released by activation of the sensory nerves has a direct effect on the tachykinin NK_1 receptors on postcapillary venular endothelium.[80] In addition to the direct effects of tachykinins on the venular endothelium, indirect mechanisms involving mast cell activation and serotonin (5-HT) release participate in the tachykinin-induced plasma exudation in the respiratory tract of some animal species. In rabbit airways, involvement of 5-HT receptors and arachidonic acid derivates in the tachykinin-induced increase in vascular permeability has been suggested.[83,84] Neurogenic plasma protein extravasation in rat airways involves the activation of tachykinin NK_1 receptors. In F344 but not in BDE rats, an additional indirect mechanism, involving mast cell activation, 5-HT release, and stimulation of $5\text{-}HT_2$ receptors, participates in this process.[85,86]

Microvascular leakage can now be measured in human airways. A particularly interesting approach is the dual-induction model: first SP is inhaled and then sputum is induced by inhalation of hypertonic saline. In this way, Van Rensen et al.[87] demonstrated that inhalation of SP induced significant increases in the levels of α_2-macroglobulin, ceruloplasmin, and albumin in induced sputum.

VIII. ROLE OF TACHYKININS IN ANIMAL MODELS OF ASTHMA AND CHRONIC OBSTRUCTIVE PULMONARY DISEASE

Tachykinins have been found to be involved in antigen-induced bronchoconstriction, airway inflammation, and enhanced bronchial responsiveness in various animal models. A combination of a tachykinin NK_1 receptor antagonist, CP-96,345,[88] and a tachykinin NK_2 receptor antagonist, SR48968,[89] inhibited bronchoconstriction produced by ovalbumin challenge in sensitized guinea pigs.[90] The NK_1 receptor antagonist, CP-96,345, was also able to limit antigen-induced plasma extravasation.[91] By using NK_1/NK_2 receptor blockade the involvement of endogenous tachykinins in antigen-induced bronchial hyperresponsiveness was demonstrated.[92]

The relative contribution of the NK_1 and NK_2 receptor in antigen-induced airway changes has been studied in guinea pigs and rats. In conscious, unrestrained guinea pigs, the NK_1 receptor is involved in both the development of antigen-induced airway hyperresponsiveness to histamine and the antigen-induced infiltration of eosinophils, neutrophils, and lymphocytes.[93] Conversely, the NK_2 receptor is involved in the development of the antigen-induced late reaction.[94] The effect of allergen challenge has also been studied in the Brown Norway (BN) rat model.[95] SP was found to increase 2.4 fold in BAL after challenge with ovalbumin. The tachykinin NK_1 receptor antagonist CP99,994 and the tachykinin NK_2 receptor antagonist SR48968 were not able to reduce the early airway response to ovalbumin, but both antagonists reduced the ovalbumin-induced late airway responses. An interesting finding in this study was that the NK_2 tachykinin receptor antagonist decreased the number of eosinophils in BAL fluid and decreased the expression of both Th1 (interferon-γ [IFN-γ]) and Th2 (IL-4 and IL-5) cytokines in BAL cells. In a mouse model of asthma, we observed no influence of the tachykinin NK_1 receptor on the development of allergic airway inflammation. However, allergen-induced goblet cell hyperplasia, one of the features of airway remodeling, was decreased in mice lacking the tachykinin NK_1 receptor.[96,97]

Thus, from animal studies, it seems that both the tachykinin NK_1 and the NK_2 receptor are involved in antigen-induced airway effects. In addition, it is possible that tachykinin NK_3 receptors also are involved in this process: administration of the tachykinin NK_3 receptor antagonist SR142801 via aerosol caused a significant reduction in neutrophil and eosinophil influx in the airways of ovalbumin-sensitized and challenged mice.[98]

In animal models, tachykinins and their receptors have been involved in airway responses to nonspecific stimuli. Both the NK_1 and the NK_2 tachykinin receptors have been involved in airway contraction induced by cold-air,[99] hyperventilation,[100] and cigarette smoke[101]; in plasma extravasation induced by hypertonic saline[102,103]; and in airway hyperresponsiveness induced by viruses,[104] IL-5, and nerve growth factor.[105,106] In addition, the tachykinin NK_3 receptor was found to be involved in citric acid-induced cough and enhanced bronchial responsiveness.[49] From studies performed in tachykinin NK_1 receptor knock-out mice, it is becoming apparent that the tachykinin NK_1 receptor plays a role in cigarette smoke-induced airway inflammation.[107]

Neurogenic mucus secretion results from the contribution of different components and shows marked variation among species. Adrenergic and cholinergic agonists might stimulate mucus secretion in the ferret and human airways. Tachykinins also cause marked mucus secretion in the ferret, an effect exclusively mediated by NK_1 receptors. Endogenous tachykinins mediate mucus secretion induced by electrical stimuli and part of the response produced by exposure to antigen via NK_1 receptor activation.[108]

IX. TACHYKININ RECEPTOR ANTAGONISTS AS A POTENTIAL NEW TREATMENT FOR OBSTRUCTIVE AIRWAY DISEASES

Studies on rodents have demonstrated that a number of strategies are possible to interfere with the action of sensory neuropeptides in the airways: (1) depletion of neuropeptides within nerves (e.g., by the neurotoxin capsaicin); (2) inhibition of the release of sensory neuropeptides (e.g., by β_2-adrenoceptor agonist, theophylline, cromoglycate, or phosphodiesterase [PDE4] inhibitors); and (3) inhibition of tachykinin receptors by receptor antagonists.[6]

In animal models tachykinins and their receptors have been involved in airway responses to nonspecific stimuli. Both the NK_1 and the NK_2 tachykinin receptors have been involved in airway contraction induced by cold-air, hyperventilation, and cigarette smoke; in plasma extravasation induced by hypertonic saline bronchoconstriction; and in airway hyperresponsiveness induced by viruses, IL-5, and nerve growth factor.[109] The tachykinin NK_1 receptor also promotes ozone-induced lung inflammation.[110] Viral infection causes an upregulation of the tachykinin NK_1 receptor, leading to enhanced neurogenic inflammation.[111]

In contrast to the extensive and overwhelming preclinical data suggesting a role for tachykinins in asthma and possibly COPD, the development of tachykinin receptor antagonists for airways diseases has been rather slow and up to now somewhat disappointing. At present, clinical trials with at least seven tachykinin antagonists have been performed and reported. Reports studying the effects of FK224, a cyclic peptide tachykinin antagonist for NK_1 and NK_2 receptors; CP99,994, a nonpeptide NK_1 tachykinin receptor antagonist; FK888, a peptidic tachykinin NK_1 receptor antagonist; and SR48968 (saredutant), a nonpeptide NK_2 tachykinin receptor antagonist, have been published. In our center, we recently completed three additional studies, one with the bicyclic peptidic tachykinin NK_2 receptor antagonist MEN 11420 (nepadutant), one with the dual NK_1/NK_2 tachykinin receptor antagonist DNK333A, and one with the triple $NK_1/NK_2/NK_3$ receptor antagonist CS003 (reviewed by Joos et al.[112]). From these studies, it has become clear that potent dual or triple tachykinin receptor antagonists are able to block the bronchoconstrictor effect of NKA in patients with asthma.[113,114] However, clinical trials performed over several weeks to months will be necessary to determine a potential clinical activity of these compounds in obstructive airways diseases. Such compounds will also allow us to determine more precisely the role of neurogenic inflammation in human airways.

FURTHER READING

1. Richardson, J.D. and Vasko, M.R., Cellular mechanisms of neurogenic inflammation, *J. Pharmacol. Exp. Ther.*, 302, 839, 2002.
2. Barnes, P.J., Neurogenic inflammation in the airways, *Respir. Physiol*, 125, 145, 2001.
3. Lembeck, F. and Holzer, P., Substance P as neurogenic mediator of antidromic vasodilatation and neurogenic plasma extravasation, *Naunyn Schmiedebergs Arch. Pharmacol.*, 310, 175, 1979.
4. Severini, C. et al., The tachykinin peptide family, *Pharmacol. Rev.*, 54, 2002.
5. Barnes, P.J., Asthma as an axon reflex, *Lancet*, 1, 242, 1986.
6. Lundberg, J.M., Pharmacology of cotransmission in the autonomic nervous system: integrative aspects on amines, neuropeptides, adenosine triphosphate, amino acids and nitric oxide, *Pharmacol. Rev.*, 48, 178, 1996.
7. Joos, G.F., Germonpre, P.R., and Pauwels, R.A., Role of tachykinins in asthma, *Allergy*, 55, 321, 2000.
8. Maggi, C.A., The effects of tachykinins on inflammatory and immune cells, *Regul. Pept.*, 70, 75, 1997.
9. Di Maria, G.U., Bellofiore, S., and Geppetti, P., Regulation of airway neurogenic inflammation by neutral endopeptidase, *Eur. Respir. J.*, 12, 1454, 1998.
10. Joos, G. and Geppetti, P., Neural mechanisms in asthma, *Eur. Respir. Mon.*, 23, 138, 2003.
11. Richardson, J.B., Nerve supply to the lungs, *Am. Rev. Respir. Dis.*, 119, 785, 1979.
12. Coburn, R.F. and Tomita, T., Evidence for nonadrenergic inhibitory nerves in the guinea pig trachealis muscle, *Am. J. Physiol.*, 224, 1072, 1973.
13. Richardson, J. and Beland, J., Nonadrenergic inhibitory nervous system in human airways, *J. Appl. Physiol.*, 41, 764, 1976.
14. Belvisi, M.G., Bronchodilator nerves, in *Asthma*, Barnes, P.J., Grunstein, M.M., Leff, A.R., and Woolcock, A.J., Eds., Lippincott Raven, Philadelphia, 1997, p. 1027.
15. Szarek, J.L. et al., Reflex activation of the nonadrenergic noncholinergic inhibitory nervous system in feline airways, *Am. Rev. Respir. Dis.*, 133, 1159, 1986.
16. Michoud M.C. et al., Reflex bronchodilatation induced by laryngeal stimulation in humans, *Am. Rev. Respir. Dis.*, 133, A172, 1986.
17. Lammers, J.W., Barnes, P.J., and Chung, K.F., Nonadrenergic, noncholinergic airway inhibitory nerves, *Eur. Respir. J.*, 5, 239, 1992.
18. Grundström, N., Andersson, R.G., and Wikberg, J.E., Prejunctional α_2 adrenoceptors inhibit contraction of tracheal smooth muscle by inhibiting cholinergic neurotransmission, *Life Sci.*, 28, 2981, 1981.
19. Karlsson, J.A. and Persson, C.G., Evidence against vasoactive intestinal polypeptide (VIP) as a dilator and in favour of substance P as a constrictor in airway neurogenic responses, *Br. J. Pharmacol.*, 79, 634, 1983.
20. Lundberg, J.M. and Saria, A., Bronchial smooth muscle contraction induced by stimulation of capsaicin-sensitive sensory neurons, *Acta Physiol. Scand.*, 116, 473, 1982.

21. Lundberg, J.M., Martling, C.-R., and Saria, A., Substance P and capsaicin-induced contraction of human bronchi, *Acta Physiol. Scand.*, 119, 49, 1983.

22. Collier, J.G. and Fuller, R.W., Capsaicin inhalation in man and the effects of sodium cromoglycate, *Br. J. Pharmacol.*, 81, 113, 1984.

23. Fuller, R.W., Dixon, C.M.S., and Barnes, P.J., Bronchoconstrictor response to inhaled capsaicin in man, *J. Appl. Physiol.*, 58, 1080, 1985.

24. Peatfield, A.C. and Richardson, P.S., Evidence for non-cholinergic, non-adrenergic nervous control of mucus secretion into the cat trachea, *J. Physiol. (Lond.)*, 342, 335, 1983.

25. Lundberg, J.M. et al., Vascular permeability changes and smooth muscle contraction in relation to capsaicin-sensitive substance P afferents in the guinea-pig, *Acta Physiol. Scand.*, 120, 217, 1984.

26. Lundberg, J.M., Brodin, E., and Saria, A., Effects and distribution of vagal capsaicin-sensitive substance P neurons with special reference to the trachea and lungs, *Acta Physiol. Scand.*, 119, 243, 1983.

27. Lundberg, J.M. and Saria, A., Capsaicin-induced desensitization of airway mucosa to cigarette smoke, mechanical and chemical irritants, *Nature*, 302, 251, 1983.

28. Lundberg, J.M. et al., Substance P-immunoreactive sensory nerves in the lower respiratory tract of various mammals including man, *Cell Tissue Res.*, 235, 251, 1984.

29. Luts, A. et al., Peptide-containing nerve fibers in human airways: distribution and coexistence pattern, *Int. Arch. Allergy Immunol.*, 101, 52, 1993.

30. Lamb, J.P. and Sparrow, M.P., Three-dimensional mapping of sensory innervation with substance P in porcine bronchial mucosa: comparison with human airways, *Am. J. Respir. Crit. Care Med.*, 166, 1269, 2002.

31. Nieber, K. et al., Substance P and β-endorphin-like immunoreactivity in lavage fluids of subjects with and without allergic asthma, *J. Allergy Clin. Immunol.*, 90, 646, 1992.

32. Heaney, L.G. et al., Neurokinin A is the predominant tachykinin in human broncho-alveolar lavage fluid in normal and asthmatic subjects, *Thorax*, 53, 357, 1998.

33. Hazbun, M.E. et al., Ozone-induced increases in substance P and 8-epi-prostaglandin $F_{2\alpha}$ in the airways of human subjects, *Am. J. Respir. Cell Mol. Biol.*, 9, 568, 1993.

34. Krishna, M.T. et al., Effects of ozone on epithelium and sensory nerves in the bronchial mucosa of healthy humans, *Am. J. Respir. Crit. Care Med.*, 156, 943, 1997.

35. Baraniuk, J.N. et al., Hypertonic saline nasal provocation stimulates nociceptive nerves, substance P release, and glandular mucous exocytosis in normal humans, *Am. J. Respir. Crit. Care Med.*, 160, 655, 1999.

36. Ollerenshaw, S.L. et al., Substance P immunoreactive nerves in airways from asthmatics and nonasthmatics, *Eur. Respir. J.*, 4, 673, 1991.

37. Howarth, P.H. et al., Neuropeptide-containing nerves in endobronchial biopsies from asthmatic and nonasthmatic subjects, *Am. J. Respir. Cell Mol. Biol.*, 3, 288, 1995.

38. Chanez, P. et al., Bronchial mucosal immunoreactivity of sensory neuropeptides in severe airway diseases, *Am. J. Respir. Crit. Care Med.*, 158, 985, 1998.

39. Lilly, C.M. et al., Neuropeptide content of lungs from asthmatic and nonasthmatic patients, *Am. J. Respir. Crit. Care Med.*, 151, 548, 1995.

40. Lucchini, R.E. et al., Increased VIP-positive nerve fibers in the mucous glands of subjects with chronic bronchitis, *Am. J. Respir. Crit. Care Med.*, 156, 1963, 1997.

41. Joos, G.F. and Pauwels, R.A., Pro-inflammatory effects of substance P: new perspectives for the treatment of airway diseases?, *Trends. Pharmacol. Sci.*, 21, 131, 2000.

42. Germonpré, P.R. et al., Presence of substance P and neurokinin 1 receptors in human sputum macrophages and U-937 cells, *Eur. Respir. J.*, 14, 776, 1999.

43. Lambrecht, B.N. et al., Endogenously produced substance P contributes to lymphocyte proliferation induced by dendritic cells and direct TCR ligation, *Eur. J. Immunol.*, 29, 3815, 1999.

44. Chu, H.W. et al., Substance P and its receptor neurokinin 1 expression in asthmatic airways, *J. Allergy Clin. Immunol.*, 106, 713, 2000.

45. Maggi, C.A., The troubled story of tachykinins and neurokinins, *Trends Pharmacol. Sci.*, 21, 173, 2000.

46. Advenier, C. et al., Role of tachykinins as contractile agonists of human airways in asthma, *Clin. Exp. Allergy*, 29, 579, 1999.

47. Naline, E. et al., Evidence for functional tachykinin NK_1 receptors on human isolated small bronchi, *Am. J. Physiol.*, 271, L763, 1996.

48. Advenier, C., Lagente, V., and Boichot, E., The role of tachykinin receptor antagonists in the prevention of bronchial hyperresponsiveness, airway inflammation and cough, *Eur. Respir. J.*, 10, 1892, 1997.

49. Daoui, S. et al., Involvement of tachykinin NK_3 receptors in citric acid-induced cough and bronchial responses in guinea pigs, *Am. J. Respir. Crit. Care Med.*, 158, 42, 1998.

50. Daoui, S. et al., Neurokinin B- and specific tachykinin NK_3 receptor agonists-induced airway hyperresponsiveness in the guinea-pig, *Br. J. Pharmacol.*, 130, 49, 2000.

51. Canning, B.J. et al., Endogenous neurokinins facilitate synaptic transmission in guinea pig airway parasympathetic ganglia, *Am. J. Physiol. Regul. Integr. Comp. Physiol.*, 283, R320, 2002.

52. Adcock, I.M. et al., Increased tachykinin receptor gene expression in asthmatic lung and its modulation by steroids, *J. Mol. Endocrinol.*, 11, 1, 1993.

53. Bai, T.R. et al., Substance P (NK_1)- and neurokinin A (NK_2)-receptor gene expression in inflammatory airway disease, *Am. J. Physiol.*, 269, L309, 1995.

54. Katsunuma, T., Mak, J.C.W., and Barnes, P.J., Glucocorticoids reduce tachykinin NK_2 receptor expression in bovine tracheal smooth muscle, *Eur. J. Pharmacol.*, 344, 99, 1998.

55. Mapp, C.E. et al., The distribution of neurokinin-1 and neurokinin-2 receptors in human central airways, *Am. J. Respir. Crit. Care Med.*, 161, 207, 2000.

56. Advenier, C. et al., Relative potencies of neurokinins in guinea-pig trachea and human bronchus, *Eur. J. Pharmacol.*, 139, 133, 1987.

57. Finney, M.J.B., Karlsson, J.A., and Persson, C.G.A, Effects of bronchoconstrictors and bronchodilators on a novel human small airway preparation, *Br. J. Pharmacol.*, 85, 29, 1985.

58. Martling, C.-R., Theodorsson-Norheim, E., and Lundberg, J.M., Occurrence and effects of multiple tachykinins; substance P, neurokinin A and neuropeptide K in human lower airways, *Life Sci.*, 40, 1633, 1987.

59. Advenier, C. et al., Effects on the isolated human bronchus of SR 48968, a potent and selective nonpeptide antagonist of the neurokinin A (NK_2) receptors, *Am. Rev. Respir. Dis.*, 146, 1177, 1992.

60. Amadesi, S. et al., NK_1 receptor stimulation causes contraction and inositol phosphate increase in medium-size human isolated bronchi, *Am. J. Respir. Crit. Care Med.*, 163, 1206, 2001.

61. Joos, G.F. et al., Sensory neuropeptides and the human lower airways: present state and future directions, *Eur. Respir. J.*, 7, 1161, 1994.

62. Crimi, N. et al., Effect of nedocromil on bronchospasm induced by inhalation of substance P in asthmatic subjects, *Clin. Allergy*, 18, 375, 1988.

63. Joos, G., Pauwels, R., and Van Der Straeten, M., The effect of nedocromil sodium on the bronchoconstrictor effect of neurokinin A in subjects with asthma, *J. Allergy Clin. Immunol.*, 83, 663, 1989.

64. Van Schoor, J., Joos, G.F., and Pauwels, R.A., Indirect bronchial hyperresponsiveness in asthma: mechanisms, pharmacology and implications for clinical research, *Eur. Respir. J.*, 16, 514, 2000.

65. Van Schoor, J., Joos, G.F., and Pauwels, R.A., Effect of inhaled fluticasone on bronchial responsiveness to neurokinin A in asthma, *Eur. Respir. J.*, 19, 997, 2002.

66. Szarek, J.L. et al., 5-HT$_2$ receptors augment cholinergic nerve-mediated contraction of rat bronchi, *Eur. J. Pharmacol.*, 231, 339, 1993.

67. Tanaka, D.T. and Grunstein, M.M., Mechanisms of substance P-induced contraction of rabbit airway smooth muscle, *J. Appl. Physiol.*, 57, 1551, 1984.

68. Tournoy, K.G. et al., Modulatory role of tachykinin NK$_1$ receptor in cholinergic contraction of mouse trachea, *Eur. Respir. J.*, 21, 3, 2003.

69. Fewtrell, C.M.S. et al., The effects of substance P on histamine and 5-hydroxytryptamine release in the rat, *J. Physiol.*, 330, 393, 1982.

70. Joos, G.F. et al., Role of 5-hydroxytryptamine and mast cells in the tachykinin-induced contraction of rat trachea *in vitro*, *Eur. J. Pharmacol.*, 338, 259, 1997.

71. Joos, G.F. and Pauwels, R.A. The *in vivo* effect of tachykinins on airway mast cells in the rat, *Am. Rev. Respir. Dis.*, 148, 922, 1993.

72. van der Kleij, H.P. et al., Functional expression of neurokinin 1 receptors on mast cells induced by IL-4 and stem cell factor, *J. Immunol.*, 171, 2074, 2003.

73. Crimi, N. et al., Influence of antihistamine (astemizole) and anticholinergic drugs (ipratropium bromide) on bronchoconstriction induced by substance P, *Ann. Allergy*, 65, 115, 1990.

74. Joos, G.F., Pauwels, R.A., and Van Der Straeten, M.E., The effect of oxitropiumbromide on neurokinin A-induced bronchoconstriction in asthmatics, *Pulm. Pharmacol.*, 1, 41, 1988.

75. Crimi, N. et al., The effect of oral terfenadine on neurokinin-A induced bronchoconstriction, *J. Allergy Clin. Immunol.*, 91, 1096, 1993.

76. Crimi, N. et al., Inhibitory effect of a leukotriene receptor antagonist (montelukast) on neurokinin A-induced bronchoconstriction, *J. Allergy Clin. Immunol.*, 111, 833, 2003.

77. Joos, G. et al., The leukotriene receptor antagonist zafirlukast inhibits neurokinin-A induced bronchoconstriction in patients with asthma, *Am. J. Respir. Crit. Care Med.*, 163, A418, 2001.

78. Joos, G.F. et al., Indirect airway challenges, *Eur. Respir. J.*, 21, 1050, 2003.

79. Saria, A. et al., Vascular protein leakage in various tissues induced by substance P, capsaicin, bradykinin, serotonin, histamine and by antigen challenge, *Naunyn Schmiedebergs Arch. Pharmacol.*, 324, 212, 1983.

80. Bowden, J.J. et al., Direct observation of substance P-induced internalization of neurokinin 1 (NK$_1$) receptors at sites of inflammation, *Proc. Natl. Acad. Sci. U.S.A.*, 91, 8964, 1994.

81. Bertrand, C. et al., Tachykinins, via NK$_1$ receptor activation, play a relevant role in plasma protein extravasation evoked by allergen challenge in the airways of sensitized guinea-pigs, *Regul. Pept.*, 46, 214, 1993.

82. Tousignant, C. et al., NK$_2$ receptors mediate plasma extravasation in guinea-pig lower airways, *Br. J. Pharmacol.*, 108, 383, 1993.

83. Delaunois, A., Gustin, P., and Ansay, M., Effects of capsaicin on the endothelial permeability in isolated and perfused rabbit lungs, *Fundam. Clin. Pharmacol.*, 7, 81, 1993.

84. Delaunois, A., Gustin, P., and Ansay, M., Role of neuropeptides in acetylcholine-induced edema in isolated and perfused rabbit lungs, *J. Pharmacol. Exp. Ther.*, 266, 483, 1993.

85. Germonpré, P.R. et al., Characterization of neurogenic inflammation in the airways of two highly inbred rat strains, *Am. J. Respir. Crit. Care Med.*, 152, 1796, 1995.

86. Germonpré, P.R. et al., Role of the 5-HT receptor in neurogenic inflammation in Fisher 344 rat airways, *Eur. J. Pharmacol.*, 324, 249, 1997.

87. Van Rensen, E.L. et al., Assessment of microvascular leakage via sputum induction: the role of substance P and neurokinin A in patients with asthma, *Am. J. Respir. Crit. Care Med.*, 165, 1275, 2002.

88. Snider, R.M. et al., A potent nonpeptide antagonist of the substance P (NK$_1$) receptor, *Science*, 251, 435, 1991.

89. Emonds-Alt, X. et al., A potent and selective non-peptide antagonist of the neurokinin A (NK$_2$) receptor, *Life Sci.*, 50, L101, 1992.

90. Bertrand, C. et al., Involvement of neurogenic inflammation in antigen-induced bronchoconstriction in guinea pigs, *Am. J. Physiol.*, 265, L507, 1993.

91. Bertrand, C. et al., Role of neurogenic inflammation in antigen-induced vascular extravasation in guinea pig trachea, *J. Immunol.*, 150, 1479, 1993.

92. Kudlacz, E.M. et al., Effect of MDL 105,212, a nonpeptide NK-1/NK-2 receptor antagonist in an allergic guinea pig model, *J. Pharmacol. Exp. Ther.*, 279, 732, 1996.

93. Schuiling, M. et al., Involvement of tachykinin NK$_1$ receptor in the development of allergen-induced airway hyperreactivity and airway inflammation in conscious, unrestrained guinea-pigs, *Am. J. Respir. Crit. Care Med.*, 159, 423, 1999.

94. Schuiling, M. et al., Role of tachykinin NK$_2$-receptor activation in the allergen-induced late asthmatic reaction, airway hyperreactivity and airway inflammation cell influx in conscious, unrestrained guinea-pigs, *Br. J. Pharmacol.*, 127, 1030, 1999.

95. Maghni, K. et al., Dichotomy between neurokinin receptor actions in modulating allergic airway responses in an animal model of helper T cell type 2 cytokine-associated inflammation, *Am. J. Respir. Crit. Care Med.*, 162, 1068, 2000.

96. De Swert, K. et al., The absence of the tachykinin NK$_1$ receptor (NK$_1$R) enhances baseline carbachol airway responsiveness but does not modulate allergen induced airway inflammation, *Am. J. Respir. Crit. Care Med.*, 163, 2001.

97. De Swert, K.O., Pauwels, R.A., and Joos, G.F, The tachykinin NK$_1$ receptor augments goblet cell hyperplasia in a mouse model of asthma, *Am. J. Respir. Crit. Care Med.*, 167, A960, 2003.

98. Nénan, S. et al., Inhibition of inflammatory cell recruitment by the tachykinin NK$_3$-receptor antagonist, SR 14280, in a murine model of asthma, *Eur. J. Pharmacol.*, 421, 210, 2001.

99. Yoshihara, S. et al., Cold air-induced bronchoconstriction is mediated by tachykinin and kinin release in guinea pigs, *Eur. J. Pharmacol.*, 296, 291, 1996.

100. Yang, X.X. et al., Hyperpnea-induced bronchoconstriction is dependent on tachykinin-induced cysteinyl leukotriene synthesis, *J. Appl. Physiol.*, 82, 538, 1997.

101. Wu, Z.X. and Lee, L.Y., Airway hyperresponsiveness induced by chronic exposure to cigarette smoke in guinea pigs: role of tachykinins, *J. Appl. Physiol.*, 87, 1621, 1999.

102. Pedersen, K.E. et al., Selective stimulation of jugular ganglion afferent neurons in guinea pig airways by hypertonic saline, *J. Appl. Physiol.*, 84, 499, 1998.

103. Piedimonte, G. et al., NK$_1$ receptors mediate neurogenic inflammatory increase in blood flow in rat airways, *J. Appl. Physiol.*, 74, 2462, 1993.

104. Piedimonte, G. et al., Respiratory syncytial virus upregulates expression of the substance P receptor in rat lungs, *Am. J. Physiol.*, 277, L831, 1999.

105. Kraneveld, A.D., Nijkamp, F.P., and Van Oosterhout, A.J.M., Role for neurokinin-2 receptor in interleukin-5-induced airway hyperresponsiveness but not eosinophilia in guinea pigs, *Am. J. Respir. Crit. Care Med.*, 156, 367, 1997.

106. De Vries, A. et al., Nerve growth factor induces a neurokinin-1 receptor-mediated airway hyperresponsiveness in guinea pigs, *Am. J. Respir. Crit. Care Med.*, 159, 1541, 1999.

107. De Swert, K.O. et al., Role of the tachykinin NK_1 receptor on smoke-induced airway inflammation in mice, *Am. J. Respir. Crit. Care Med.*, 167, A146, 2003.

108. Khan, S. et al., Effect of the long-acting tachykinin NK_1 receptor antagonist MEN 11467 on tracheal mucus secretion in allergic ferrets, *Br. J. Pharmacol.*, 132, 189, 2001.

109. Joos, G.F., De Swert, K.O., and Pauwels, R.A., Airway inflammation and tachykinins: prospects for the development of tachykinin receptor antagonists, *Eur. J. Pharmacol.*, 429, 239, 2001.

110. Graham, R.M., Friedman, M., and Hoyle, G.W., Sensory nerves promote ozone-induced lung inflammation in mice, *Am. J. Respir. Crit. Care Med.*, 164, 313, 2001.

111. Piedimonte, G., Neural mechanisms of respiratory syncytial virus-induced inflammation and prevention of respiratory syncytial virus sequelae, *Am. J. Respir. Crit. Care Med.*, 163, S18, 2001.

112. Joos, G.F. and Pauwels, R.A., Tachykinin receptor antagonists: potential in airways diseases, *Curr. Opin. Pharmacol.*, 1, 235, 2001.

113. Joos, G.F. et al., Dual tachykinin NK_1/NK_2 antagonist DNK333 inhibits neurokinin A-induced bronchoconstriction in asthma patients, *Eur. Respir. J.*, 23, 76, 2004.

114. Schelfhout, V. et al., The triple neurokinin receptor antagonist CS-003 inhibits neurokinin A (NKA)-induced bronchoconstriction in patients with asthma, *Eur. Respir. J.*, 22, Suppl. 45, 415s, 2003.

14 Cytokines and Chemokines in Airway Inflammation

Suzanne L. Traves and Louise E. Donnelly

CONTENTS

0-415-32465-3/05/$0.00+$1.50
© 2005 by CRC Press LLC

I. INTRODUCTION

Cytokines and chemokines are secreted proteins that regulate the immune response. They are critical in orchestrating the immune response. They are involved in innate immunity, differentiation, antigen presentation, recruitment, activation, and adhesion molecule expression. The primary function of the lung is to mediate gas exchange, and, as such, it has a unique relationship with the environment. This means that the lung is susceptible to infection and damage from inhaled particles and must therefore mount protective mechanisms to combat these dangers. A variety of factors, including cytokines and chemokines, are involved in the defense mechanisms to protect the lung; however, excessive production or dysregulation of these mediators can lead to chronic inflammation and the development of chronic inflammatory lung diseases such as asthma and chronic obstructive pulmonary disease (COPD).

II. CYTOKINES

Cytokines are extracellular signaling proteins that play a pivotal role in the regulation of inflammation. Currently, there are about 50 known cytokines[1] consisting of 120 to 200 amino acids. They all have a four-helix bundle, in which four helices are arranged in an up-up-down-down topology connected by long-short-long loops[2] (Figure 14.1).[3] Cytokines bind to specific cell-surface receptors and regulate many cellular functions, including cell migration, activation, differentiation, proliferation, apoptosis, and production and secretion of other cytokines. Many cytokines and chemokines have been implicated in the underlying pathophysiology of airway

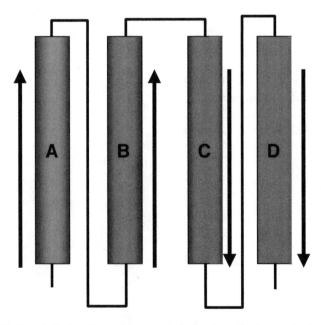

FIGURE 14.1 Four-helix bundle cytokine structure. A schematic diagram to show the up-up-down-down topology of the four-helix bundle characteristic of many cytokines.

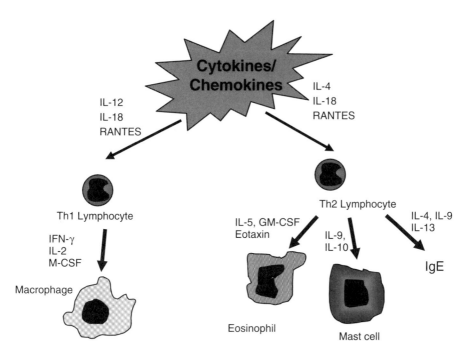

FIGURE 14.2 Overview of the role of cytokines. A schematic of the actions of cytokines. Th1-like cells produce IFN-γ and contribute to cellular immunity; Th2-like cells are characterized by production of IL-4, IL-5, Il-9, and IL-13, and are primarily concerned with humeral and allergic responses.

inflammatory diseases.[4] Cytokine receptors are multi-subunit complexes, with many cytokines sharing a receptor subunit, indicating some redundancy in the function of individual cytokines. Cytokines can be grouped according to functions as proinflammatory cytokines, T-lymphocyte-derived cytokines, anti-inflammatory cytokines, growth factors, and chemokines. Interest in inflammatory cytokines has been based around T-cell-derived cytokines (termed lymphokines); however, it is now acknowledged that many lymphokines can be synthesized by many other cell types. T lymphocytes can be subdivided on the basis of their secretion of specific cytokines (Figure 14.2). CD4+ T lymphocytes can be divided into T-helper (Th)-1 and Th2 cells. Th1 cytokines are important in the activation of macrophages and neutrophils and provide immunity against invading pathogens. Th1 cytokines include interferon (IFN)-γ, interleukin (IL)-2, IL-12, IL-18, and tumor necrosis factor (TNF). Th2 cytokines tend to inhibit innate host responses promoting adaptive immune responses, including allergic inflammation. Th2 cytokines include IL-4, IL-5, IL-6, IL-10, and IL-13. Similarly, CD8+ T lymphocytes can be divided into T-cytotoxic (Tc)-1 and Tc2 subgroups and essentially express similar profiles of cytokines as Th1 and Th2 cells. The balance of Th1/Tc1 and Th2/Tc2 responses are thought to be critical in the development of many inflammatory lung diseases. All of these groups of cytokines might be involved in the lung inflammatory processes associated with disease; however, it would be beyond the scope of this chapter to discuss every cytokine in depth. This chapter is restricted to families of cytokines that currently are thought to have relevance in lung disease.

A. TUMOR NECROSIS FACTORS

There are two major isoforms of TNFs: TNF-α (cachectin) and TNF-β (lymphotoxin). The two isoforms share 35% amino acid identity and bind to similar receptors. TNF-α is synthesized as a 26-kDa membrane-bound protein and is cleaved by TNF-α converting enzyme (TACE) to form the active 17-kDa molecule,[5] and was first described in macrophages and monocytes[6] but can be produced by a variety of cell types including eosinophils,[7] epithelial cells,[8] and mast cells.[9] There are two specific receptors for this cytokine that mediate its cellular effects.[5] TNF-α is cytotoxic for many tumors and produces systemic fever and cachexia.[10,11]

The relevance of TNF-α in airway inflammation has arisen from a number of studies. In asthma, following allergen challenge, there is an increase in the levels of TNF-α produced by macrophages and monocytes.[12] Moreover, inhalation of TNF-α by normal subjects induced sputum neutrophilia and airway reactivity.[13] Lipopolysaccharide (LPS) stimulation of monocytes and activation of lavage leukocytes also led to increases in production of TNF-α.[12,14,15] TNF-α also has been implicated in the pathogenesis of COPD, given that TNF-α gene polymorphisms have been associated with this disease.[16,17]

At the cellular level, increased TNF-α production can have many effects that are relevant to lung inflammation. TNF-α upregulates adhesion molecules, including E-selectin, vascular cell adhesion molecule (VCAM)-1, and intercellular adhesion molecule (ICAM)-1 on the pulmonary endothelium and airway epithelial cell layer, thus mediating the inflammatory cell influx.[5] Moreover, it can stimulate neutrophil degranulation and stimulate the respiratory burst.[18] TNF-α also stimulates mucus production via induction of mucous cell hyperplasia and hypersecretion[19,20] and thus can contribute to increased mucus production observed in chronic bronchitis. TNF-α in combination with other cytokines also can mediate nitric oxide production from human airway epithelial cells[21] and hence might regulate airway tone. Therefore, TNF-α is thought to have a pivotal role in mediating lung inflammation.

B. INTERFERONS

Interferons (IFNs) are categorized into three classes: α, β, and γ. IFN-α and IFN-β are type I interferons, have a globular structure, and are secreted by virus-infected cells.[22] In contrast, IFN-γ is a type II interferon secreted mainly by T lymphocytes, natural killer (NK) cells, and macrophages.[22] IFN-γ is a Th1 cytokine and has aroused interest in the development of COPD, many features of which are thought to be mediated via Th1 cytokines.[23] IFN-γ stimulates epithelial cells and macrophages to produce CX3C chemokines including inducible T-cell α chemoattractant (ITAC), monokine-induced by IFN-γ (MIG), and interferon inducible protein (IP)-10. These, in turn, lead to the recruitment of T lymphocytes and may be responsible for the increased number of CD8+ lymphocytes observed at the sites of parenchymal destruction in COPD.[24] Moreover, these cells are coincident with $CXCR_3$ expression and IFN-γ production in these subjects,[25] suggesting a role for this cytokine in the orchestration of the inflammatory response in COPD.

C. COLONY-STIMULATING FACTORS

There are three colony-stimulating factors (CSF) expressed in humans: granulocyte-macrophage colony-stimulating factor (GM-CSF), granulocyte colony-stimulating factor (G-CSF), and macrophage colony-stimulating factor (M-CSF). The role of these proteins is to promote the differentiation and proliferation of immature myeloid cells. G-CSF acts primarily on neutrophils, M-CSF acts on cells of a monocytic/macrophage lineage, whereas GM-CSF has a broader spectrum activity on cells of monocyte, neutrophil, or granulocyte lineage.[26] The importance of these cytokines in promoting cell survival predicts that regulation of their respective concentrations in the lung is critical in the progression and resolution of inflammation. Levels of GM-CSF are elevated in the BAL fluid of asthmatic subjects compared with control subjects and this is correlated with eosinophil numbers.[27] Moreover, GM-CSF regulates the survival of eosinophils from bronchoalveolar lavage (BAL) and blood.[28] Elevated levels of GM-CSF also are found in BAL from patients with chronic bronchitis compared with healthy controls, and these concentrations increased during an exacerbation.[29] Taken together, these studies indicate that regulation of CSFs is important in the inflammatory response.

GM-CSF is produced by a variety of cell types, including macrophages,[30] airway epithelial cells,[21] airway smooth muscle cells,[31] and lung fibroblasts.[32] Stimuli include LPS, cigarette smoke, and a variety of cytokines, including IL-1β. Moreover, glucocorticosteroids inhibit synthesis of GM-CSF but not G-CSF from bronchial epithelial cells,[33,34] indicating that differential regulation of CSF in airway disease might prolong leukocyte infiltration and hence the inflammatory response.

D. INTERLEUKINS

1. Interleukin-1 Family

IL-1 is a proinflammatory cytokine that consists of two distinct isoforms, α and β, that are produced from two separate genes. There is only a 20% amino acid sequence identity between IL-1α and IL-β, yet they share the same receptor. Both isoforms are glycosylated, with molecular weights of 31 to 33 kDa.[35] IL-1α is retained within the cell, whereas IL-1β is secreted and is thought to mediate many of the effects of IL-1. IL-1β is synthesized as a 31-kDa peptide that is cleaved to the active 17.5-kDa cytokine via IL-1 converting enzyme (ICE).[36] IL-1 is produced by a variety of cell types, including monocytes and macrophages, eosinophils, endothelial cells, smooth muscle cells, and airway epithelial cells. The effects of IL-1 are numerous. It can induce fever akin to that seen with TNF, but, at a cellular level, IL-1β can act as a growth factor for Th2 cells and B cells.[37] This cytokine is instrumental in the production of many other cytokines, including IL-2, IL-3, IL-4, IL-5, IL-6, IL-8, GM-CSF, INF-γ, and TNF, from a variety of cell types.[38] Moreover, IL-1β can induce matrix metalloproteinase (MMP) production by alveolar macrophages.[30,39] Other inflammatory mediators upregulated by IL-1 include prostaglandin (PG) E_2, platelet-derived growth factor (PDGF), ICAM-1, and VCAM-1.[37] Elevated levels of IL-1β have been found in BAL fluid of asthmatic subjects[40] and smokers compared with normal subjects.[41] IL-1β is released from bronchial epithelial cells in response to cigarette smoke[42] and this response is enhanced in cells derived from subjects with COPD compared with asymptomatic smokers, again indicating a role for this cytokine in inflammatory lung diseases.

There are two other members of the IL-1 family: IL-1 receptor antagonist (IL-1ra) and IL-18. IL-1ra is a 25-kDa protein with amino acid sequence similarity to IL-1α of 19% and IL-1β of 26%.[43] IL-1ra is released from a variety of cell types including mononuclear cells and epithelial cells.[44,45] It is a natural inhibitor of IL-1 and, as such, there has been much interest in this molecule as an anti-inflammatory agent.[43] IL-18 is synthesized as a 24-kDa protein that is processed by proteolytic cleavage by ICE, producing the 18-kDa mature molecule.[46] IL-18 is not only produced by Th1/Tc1 cells but is expressed constitutively in airway epithelial cells and can stimulate the release of IL-8, monocyte chemotactic protein (MCP)-1, and eotaxin. IL-18 is a potent inducer of IFN-γ production from Th1 lymphocytes.[47]

2. Interleukin-2

IL-2 is a glycosylated protein of approximately 15 to 18 kDa.[48] IL-2 is produced predominantly by Th0 and Th1 cells but also by eosinophils and airway epithelial cells.[38] IL-2 promotes the proliferation of T cells, B cells, and monocytes, but also can stimulate monocytes to secrete IL-1β and enhance the production of IL-4 and IL-5 from peripheral-blood mononuclear cells (PBMC) derived from asthmatic subjects. Moreover, IL-2 is elevated in the BAL fluid of asthmatic subjects.[49,50] In addition, BAL cells from steroid-insensitive asthmatics express increased levels of IL-2 mRNA when compared with cells derived from steroid-sensitive asthmatics.[51] This might be associated with the observation that IL-2 and IL-4 can reduce glucocorticoid receptor binding affinity of PBMC and hence reduce the steroid responsiveness.[52]

3. Interleukins-4 and -13

IL-4 is synthesized by Th2 cells and is important in the development of the Th2 phenotype. Synthesis can be induced via CD40 signaling and stimulation of the T-cell antigen receptor.[38] Alternatively, IL-4 can be expressed by mast cells through activation of the immunoglobulin (Ig)E receptor.[53] The IL-4 receptor consists of two chains, the high IL-4 binding affinity α-chain and the IL-2 receptor γ-chain. IL-4 receptors are located on activated B and T cells but are also expressed on mast cells, macrophages, endothelial cells, epithelial cells, muscle cells, and fibroblasts.[54,55] IL-4 signals are mediated via signal transducers and activators of transcription (STAT) leading to cellular responses.

IL-4 enhances the Th2 CD4+ response and diminishes the development of Th1 cells[56]; however, IL-4 also inhibits the release of Th1-like cytokines from macrophages.[38] The role of IL-4 in COPD is supported by reports of elevated plasma levels of IL-4 in patients with COPD compared with normal controls; moreover, this correlated inversely with lung function.[57] Enhanced IL-4 mRNA expression has been associated with the submucosal glands of subjects with chronic bronchitis but reduced in subjects with both chronic bronchitis and airways obstruction, indicating a role in mucus hypersecretion.[58]

IL-13 shares a receptor with IL-4 and, as such, shares many of the responses associated with IL-4.[59] IL-13 is secreted as a 10-kDa protein sharing 25% amino acid identity with IL-4.[60] IL-13 is produced by both CD4+ and CD8+ cells together with a variety of other cell types, including eosinophils and human airway smooth muscle cells,[61] and has been identified as a regulator of the allergic asthmatic response.[62] There is evidence that IL-13 can mediate the mucus hypersecretion associated with asthma,[63] and it is also implicated in airway hyperresponsiveness by impairment of β_2-adrenoceptor responses in airway smooth muscle,[64] increased mucus production,[63] and modulation of the extracellular matrix via the upregulation of transforming growth factor (TGF)-β.[65] Moreover, IL-13 is increased in the BAL fluid of asthmatic patients[66] and there are several IL-13 genetic polymorphisms associated with the asthmatic phenotype.[67,68]

Although not as well defined, IL-13 is also implicated in the development of COPD. There is an IL-13 promoter polymorphism associated with an enhanced risk of COPD.[69] Targeting of IL-13 expression in murine lungs has been demonstrated to MMP- and cathepsin-mediated emphysema,[70] again implicating this cytokine in lung remodeling.

4. Interleukin-5

IL-5 is a 12.5-kDa protein produced by T cells and eosinophils but it is heavily glycosylated, giving it a molecular weight of 22-kDa.[71] Monomeric IL-5 is inactive, but the functional molecule is a 40- to 50-kDa homodimer linked by disulfide bonds.[71] The IL-5 receptor is expressed by eosinophils, basophils, and B cells. The role of IL-5 is to regulate eosinophil maturation and activation[72] but it also can prolong the survival of eosinophils.[73,74] IL-5 might also act to regulate eosinophil migration into tissues.[75] Levels of mRNA and protein for IL-5 are increased in the induced sputum of asthmatic subjects[76,77] and elevated levels of protein have been observed in the BAL fluid of symptomatic asthmatics.[78] Furthermore, the percentage of CD4+ cells expressing IL-5 is increased in subjects with atopic asthma when compared with those of healthy controls.[79] Given this information, IL-5 has been suggested as a target for the treatment of asthma.[80] Treatment of asthmatic patients with anti-IL-5 antibodies reduced sputum eosinophilia but this was not associated with an alteration in airway hyperreactivity, thus leading to the speculation that eosinophilia is not critical for airway hyperresponsiveness in humans.[81]

5. Interleukin-6

IL-6 is a 22- to 27-kDa glycoprotein that has been implicated in COPD. It is elevated in BAL fluid from patients with COPD[82] and is thought be derived from alveolar macrophages. Sputum and plasma IL-6 levels are also elevated in COPD patients undergoing exacerbation, the latter leading to a concomitant increase in plasma fibrinogen levels.[83,84] Airway epithelial cells release IL-6 and following stimulation with TNF-α, cells derived from patients with COPD release increased levels of IL-6.[85] TNF-α dependent release of IL-6 from airway epithelial cells can be attenuated by treatment with IL-4 and IL-13 but will augment IFN-γ-mediated IL-6 release.[86] Blood-derived mononuclear cells from asthmatic subjects also produce IL-6[87] and both BAL and plasma from asthmatic subjects also contained increased concentrations of IL-6.[88,89] Studies using IL-6 knock-out mice have demonstrated that IL-6 has a role in pulmonary injury following exposure to environmental air pollutants[90] and following lipoteichoic acid and peptidoglycan from *Staphylococcus aureus*, there was reduced neutrophilic infiltrate in the lungs of the knock-out mice compared with wild-type control animals.[91] The role of IL-6 in mediating lung injury may be associated with a recent observation whereby IL-6 exposure of A549 epithelial cells led to an increased expression of cysteine protease, cathepsin L. Taken together, these studies indicate that IL-6 might have an important role in the development of inflammatory lung disease.

6. Interleukin-9

IL-9 is a Th2 cytokine that has been suggested to play a role in allergic airway disease.[92] IL-9 promotes the differentiation and survival of eosinophils, regulates IL-5 cell surface expression,[93] and can enhance the proliferation of mast cell progenitors,[94] hence its importance in asthma. It also is a growth factor for T cells[95] and promotes mucus hypersecretion and goblet cell hyperplasia.[96,97] Further evidence of the role of IL-9 in asthma has come from animal studies. Transgenic mice that overexpress IL-9 demonstrate increased bronchial hyperresponsiveness in a murine model of asthma,[98] and anti-IL-9 treatment inhibits airway inflammation and hyperreactivity.[99] A recent study using human airway smooth muscle cells showed that IL-9 synergizes with TNF-α, leading to the induction of IL-8.[92] IL-9 also can stimulate the release of T-cell chemotactic factors, including IL-16 and regulated on activation normal T-cell expressed and secreted (RANTES) from bronchial epithelial cells.[100] Elevated expression of IL-9 mRNA has been described in bronchial mucosa of asthmatic patients compared with that of normal controls.[101] Taken together, these studies suggest a role for IL-9 in mediating the allergic inflammatory response.

7. Interleukin-10 Family

IL-10 is an 18-kDa protein and also is known as cytokine synthesis inhibitory factor. T lymphocytes, monocytes/macrophages, NK cells, and eosinophils express IL-10. IL-10 is considered an anti-inflammatory cytokine by inhibiting neutrophil secretion of macrophage inhibitory protein (MIP)-1α, MIP-1β, and IL-8 and reduces the release of GM-CSF from monocytes.[102] IL-10 mRNA and protein expression is increased in BAL cells in atopic allergy and asthma,[103,104] but another study demonstrated decreased levels of IL-10 protein in the BAL fluid of asthmatics compared with that of healthy controls.[105] Similarly, IL-10 concentrations are reduced in the sputum of asthmatic subjects compared with that of healthy controls.[106] Moreover, PBMCs from asthmatics released less IL-10 than did cells from healthy subjects.[105,107]

Polymorphisms in the promoter of the IL-10 gene are associated with allergy and asthma.[108] Glucocorticosteroids are potent anti-inflammatory therapies used for the treatment of asthma. Exposure of whole blood cells to steroids upregulates IL-10 release[109] and inhaled steroids stimulate alveolar macrophage expression of IL-10.[110] This would suggest that some of the anti-inflammatory effects of glucocorticosteroids might be mediated via induction of IL-10. Studies comparing IL-10 knock-out mice with their wild-type counterparts showed that endogenous IL-10 suppressed allergen-induced airway inflammation and nonspecific airway hyperresponsiveness.[111] Although there appears to be a clear role for IL-10 in mediating the airway inflammation associated with asthma, its role in COPD is less clear. IL-10 will stimulate alveolar macrophages to release increased levels of tissue inhibitor of metalloproteinase (TIMP)-1 but not MMP-9, hence favoring an antiprotease phenotype.[112] IL-10 levels in induced sputum of both COPD patients and smokers without COPD are reduced compared with sputum from healthy controls,[106] again favoring a proinflammatory phenotype.

Recently, more members of the IL-10 family have been identified. These include IL-19, IL-20, IL-22, IL-26 (AK55), and melanoma differentiation-associated gene (*mda*)-7.[113] These related cytokines share ~30% identity with IL-10 but little is known regarding their function, although IL-19 induces IL-6 and TNF-α production and apoptosis in epithelial cells.[114]

8. Interleukin-12 Family

IL-12 is produced by dendritic cells, monocytes, macrophages, and eosinophils.[115,116] This cytokine regulates Th1 differentiation and decreases the Th2-mediated responses, including IL-4 expression. Moreover, IL-12 stimulates the production of IFN-γ from Th1 cells. IL-18 is also a Th1/Tc1 cytokine and a potent inducer of IFN-γ production from activated T-cells. Together with IL-12, it can regulate Th1 cell differentiation.[115] IL-12 is a heterodimer of subunits p40 and p35.[117] There are now two more members of the IL-12 family, IL-23 and IL-27,[118] both of which are produced by antigen-presenting cells. IL-23 has a role in T memory cell proliferation and can induce IL-12 production from dendritic cells.[119] IL-27 also is produced by antigen-presenting cells, induces the proliferation of T cells, and promotes Th1 cell differentiation.[118] The release of IL-12 is inhibited by both IL-10 and IL-13, and release of IL-12 from blood cells is reduced in patients with asthma,[107,120] which might reflect the Th2 nature of this disease.

9. Interleukin-17

IL-17 is a 20- to 30-kDa glycosylated protein secreted by CD4+ cells.[121,122] IL-17 is thought to play a role in early immune responses, given that it is produced by activated T-cells.[121] The receptor for IL-17 is expressed widely and intratracheal instillation of IL-17 increased neutrophil numbers in the mouse airway.[123,124] This mechanism of IL-17-driven neutrophil recruitment might be due to the increased expression of IL-8 and IL-6 from airway epithelial cells following exposure to IL-17.[125] These studies have led to the suggestion that IL-17 might mediate airway neutrophilia and hence might have a critical role in the development of airway inflammation. Although sputum neutrophilia is a feature of COPD, levels of IL-17 were not enhanced in the sputum of these subjects compared with that of healthy controls and asthmatic subjects.[126] Moreover, sputum IL-17 correlated with airway hyperresponsiveness, suggesting a role for this chemokine in asthma rather than COPD.[126]

E. Transforming Growth Factors

The TGFs (TGF-β1, TGF-β2, and TGF-β3) are a family of dimeric proteins that regulate differentiation, proliferation, wound healing, and angiogenesis. In the lung TGFs are thought to be involved in airway modeling, a pathological feature of many chronic inflammatory diseases. TGF-β is secreted in an inactive form and stored within the extracellular matrix in a complex with latency-associated peptide.[127] Active TGF-β is released via the action of thrombospondin-1 and plasmin.[127]

Cigarette smoking enhances TGF-β1 release from airway epithelial cells; increased expression has been reported in biopsy samples from smokers and patients with COPD when compared with samples from nonsmokers.[128] However, exposure of airway epithelial cells to cigarette smoke extract inhibited the ability of these cells to produce TGF-β.[129] Moreover, TNF-α and IL-4 significantly reduce TGF-β1 production from airway epithelial cells,[130] leading to the supposition that TGF-β1 is required for lung repair processes and that reduction of this growth factor in inflammatory diseases leads to compromised repair mechanisms. TGF-β1 is chemotactic for macrophages and levels of expression are associated with and increased number of macrophages in the lung of patients with COPD.[131] Furthermore, T lymphocytes isolated from peripheral blood of patients with COPD release increased levels of TGF-β compared with that from control subjects.[132]

TGF-β1 expression also is elevated in lung samples from asthmatic subjects compared with those from controls.[133–135] TGF-β1 will act synergistically with IL-13 to increase eotaxin release from airway fibroblasts[136] and can stimulate mitogen-activated protein kinases in human airway epithelial cells[137] that lead to induction of proinflammatory mediators, including IL-8 and GM-CSF.

F. Cytokine Summary

The multitude of cytokines and their respective signaling pathways contribute to the complexity of the inflammatory response. They are produced in response to external stimuli such as damage to the epithelium or invasion of micro-organisms. They are then involved in the recruitment and maintenance of leukocytes and in the resolution of the inflammatory response. The targeting of a single cytokine as a therapeutic target for intervention in inflammatory disease might not be appropriate but the targeting of a limited set of cytokines (e.g., IL-4, IL-5, IL-9, and IL-13 in asthma) might be a more attractive strategy. More information regarding the expression and regulation of cytokines and their interactions in the inflammatory processes involved in human lung disease therefore needs to be elucidated.

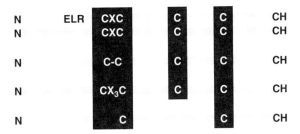

FIGURE 14.3 Overview of the structure of the chemokines. CXC chemokines consist of an NH$_2$-terminus (N), four cysteines (C), the first two of which are separated by an amino acid (X), and a COOH-terminus (CH). A subset of CXC chemokines has an ELR motif adjacent to the first cysteine. CC chemokines consist of an NH$_2$-terminus (N), four cysteines (C), the first two of which are juxtaposed (C-C), and a COOH-terminus (CH). CX$_3$C chemokines consist of an NH$_2$-terminus (N), four cysteines (C), the first two of which are separated by three amino acids (X$_3$), and a COOH-terminus (CH). C chemokines consist of an NH$_2$-terminus (N), two cysteines (C), and a COOH-terminus (CH).

III. CHEMOKINES

Recruitment of inflammatory cells into the airways is a critical event that triggers and sustains the clinical manifestations of inflammation.[138] The discovery of a family of chemotactic cytokines, known as chemokines, which regulate cell trafficking within the immune system, has led to these molecules taking center stage in the field of inflammation.[138] Chemokines, like cytokines, are secretory proteins produced by leukocytes and tissue cells either constitutively or after induction, and exert their effects locally in a paracrine or autocrine fashion.[139] They are smaller proteins than cytokines and act via heptahelical G-protein-coupled receptors (GPCR).[139] Chemokines consist of 70 to 130 amino acids[139] and are 8 to 10 kDa, with four conserved cysteine residues linked by disulfide bonds.[140] They are subclassified into four groups according to structure and spacing of the conserved cysteines: CXC, CC, C, and CX$_3$C (Figure 14.3).[141] CXC, CC, and CX$_3$C chemokines have four conserved cysteine residues, whereas C chemokines have two conserved cysteine residues. CXC and CX$_3$C chemokines are distinguished by the presence of one (CXC) or three (CX$_3$C) amino acids between the first and second cysteine residues,[142] whereas the first two cysteine residues of CC chemokines are juxtaposed (Figure 14.3).[141] CXC chemokines can be further divided into ELR+ and ELR− chemokines based on the presence or absence of the tripeptide motif glutamic acid-leucine-arginine (ELR) between the amino (NH$_2$)-terminus and the first cysteine residue[143,144] (Figure 14.3). Chemokines have a low level of sequence identity; however, their three-dimensional structure shows a remarkable homology in that they all have the same monomeric fold.[145] This fold, a carboxy (COOH)-terminal helix and a flexible NH$_2$-terminal region, is conferred on these proteins by a four-cysteine motif that forms two disulfide bridges (Figure 14.3). The flexible NH$_2$-terminal region is believed to be important in receptor activation, given that modification of this region has been shown to affect activity.[113,144,146]

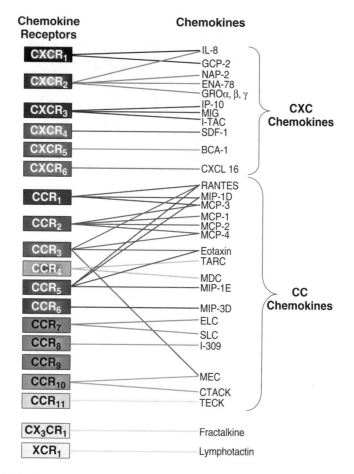

FIGURE 14.4 An overview of the chemokines and their receptors to date. Chemokines are divided into CXC, CC, C, and CX_3C subfamilies based on the spacing of the NH_2-terminal cysteines residues. The abbreviations for the chemokines are as follows: BCA-1, B-cell-attracting chemokine 1; CTACK, cutaneous T-cell attracting chemokine; ELC, Epstein-Barr-virus-induced gene 1 ligand chemokine; GCP-2, granulocyte chemotactic protein; MEC, mucosae-associated epithelial chemokine; SLC, secondary lymphoid-tissue chemokine; TECK, thymus-expressed chemokine. (From Proudfoot, A.E., *Nature Rev. Immunol.*, 2, 106, 2002. With permission.)

To date, approximately 50 human chemokines but only 19 receptors have been discovered (Figure 14.4).[139] The majority of CXC and CC chemokines have been mapped to chromosomes 4 and 17, respectively, in humans. A number of chemokines has been implicated in inflammatory diseases. The role of the CC chemokines, including eotaxin-1, eotaxin-2, eotaxin-3, RANTES, MIP-1α, and monocyte chemoattractant protein (MCP)-2, -3, and -4 are of particular interest in asthma because they are potent chemoattractants for eosinophils, basophils, monocytes, and T lympho-cytes.[116] The role of CXC and CC chemokines also has been implicated in COPD, with IL-8,[147,148] growth-related oncogene (GRO)-α, and MCP-1[149] being elevated in the sputum from these patients. These chemokines are important because they can recruit inflammatory cells, and IL-8 has been shown to cause elevated migration of neutrophils from patients with COPD when compared with control subjects.[150] Although a proinflammatory role of chemokines is mainly linked to their ability to promote leukocyte migration, there is increasing evidence that suggests an important role for chemokines in the control of cellular proliferation, differentiation, and survival.[138]

A. CXC CHEMOKINES

The first CXC chemokine to be characterized was platelet factor 4 (PF4) in 1977, 10 years before the discovery of IL-8.[151] CXC chemokines can be divided into ELR+ chemokines and ELR– chemokines. The ELR+ chemokines have a uniformity of function that allows classification as a family of neutrophil chemoattractants and activators, whereas the ELR– CXC chemokines display a mixture of disparate activities, with (to date) no clear underlying theme.[152]

1. Interleukin-8, Growth-Related Oncogene, Neutrophil-Activating Peptide-2, and Epithelial-Cell-Derived Neutrophil-Activating Peptide-78

IL-8 (CXCL8) was originally isolated from the culture supernatants of stimulated human blood monocytes and was identified as a protein of 72 amino acids with a molecular weight of 8.3 kDa. IL-8 exists in two forms, a 72-amino acid protein that predominates in cultures of monocytes and macrophages, and a 77-amino acid protein that predominates in cultures of tissue cells such as endothelial cells and fibroblasts.[151] Lymphocytes, granulocytes, bronchial epithelial cells, smooth muscle cells, keratinocytes, hepatocytes, mesangial cells, and chondrocytes also produce IL-8. It is an inflammatory cytokine, which functions mainly as a neutrophil chemoattractant and activating factor. IL-8 stimulation of neutrophils via $CXCR_1$ and $CXCR_2$ receptors causes an immediate increase in intracellular calcium.[153] High levels of IL-8 are found in acute inflammatory conditions of the lung, including adult respiratory distress syndrome (ARDS), in which IL-8 and neutrophil numbers are reported to correlate with mortality, and in emphysema.[151] Studies by Goodman et al.[154] have shown that IL-8 is produced in higher quantities than other CXC chemokines by human alveolar macrophages upon stimulation with LPS, suggesting that this might be one source of enhanced levels of IL-8. IL-8 expression is increased in the induced sputum from patients with COPD,[147,148] and it has been shown that neutrophils from patients with COPD migrate in higher numbers toward IL-8 than do neutrophils from nonsmokers.[150]

GROα (CXCL1) was originally reported as an endogenous growth factor for human melanoma cells and termed melanoma growth stimulatory activity (MGSA).[155] The GROα gene was identified in transformed Chinese hamster and human fibroblasts, where its expression was found to be growth regulated. It was subsequently shown to be expressed by melanoma and glioblastoma cells as well as renal, prostatic, and bladder carcinoma cells.[155] Monocytes, endothelial cells, fibroblasts, and synovial cells also produced GROα after stimulation with LPS, IL-1β, or TNFα.[155] GROα is structurally related to IL-8 and is a powerful activator of neutrophils, with chemotactic ability for neutrophils, basophils, and freshly isolated T lymphocytes.[156,157] GROβ and GROγ were identified subsequently in cDNA libraries from activated monocytes and neutrophils. They share 90 and 86% amino acid identity with GROα, respectively, and all three GRO proteins share 33 to 40% identity with IL-8. GROβ and GROγ also can induce chemotaxis, shape change, and a transient increase in cytosolic intracellular calcium, granule exocytosis, and the respiratory burst.

Neutrophil-activating peptide (NAP)-2 (CXCL7) originally was isolated from stimulated mononuclear cells.[158] NAP-2 is produced by proteolytic processing from inactive precursors released from platelet α-granules and occurs in the presence of monocytes and purified proteases, such as cathepsin G.[158] The formation of NAP-2 depends on the presence of platelets in monocyte cultures.[158] NAP-2 is chemotactic for neutrophils *in vitro* and *in vivo*, and can induce cytosolic calcium increases, exocytosis, and respiratory burst.[158] It has equipotent activity with IL-8 and GROα as a stimulus of chemotaxis and changes in cytosolic free calcium.[158] NAP-2 is the only neutrophil-activating chemokine that is not induced by gene activation; it is generated by the proteolysis of inactive precursors. Cathepsin G and other serine proteases that are released from monocytes are responsible for this conversion.

Epithelial-cell-derived neutrophil-activating peptide (ENA)-78 (CXCL5) was first isolated from the human type II-like epithelial cell line, A549.[159] It is a 78-amino acid protein,[160] with a molecular weight of 8.4 kDa.[159] Unstimulated epithelial cells produce low levels of ENA-78, although in the presence of TNFα or IL-1β, a rapid induction of ENA-78 is observed.[159] ENA-78 mRNA is produced by lung fibroblasts, monocytes, endothelial cells, and mesothelial cells following stimulation with LPS or IL-1β.[159] Furthermore, LPS also can induce ENA-78 peptide production from monocytes.[159] ENA-78 has only 22% sequence identity to IL-8, but shares 53 and 52% sequence identity with NAP-2 and GROα, respectively.[159] ENA-78 is a potent activator of neutrophil function,[160] inducing concentration-dependent chemotaxis between 0.1 and 100 nM *in vitro*.[159] This response is identical to NAP-2, but somewhat reduced compared with that of IL-8.[159] However, when ENA-78 is released from type II-like epithelial cells, it can be processed by alveolar macrophages through the release of cathepsin G to molecules that are equipotent with IL-8. ENA-78 might contribute significantly to the recruitment of neutrophils into the lung,[159] however, ENA-78 is also chemotactic for monocytes;[161] therefore, this chemokine is important in sustaining airway inflammation.

2. Other CXC Chemokines

Stromal-cell-derived factor (SDF)-1 (CXCL12) and its receptor CXCR$_4$ are ubiquitously expressed,[138] with CXCR$_4$ expression on T lymphocytes being upregulated by IL-4, suggesting a predominant expression on Th2 cells.[138] Th2 cells are believed to play a crucial role in orchestrating the airway inflammation associated with asthma by regulating the production of IgE, as well as the growth and differentiation of mast cells, basophils, and eosinophils.[138] Neutralization of $CXCR_4$ by antibodies and small molecule antagonists attenuates airway hyperresponsiveness and eosinophil infiltration during ovalbumin-allergic airway responses.[138]

The CX3C chemokines include ITAC, MIG, and IP-10. The receptor for these chemokines, $CXCR_3$, is preferentially expressed on the surface of Th1 cells.[162] Moreover ITAC, MIG, and IP-10 can all act as antagonists at the CCR_3 receptor that promotes Th2 cell migration.[162] Hence, expression of these chemokines would favor a more polarized Th1 response. Enhanced levels of $CXCR_3$ expression associated with increased numbers of CD8+ cells has been reported in the lungs of patients with COPD,[25] indicating that this might be the mechanism of CD8+ cell recruitment into the lungs of these patients. This evidence supports a mechanism by which the airway inflammation in the lungs of patients with COPD is maintained and amplified.[138] The other CXC chemokines, although involved in the recruitment of inflammatory cells, have not been reported to be involved in airway inflammation.[163]

B. CC CHEMOKINES

The first CC chemokine was identified after cloning by differential hybridization from human tonsillar lymphocytes and was termed LD78.[151] Several cDNA isoforms of a closely related chemokine, Act-2, were later identified. Two similar proteins, MIP-1α and MIP-1β, were purified from the culture medium of murine macrophages stimulated with LPS and subsequently cloned.[151] The murine proteins are considered as the homologues of LD28 and Act-2 because of their amino acid identity of more than 70%, and the terms human MIP-1α and MIP-1β are commonly used instead of LD28 and Act-2.[151] The best-characterized CC chemokine is MCP-1, which was purified from culture supernatants of blood mononuclear cells, as well as glioma and myelomonocytic cell lines, and was cloned from different sources.[151] Other CC chemokines, I-309, regulated on activation, RANTES, and MCP-2 were purified or cloned as products of activated T lymphocytes. MCP-2 was purified along with MCP-3 from cultures of osteosarcoma cells.[151] Eotaxin is a potent stimulus for eosinophils, inducing eosinophil migration *in vitro* and accumulation *in vivo*.[164]

1. Monocyte Chemotactic Proteins

MCP-1 (CCL2) is an 8.7-kDa chemokine produced by monocytes, T lymphocytes, fibroblasts, endothelial cells, epithelial cells, smooth muscle cells, and keratinocytes.[153] It was first purified from conditioned medium of baboon aortic smooth muscle cells in culture on the basis of its ability to attract monocytes but not neutrophils *in vitro*.[152] MCP-1 is a potent chemoattractant for monocytes *in vitro* and can induce the expression of integrins required for chemotaxis.[152] In transendothelial migration assays, MCP-1 is equipotent for activated CD4+ and CD8+ T lymphocytes,[152] but not B lymphocytes or NK cells.[152] MCP-1 generally has been observed to be a more potent and efficacious monocyte chemoattractant than MCP-2, MCP-3,[140] or MCP-4.[152] MCP-5 has so far only been identified in mice.[152] MCP-1 is expressed in various tissues, including human lungs, where it occurs in macrophages, and endothelial, bronchial epithelial, and smooth muscle cells.[165] MCP-1 mediates its cellular effects by binding to CCR_2,[166] which mainly is expressed by monocytes, macrophages, and T lymphocytes.[165] MCP-1 activation of monocytes results in a calcium flux via a specific GPCR.[153] MCP-1 has been implicated in diseases that have a mononuclear cell inflammatory component.[167] COPD is associated with an increase in inflammatory cells (in particular, macrophages).[168] Monocytes are the precursor cells for macrophages;[169] therefore, MCP-1 might be an important chemokine in the pathogenesis of airway inflammation in COPD. MCP-2, MCP-3, and MCP-4 are potent chemoattractants for eosinophils,[38] which have been shown to be central to the airway inflammation associated with asthma.[170]

2. Eotaxin

Eotaxin was first described as a novel eosinophil chemoattractant that is present in the BAL fluid of asthmatic subjects.[116] The eotaxins are a group of three chemokines that mediate the recruitment of eosinophils via interaction with CCR_3.[171] Increased expression of mRNA and protein for eotaxin and eotaxin-2 can be demonstrated in bronchial biopsies from asthmatic subjects when compared with controls, indicating that it is indicative of an ongoing airway inflammatory response.[116] Increased levels of eotaxin also are found in bronchial mucosa and there is a correlation between eotaxin expression and airway hyperresponsiveness.[138] Soluble eotaxin has been measured in the serum of asthmatics and eotaxin levels correlate with disease severity, especially during acute asthma.[171] Eotaxin-3 is chemotactic for eosinophils and basophils but is 10-fold less potent than the other two eotaxins.[171] Recently, it was shown that eotaxin-1 and eotaxin-2 expression was increased in asthmatics compared with controls, but only eotaxin-3 expression was significantly increased following allergen challenge, indicating that eotaxin-3 might account for the ongoing eosinophil recruitment into the asthmatic airways in the later stages following allergen challenge,[171] thus prolonging airway inflammation.

3. Other CC Chemokines

RANTES also is elevated in the bronchial biopsies from mild asymptomatic asthmatic subjects compared with controls.[116] The number of cells that express mRNA for RANTES is significantly increased in mild to moderate symptomatic asthmatic subjects compared with controls.[116] RANTES is also chemoattractant for memory T lymphocytes *in vitro*; however, it is the most effective basophil chemoattractant.[38] The expression of thymus- and activation-regulated chemokine (TARC) also was increased in the bronchial epithelium from asthmatic subjects when compared with controls.[116] TARC and macrophage-derived chemokine (MDC) are produced by airway epithelial cells of asthmatic patients upon allergen challenge. Th2 cytokines, including IL-4 and IL-13, upregulate TARC and MDC production by monocytes and airway epithelial cells. This supports the hypothesis that CCR_4 ligands induced by IL-4 attract T lymphocytes, which in turn secrete more IL-4, thus amplifying Th2 lymphocyte recruitment and airway inflammation.[138] MIP-3α (which binds CCR_6) expression is increased after allergen challenge in sensitized mice. However, CCR_6-deficient mice have an attenuated airway inflammatory response with reduced eosinophil infiltration, decreased IL-5 in the lung, and decreased serum levels of IgE,[138] suggesting that CCR_6 and MIP3α are important in airway inflammation. MIP-1α and MIP-1β were purified from LPS-treated monocytic cell lines. MIP-1α attracts and activates monocytes more efficiently than MIP-1β but less so than MCP-1.[152] However the MIP proteins might still be important in airway inflammation because they can recruit inflammatory cells, including dendritic cells, NK cells, basophils, and eosinophils.[152]

C. CHEMOKINE SUMMARY

Although there are more than 50 chemokines, only 19 receptors have been identified to date;[139] therefore, one receptor can bind a number of chemokines, suggesting a level of redundancy. This finding poses the question of how the chemokines cooperate to bring about an inflammatory response. Early thinking suggested that a single chemokine could attract a specific cell type.[172] However, receptor expression studies on various cells have disproved this theory.[142,173] For example, it is known that both $CXCR_1$ and $CXCR_2$, which bind ELR+ CXC chemokines, are present on both neutrophils and monocytes.[142,161,173] These receptors are functional on both cell types and are responsible for the observed migration of neutrophils[174] and monocytes[161] toward CXC chemokines. This is important in inflammatory diseases such as COPD because CXC chemokines (e.g., IL-8) are elevated in the lungs of these patients.[147,148] IL-8 can attract both neutrophils[174] and monocytes;[161] therefore, deciding on a single receptor or chemokine as a therapeutic target for reducing the inflammatory load in the lungs will be complex. The matter is further complicated by the observation that chemokines also might act as antagonists at some receptors. Chemokines have been thought to be purely agonistic but recent studies have shown that they also can be antagonistic[164,175] and thus might play a role in reducing airway inflammation. Eotaxin is a potent inducer of eosinophil chemotaxis via CCR_3; however, it is also antagonistic for CCR_2.[164] The antagonism toward CCR_2 is sufficient to reduce the main functional responses of monocytes, chemotaxis, and enzyme release to minimal levels.[164] Not only can chemokines act as antagonists, but metabolized chemokines also can have antagonistic activity. MCP-2 is cleaved by MMP-3, whereas MCP-4 is cleaved by MMP-3 and MMP-1.[175] Once these chemokines have been cleaved, they become antagonistic for CCR_2[175] again reducing monocyte chemotaxis. Agonistic activity of chemokines is dependent on the NH_2-terminal region.[176] Modifications of the NH_2-terminus can lead to derivatives that still recognize the receptor but do not signal and thus act as antagonists. The first such antagonist was obtained by NH_2-terminal truncation of IL-8.[177] MCP-1 lacking the first eight NH_2-terminal residues blocks CCR_2 and prevents responses induced by MCP-1, MCP-2, and MCP-3.[178] These natural antagonists might help regulate leukocyte recruitment to inflammatory lesions *in vivo*. However, proteolytic degradation of chemokines might also increase potency. MMP-9 can truncate IL-8 at the NH_2-terminus, producing a 10-fold more potent chemokine.[179] Therefore, the role of chemokines in airway inflammation is extremely complex and requires further investigation before their complete role can be fully elucidated.

IV. SUMMARY

Cytokines and chemokines are important in the pathophysiology of allergic disease and chronic inflammatory diseases. Differences in expression and regulation of various cytokines and/or chemokines will contribute to the underlying pathophysiologies. IL-1β, TNF-α, and IFN-γ all will increase adhesion molecule expression and stimulate the production of chemokines, including IL-8 and eotaxin, thus promoting the recruitment of leukocytes. Once in the lung, leukocytes can be activated by cytokines, including IL-1β, or in the case of GM-CSF, promote their survival. Finally, cytokines such as IL-13 or TGF-β are important in promoting fibrosis and airway remodeling, a key feature of chronic inflammatory diseases including asthma and COPD. The elucidation of the pathways controlling the expression of cytokines and chemokines not only will improve our understanding of the mechanisms underlying inflammatory lung diseases but also will aid in the design of novel therapies for the treatment of these diseases.

FURTHER READING

1. Rose-John, S., Cytokines come of age, *Biochim. Biophys. Acta,* 1592, 213, 2002
2. Grotzinger, J., Molecular mechanisms of cytokine receptor activation, *Biochim. Biophys. Acta*, 1592, 215, 2002.
3. Kelley, J., Cytokines of the lung, *Am. Rev. Respir. Dis.*, 141, 765, 1990.
4. Barnes, P.J., Cytokine modulators as novel therapies for airway disease, *Eur. Respir. J. Suppl.*, 34, 67s, 2001.
5. Thomas, P.S., Tumour necrosis factor-α: the role of this multifunctional cytokine in asthma, *Immunol. Cell Biol.*, 79, 132, 2001.
6. Pennica, D. et al., Human tumour necrosis factor: precursor structure, expression and homology to lymphotoxin, *Nature*, 312, 724, 1984.
7. Costa, J.J. et al., Human eosinophils can express the cytokines tumor necrosis factor-α and macrophage inflammatory protein-1 α, *J. Clin. Invest.*, 91, 2673, 1993.
8. Khair, O.A. et al., Effect of *Haemophilus influenzae* endotoxin on the synthesis of IL-6, IL-8, TNF-α and expression of ICAM-1 in cultured human bronchial epithelial cells, *Eur. Respir. J.*, 7, 2109, 1994.
9. Thomas, P.S. et al., Authentic 17 kDa tumour necrosis factor α is synthesized and released by canine mast cells and up-regulated by stem cell factor, *Clin. Exp. Allergy*, 26, 710, 1996.
10. Carswell, E.A. et al., An endotoxin-induced serum factor that causes necrosis of tumors, *Proc. Natl. Acad. Sci. U.S.A.*, 72, 3666, 1975.
11. Beutler, B. and Cerami, A., Cachectin and tumour necrosis factor as two sides of the same biological coin, *Nature*, 320, 584, 1986.
12. Gosset, P. et al., Tumor necrosis factor α and interleukin-6 production by human mononuclear phagocytes from allergic asthmatics after IgE-dependent stimulation, *Am. Rev. Respir. Dis.*, 146, 768, 1992.
13. Thomas, P.S., Yates, D.H., and Barnes, P.J., Tumor necrosis factor-α increases airway responsiveness and sputum neutrophilia in normal human subjects, *Am. J. Respir. Crit. Care Med.*, 152, 76, 1995.

14. Gosset, P. et al., Production of tumor necrosis factor-α and interleukin-6 by human alveolar macrophages exposed *in vitro* to coal mine dust, *Am. J. Respir. Cell Mol. Biol.*, 5, 431, 1991.

15. Ying, S. et al., TNF α mRNA expression in allergic inflammation, *Clin. Exp. Allergy*, 21, 745, 1991.

16. Kucukaycan, M. et al., Tumor necrosis factor-α +489G/A gene polymorphism is associated with chronic obstructive pulmonary disease, *Respir. Res.*, 3, 29, 2002.

17. Ferrarotti, I. et al., Tumour necrosis factor family genes in a phenotype of COPD associated with emphysema, *Eur. Respir. J.*, 21, 444, 2003.

18. de Boer, W.I., Cytokines and therapy in COPD: a promising combination?, *Chest*, 121, 209S, 2002.

19. Takeyama, K. et al., Epidermal growth factor system regulates mucin production in airways, *Proc. Natl. Acad. Sci. U.S.A.*, 96, 3081, 1999.

20. Takeyama, K., Fahy, J.V., and Nadel, J.A., Relationship of epidermal growth factor receptors to goblet cell production in human bronchi, *Am. J. Respir. Crit. Care Med.*, 163, 511, 2001.

21. Donnelly, L.E and Barnes, P.J., Expression and regulation of inducible nitric oxide synthase from human primary airway epithelial cells, *Am. J. Respir. Cell Mol. Biol.*, 26, 144, 2002.

22. Antoniou, K.M., Ferdoutsis, E., and Bouros, D., Interferons and their application in the diseases of the lung, *Chest*, 123, 209, 2003.

23. Majori, M. et al., Predominant TH1 cytokine pattern in peripheral blood from subjects with chronic obstructive pulmonary disease, *J. Allergy Clin. Immunol.*, 103, 458, 1999.

24. Jeffery, P.K, Differences and similarities between chronic obstructive pulmonary disease and asthma, *Clin. Exp. Allergy*, 29, Suppl. 2, 14, 1999.

25. Saetta, M. et al., Increased expression of the chemokine receptor CXCR3 and its ligand CXCL10 in peripheral airways of smokers with chronic obstructive pulmonary disease, *Am. J. Respir. Crit. Care Med.*, 165, 1404, 2002.

26. Nemunaitis, J., A comparative review of colony-stimulating factors, *Drugs*, 54, 709, 1997.

27. Woolley, K.L. et al., Granulocyte-macrophage colony-stimulating factor, eosinophils and eosinophil cationic protein in subjects with and without mild, stable, atopic asthma, *Eur. Respir. J.*, 7, 1576, 1994.

28. Park, C.S. et al., Granulocyte macrophage colony-stimulating factor is the main cytokine enhancing survival of eosinophils in asthmatic airways, *Eur. Respir. J.*, 12, 872, 1998.

29. Balbi, B., et al., Increased bronchoalveolar granulocytes and granulocyte/macrophage colony-stimulating factor during exacerbations of chronic bronchitis, *Eur. Respir. J.*, 10, 846, 1997.

30. Culpitt, S.V. et al., Impaired inhibition by dexamethasone of cytokine release by alveolar macrophages from patients with chronic obstructive pulmonary disease, *Am. J. Respir. Crit. Care Med.*, 167, 24, 2003.

31. Saunders, M.A. et al., Release of granulocyte-macrophage colony stimulating factor by human cultured airway smooth muscle cells: suppression by dexamethasone, *Br. J. Pharmacol.*, 120, 545, 1997.

32. Sato, E. et al., Smoke extract stimulates lung fibroblasts to release neutrophil and monocyte chemotactic activities, *Am. J. Physiol.*, 277, L1149, 1999.

33. Newton, R. et al., GM-CSF expression in pulmonary epithelial cells is regulated negatively by posttranscriptional mechanisms, *Biochem. Biophys. Res. Commun.*, 287, 249, 2001.

34. Levine, S.J. et al., Corticosteroids differentially regulate secretion of IL-6, IL-8, and G-CSF by a human bronchial epithelial cell line, *Am. J. Physiol.*, 265, L360, 1993.

35. March, C.J. et al., Cloning, sequence and expression of two distinct human interleukin-1 complementary DNAs, *Nature*, 315, 641, 1985.

36. Thornberry, N.A. et al., A novel heterodimeric cysteine protease is required for interleukin-1β processing in monocytes, *Nature*, 356, 768, 1992.

37. Borish, L.C. and Steinke, J.W., 2. Cytokines and chemokines, *J. Allergy Clin. Immunol.*, 111, S460 2003.

38. Barnes, P.J., Chung K.F., and Page, C.P., Inflammatory mediators of asthma: an update, *Pharmacol. Rev.*, 50, 515, 1998.

39. Russell, R.E. et al., Alveolar macrophage-mediated elastolysis: roles of matrix metalloproteinases, cysteine, and serine proteases, *Am. J. Physiol. Lung Cell Mol. Physiol.*, 283, L867, 2002.

40. Borish, L. et al., Detection of alveolar macrophage-derived IL-1β in asthma. Inhibition with corticosteroids, *J. Immunol.*, 149, 3078, 1992.

41. Ekberg-Jansson, A. et al., Respiratory symptoms relate to physiological changes and inflammatory markers reflecting central but not peripheral airways. A study in 60-year-old "healthy" smokers and never-smokers, *Respir. Med.*, 95, 40, 2001.

42. Rusznak, C. et al., Effect of cigarette smoke on the permeability and IL-1β and sICAM-1 release from cultured human bronchial epithelial cells of never-smokers, smokers, and patients with chronic obstructive pulmonary disease, *Am. J. Respir. Cell Mol. Biol.*, 23, 530, 2000.

43. Arend, W.P. et al., Interleukin-1 receptor antagonist: role in biology, *Annu. Rev. Immunol.*, 16, 27, 1998.

44. Corradi, A. et al., Production and secretion of interleukin 1 receptor antagonist in monocytes and keratinocytes, *Cytotechnology*, 11, Suppl. 1, S50, 1993.

45. Haskill, S. et al., cDNA cloning of an intracellular form of the human interleukin 1 receptor antagonist associated with epithelium, *Proc. Natl. Acad. Sci. U.S.A.*, 88, 3681, 1991.

46. Liu, B. et al., Production of a biologically active human interleukin 18 requires its prior synthesis as PRO-IL-18, *Cytokine*, 12, 1519, 2000.

47. Jordan, J.A. et al., Role of IL-18 in acute lung inflammation, *J. Immunol.*, 167, 7060, 2001.

48. Smith, K.A., Interleukin-2: inception, impact, and implications, *Science*, 240, 1169, 1988.

49. Park, C.S. et al., Interleukin-2 and soluble interleukin-2 receptor in bronchoalveolar lavage fluid from patients with bronchial asthma, *Chest*, 106, 400, 1994.

50. Park, C.S. et al., Soluble interleukin-2 receptor and cellular profiles in bronchoalveolar lavage fluid from patients with bronchial asthma, *J. Allergy Clin. Immunol.*, 91, 623, 1993.

51. Leung, D.Y. et al., Dysregulation of interleukin 4, interleukin 5, and interferon γ gene expression in steroid-resistant asthma, *J. Exp. Med.*, 181, 33, 1995.

52. Sher, E.R. et al., Steroid-resistant asthma. Cellular mechanisms contributing to inadequate response to glucocorticoid therapy, *J. Clin. Invest.*, 93, 33, 1994.

53. Plaut, M. et al., Mast cell lines produce lymphokines in response to cross-linkage of Fc epsilon RI or to calcium ionophores, *Nature*, 339, 64, 1989.

54. Park, L.S. et al., Characterization of the human B cell stimulatory factor 1 receptor, *J. Exp. Med.*, 166, 476, 1987.

55. Ohara, J. and Paul, W.E., Up-regulation of interleukin 4/B-cell stimulatory factor 1 receptor expression, *Proc. Natl. Acad. Sci. U.S.A.*, 85, 8221, 1988.

56. van Roon, J.A. et al., Proinflammatory cytokine production and cartilage damage due to rheumatoid synovial T helper-1 activation is inhibited by interleukin-4, *Ann. Rheum. Dis.*, 54, 836, 1995.

57. Zhang, N. et al., Effects of theophylline on plasma levels of interleukin-4, cyclic nucleotides and pulmonary functions in patients with chronic obstructive pulmonary disease, *J. Tongji Med. Univ.*, 19, 15, 1999.

58. Zhu, J. et al., Interleukin-4 and interleukin-5 gene expression and inflammation in the mucus-secreting glands and subepithelial tissue of smokers with chronic bronchitis. Lack of relationship with CD8(+) cells, *Am. J. Respir. Crit. Care Med.*, 164, 2220, 2001.

59. Mueller, A., Kelly, E., and Strange, P.G., Pathways for internalization and recycling of the chemokine receptor CCR5, *Blood*, 99, 785, 2002.

60. Hershey, G.K., IL-13 receptors and signaling pathways: an evolving web, *J. Allergy Clin. Immunol.*, 111, 677, 2003.

61. Wills-Karp, M. and Chiaramonte, M., Interleukin-13 in asthma, *Curr. Opin. Pulm. Med.*, 9, 21, 2003.

62. Wills-Karp, M. et al., Interleukin-13: central mediator of allergic asthma, *Science*, 282, 2258, 1998.

63. Kuperman, D.A. et al., Direct effects of interleukin-13 on epithelial cells cause airway hyperreactivity and mucus overproduction in asthma, *Nat. Med.*, 8, 885, 2002.

64. Laporte, J.C. et al., Direct effects of interleukin-13 on signaling pathways for physiological responses in cultured human airway smooth muscle cells, *Am. J. Respir. Crit. Care Med.*, 164, 141, 2001.

65. Wen, F.Q. et al., Interleukin-4- and interleukin-13-enhanced transforming growth factor-$\beta2$ production in cultured human bronchial epithelial cells is attenuated by interferon-γ, *Am. J. Respir. Cell Mol. Biol.*, 26, 484, 2002.

66. Prieto, J. et al., Increased interleukin-13 mRNA expression in bronchoalveolar lavage cells of atopic patients with mild asthma after repeated low-dose allergen provocations, *Respir. Med.*, 94, 806, 2000

67. Arima, K. et al., Upregulation of IL-13 concentration *in vivo* by the IL13 variant associated with bronchial asthma, *J. Allergy Clin. Immunol.*, 109, 980, 2002.

68. Howard, T.D. et al., Identification and association of polymorphisms in the interleukin-13 gene with asthma and atopy in a Dutch population, *Am. J. Respir. Cell Mol. Biol.*, 25, 377, 2001.

69. van der Pouw Kraan, T.C. et al., Chronic obstructive pulmonary disease is associated with the -1055 IL-13 promoter polymorphism, *Genes Immun.*, 3, 436, 2002.

70. Zheng, T. et al., Inducible targeting of IL-13 to the adult lung causes matrix metalloproteinase- and cathepsin-dependent emphysema, *J. Clin. Invest.*, 106, 1081, 2000.

71. Tavernier, J. et al., Expression of human and murine interleukin-5 in eukaryotic systems, *DNA*, 8, 491, 1989.

72. Clutterbuck, E.J., Hirst, E.M., and Sanderson, C.J., Human interleukin-5 (IL-5) regulates the production of eosinophils in human bone marrow cultures: comparison and interaction with IL-1, IL-3, IL-6, and GMCSF, *Blood*, 73, 1504, 1989.

73. Hirai, K. et al., Regulation of the function of eosinophils and basophils, *Crit. Rev. Immunol.*, 17, 325, 1997.

74. Ohnishi, T. et al., Eosinophil survival activity identified as interleukin-5 is associated with eosinophil recruitment and degranulation and lung injury twenty-four hours after segmental antigen lung challenge, *J. Allergy Clin. Immunol.*, 92, 607, 1993.

75. Mould, A.W. et al., Relationship between interleukin-5 and eotaxin in regulating blood and tissue eosinophilia in mice, *J. Clin. Invest.*, 99, 1064, 1997.

76. Gelder, C.M. et al., Cytokine expression in normal, atopic, and asthmatic subjects using the combination of sputum induction and the polymerase chain reaction, *Thorax*, 50, 1033, 1995.

77. Park, S.W. et al., Association of interleukin-5 and eotaxin with acute exacerbation of asthma, *Int. Arch. Allergy Immunol.*, 131, 283, 2003.

78. Ohnishi, T. et al., IL-5 is the predominant eosinophil-active cytokine in the antigen-induced pulmonary late-phase reaction, *Am. Rev. Respir. Dis.*, 147, 901, 1993.

79. Shiota, Y. et al., Intracellular IL-5 and T-lymphocyte subsets in atopic and nonatopic bronchial asthma, *J. Allergy Clin. Immunol.*, 109, 294, 2002.

80. Blumchen, K., Kallinich, T., and Hamelmann, E., Interleukin-5: a novel target for asthma therapy, *Expert Opin. Biol. Ther.*, 1, 433, 2001.

81. Leckie, M.J. et al., Effects of an interleukin-5 blocking monoclonal antibody on eosinophils, airway hyper-responsiveness, and the late asthmatic response, *Lancet*, 356, 2144, 2000.

82. Song, W., Zhao, J., and Li, Z., Interleukin-6 in bronchoalveolar lavage fluid from patients with COPD, *Chin. Med. J. (Engl.)*, 114, 1140, 2001.

83. Bhowmik, A. et al., Relation of sputum inflammatory markers to symptoms and lung function changes in COPD exacerbations, *Thorax*, 55, 114, 2000.

84. Wedzicha, J.A. et al., Acute exacerbations of chronic obstructive pulmonary disease are accompanied by elevations of plasma fibrinogen and serum IL-6 levels, *Thromb. Haemost.*, 84, 210, 2000.

85. Patel, I.S. et al., Airway epithelial inflammatory responses and clinical parameters in COPD, *Eur. Respir. J.*, 22, 94, 2003.

86. Striz, I., et al., Th2-type cytokines modulate IL-6 release by human bronchial epithelial cells, *Immunol. Lett.*, 70, 83, 1999.

87. Stankiewicz, W. et al., Cellular and cytokine immunoregulation in patients with chronic obstructive pulmonary disease and bronchial asthma, *Mediators Inflamm.*, 11, 307, 2002.

88. Tonnel, A.B., Gosset, P., and Tillie-Leblond, I., Characteristics of the inflammatory response in bronchial lavage fluids from patients with status asthmaticus, *Int. Arch. Allergy Immunol.*, 124, 267, 2001.

89. Yokoyama, A. et al., Circulating interleukin-6 levels in patients with bronchial asthma, *Am. J. Respir. Crit. Care Med.*, 151, 1354, 1995.

90. Yu, M. et al., The role of interleukin-6 in pulmonary inflammation and injury induced by exposure to environmental air pollutants, *Toxicol. Sci.*, 68, 488, 2002.

91. Leemans, J.C. et al., Differential role of interleukin-6 in lung inflammation induced by lipoteichoic acid and peptidoglycan from *Staphylococcus aureus*, *Am. J. Respir. Crit. Care Med.*, 165, 1445, 2002.

92. Baraldo, S. et al., Interleukin-9 influences chemokine release in airway smooth muscle: role of ERK, *Am. J. Physiol. Lung Cell Mol. Physiol.*, 284, L1093, 2003.

93. Gounni, A.S. et al., IL-9 expression by human eosinophils: regulation by IL-1β and TNF-α, *J. Allergy Clin. Immunol.*, 106, 460, 2000.

94. Matsuzawa, S. et al., IL-9 enhances the growth of human mast cell progenitors under stimulation with stem cell factor, *J. Immunol.*, 170, 3461, 2003.

95. Houssiau, F.A. et al., Human T cell lines and clones respond to IL-9, *J. Immunol.*, 150, 2634, 1993.

96. Longphre, M. et al., Allergen-induced IL-9 directly stimulates mucin transcription in respiratory epithelial cells, *J. Clin. Invest.*, 104, 1375, 1999.

97. Louahed, J. et al., Interleukin-9 upregulates mucus expression in the airways, *Am. J. Respir. Cell Mol. Biol.*, 22, 649, 2000.

98. McLane, M.P. et al., Interleukin-9 promotes allergen-induced eosinophilic inflammation and airway hyperresponsiveness in transgenic mice, *Am. J. Respir. Cell Mol. Biol.*, 19, 713, 1998.

99. Cheng, G. et al., Anti-interleukin-9 antibody treatment inhibits airway inflammation and hyperreactivity in mouse asthma model, *Am. J. Respir. Crit. Care Med.*, 166, 409, 2002.

100. Little, F.F., Cruikshank, W.W., and Center, D.M., IL-9 stimulates release of chemotactic factors from human bronchial epithelial cells, *Am. J. Respir. Cell Mol. Biol.*, 25, 347, 2001.

101. Ying, S. et al., Elevated expression of interleukin-9 mRNA in the bronchial mucosa of atopic asthmatics and allergen-induced cutaneous late-phase reaction: relationships to eosinophils, mast cells and T lymphocytes, *Clin. Exp. Allergy*, 32, 866, 2002.

102. Pretolani, M. and Goldman, M., IL-10: a potential therapy for allergic inflammation?, *Immunol. Today*, 18, 277, 1997.

103. Robinson, D.S. et al., Increased interleukin-10 messenger RNA expression in atopic allergy and asthma, *Am. J. Respir. Cell Mol. Biol.*, 14, 113, 1996.

104. Magnan, A. et al., Alveolar macrophage interleukin (IL)-10 and IL-12 production in atopic asthma, *Allergy*, 53, 1092, 1998.

105. Borish, L. et al., Interleukin-10 regulation in normal subjects and patients with asthma, *J. Allergy Clin. Immunol.*, 97, 1288, 1996.

106. Takanashi, S. et al., Interleukin-10 level in sputum is reduced in bronchial asthma, COPD and in smokers, *Eur. Respir. J.*, 14, 309, 1999.

107. Tomita, K. et al., Attenuated production of intracellular IL-10 and IL-12 in monocytes from patients with severe asthma, *Clin. Immunol.*, 102, 258, 2002.

108. Hobbs, K. et al., Interleukin-10 and transforming growth factor-β promoter polymorphisms in allergies and asthma, *Am. J. Respir. Crit. Care Med.*, 158, 1958, 1998.

109. Hodge, S. et al., Methyl-prednisolone up-regulates monocyte interleukin-10 production in stimulated whole blood, *Scand. J. Immunol.*, 49, 548, 1999.

110. John, M. et al., Inhaled corticosteroids increase interleukin-10 but reduce macrophage inflammatory protein-1α, granulocyte-macrophage colony-stimulating factor, and interferon-γ release from alveolar macrophages in asthma, *Am. J. Respir. Crit. Care Med.*, 157, 256, 1998.

111. Tournoy, K.G. et al., Endogenous interleukin-10 suppresses allergen-induced airway inflammation and nonspecific airway responsiveness, *Clin. Exp. Allergy*, 30, 775, 2000.

112. Lim, S. et al., Balance of matrix metalloprotease-9 and tissue inhibitor of metalloprotease-1 from alveolar macrophages in cigarette smokers. Regulation by interleukin-10, *Am. J. Respir. Crit. Care Med.*, 162, 1355, 2000.

113. Wolk, K. et al., Cutting edge: immune cells as sources and targets of the IL-10 family members?, *J. Immunol.*, 168, 5397, 2002.

114. Liao, Y.C. et al., IL-19 induces production of IL-6 and TNF-α and results in cell apoptosis through TNF-α, *J. Immunol.*, 169, 4288, 2002.

115. Chung, K.F., Cytokines in chronic obstructive pulmonary disease. *Eur. Respir. J.*, *Suppl.* 34, 50s, 2001.

116. Riffo-Vasquez, Y. and Spina, D., Role of cytokines and chemokines in bronchial hyperresponsiveness and airway inflammation, *Pharmacol. Ther.*, 94, 185, 2002.

117. Gately MK, Desai BB, Wolitzky AG, et al: Regulation of human lymphocyte proliferation by a heterodimeric cytokine, IL-12 (cytotoxic lymphocyte maturation factor). *J. Immunol.* 147, 874, 1991

118. Gadina, M., Ferguson, P.R., and Johnston, J.A., New interleukins: are there any more?, *Curr. Opin. Infect. Dis.*, 16, 211, 2003.

119. Belladonna, M.L. et al., IL-23 and IL-12 have overlapping, but distinct, effects on murine dendritic cells, *J. Immunol.*, 168, 5448, 2002.

120. van der Pouw Kraan, T.C. et al., Reduced production of IL-12 and IL-12-dependent IFN-γ release in patients with allergic asthma, *J. Immunol.*, 158, 5560, 1997.

121. Yao, Z. et al., Human IL-17: a novel cytokine derived from T cells, *J. Immunol.*, 155, 5483, 1995.

122. Fossiez, F. et al., T cell interleukin-17 induces stromal cells to produce proinflammatory and hematopoietic cytokines, *J. Exp. Med.*, 183, 2593, 1996.

123. Laan, M. et al., Neutrophil recruitment by human IL-17 via C-X-C chemokine release in the airways, *J. Immunol.*, 162, 2347, 1999.

124. Hoshino, H. et al., Increased elastase and myeloperoxidase activity associated with neutrophil recruitment by IL-17 in airways *in vivo*, *J. Allergy Clin. Immunol.*, 105, 143, 2000.

125. Laan, M. et al., IL-17-induced cytokine release in human bronchial epithelial cells *in vitro*: role of mitogen-activated protein (MAP) kinases, *Br. J. Pharmacol.*, 133, 200, 2001.

126. Barczyk, A., Pierzchala, W., and Sozanska, E, Interleukin-17 in sputum correlates with airway hyperresponsiveness to methacholine, *Respir. Med.*, 97, 726, 2003.

127. Dhainaut, J.F., Charpentier, J., and Chiche, J.D., Transforming growth factor-β: a mediator of cell regulation in acute respiratory distress syndrome, *Crit. Care Med.*, 31, S258, 2003.

128. Takizawa, H. et al., Increased expression of transforming growth factor-$\beta 1$ in small airway epithelium from tobacco smokers and patients with chronic obstructive pulmonary disease (COPD), *Am. J. Respir. Crit. Care Med.*, 163, 1476, 2001.

129. Wang, H. et al., Cigarette smoke inhibits human bronchial epithelial cell repair processes, *Am. J. Respir. Cell Mol. Biol.*, 25, 772, 2001.

130. Hodge, S. et al., Interleukin-4 and tumour necrosis factor-α inhibit transforming growth factor-β production in a human bronchial epithelial cell line: possible relevance to inflammatory mechanisms in chronic obstructive pulmonary disease, *Respirology*, 6, 205, 2001.

131. de-Boer, W.I. et al., Transforming growth factor $\beta 1$ and recruitment of macrophages and mast cells in airways in chronic obstructive pulmonary disease, *Am. J. Respir. Crit. Care Med.*, 158, 1951, 1998.

132. Hodge, S.J. et al., Increased production of TGF-β and apoptosis of T lymphocytes isolated from peripheral blood in COPD, *Am. J. Physiol. Lung Cell Mol. Physiol.*, 285, L492, 2003.

133. Vignola, A.M. et al., Transforming growth factor-β expression in mucosal biopsies in asthma and chronic bronchitis, *Am. J. Respir. Crit. Care Med.*, 156, 591, 1997.

134. Redington, A.E. et al., Transforming growth factor-β 1 in asthma. Measurement in bronchoalveolar lavage fluid, *Am. J. Respir. Crit. Care Med.*, 156, 642, 1997.

135. Magnan, A. et al., Altered compartmentalization of transforming growth factor-β in asthmatic airways, *Clin. Exp. Allergy*, 27, 389, 1997.

136. Wenzel, S.E. et al., TGF-β and IL-13 synergistically increase eotaxin-1 production in human airway fibroblasts, *J. Immunol.*, 169, 4613, 2002.

137. Pelaia, G. et al., Effects of transforming growth factor-β and budesonide on mitogen-activated protein kinase activation and apoptosis in airway epithelial cells, *Am. J. Respir. Cell Mol. Biol.*, 29, 12, 2003.

138. Panina-Bordignon, P. and D'Ambrosio, D., Chemokines and their receptors in asthma and chronic obstructive pulmonary disease, *Curr. Opin. Pulm. Med.*, 9, 104, 2003.

139. Baggiolini, M., Chemokines in pathology and medicine, *J. Intern. Med.*, 250, 91, 2001.

140. Uguccioni, M. et al., Actions of the chemotactic cytokines MCP-1, MCP-2, MCP-3, RANTES, MIP-1α and MIP-1β on human monocytes, *Eur. J. Immunol.*, 25, 64, 1995.

141. Chantry, D. et al., Macrophage-derived chemokine is localized to thymic medullary epithelial cells and is a chemoattractant for CD3(+), CD4(+), CD8(low) thymocytes, *Blood*, 94, 1890, 1999.

142. Murphy, P.M. et al., International union of pharmacology. XXII. Nomenclature for chemokine receptors, *Pharmacol. Rev.*, 52, 145, 2000.

143. Clark-Lewis, I. et al., Structure-activity relationships of interleukin-8 determined using chemically synthesized analogs. Critical role of NH2-terminal residues and evidence for uncoupling of neutrophil chemotaxis, exocytosis, and receptor binding activities, *J. Biol. Chem.*, 266, 23128, 1991.

144. Hebert, C.A., Vitangcol, R.V., and Baker, J.B., Scanning mutagenesis of interleukin-8 identifies a cluster of residues required for receptor binding, *J. Biol. Chem.*, 266, 18989, 1991.

145. Proudfoot, A.E., Chemokine receptors: multifaceted therapeutic targets, *Nature Rev. Immunol.*, 2, 106, 2002.

146. Proudfoot, A.E. et al., Extension of recombinant human RANTES by the retention of the initiating methionine produces a potent antagonist, *J. Biol. Chem.*, 271, 2599, 1996.

147. Culpitt, S.V. et al., Effect of high dose inhaled steroid on cells, cytokines, and proteases in induced sputum in chronic obstructive pulmonary disease, *Am. J. Respir. Crit. Care Med.*, 160, 1635, 1999.

148. Keatings, V.M. et al., Differences in interleukin-8 and tumor necrosis factor-α in induced sputum from patients with chronic obstructive pulmonary disease or asthma, *Am. J. Respir. Crit. Care Med.*, 153, 530, 1996.

149. Traves, S.L. et al., Elevated levels of the chemokines GRO and MCP-1 in sputum samples from COPD patients, *Thorax*, 57, 586, 2002.

150. Culpitt, S.V. et al., Effect of theophylline on induced sputum inflammatory indices and neutrophil chemotaxis in chronic obstructive pulmonary disease, *Am. J. Respir. Crit. Care Med.*, 165, 1371, 2002.

151. Baggiolini, M. et al., Interleukin-8 and related chemotactic cytokines — CXC and CC chemokines, *Adv. Immunol.*, 55, 97, 1994.

152. Rollins, B.J., Chemokines, *Blood*, 90, 909, 1997.

153. Callard, R. and Gearing, A., *The Cytokine Facts Book*, Academic Press Limited, London, 1994.

154. Goodman, R.B. et al., Quantitative comparison of C-X-C chemokines produced by endotoxin-stimulated human alveolar macrophages, *Am. J. Physiol.*, 275, L87, 1998.

155. Geiser, T. et al., The interleukin-8-related chemotactic cytokines GRO α, GRO β, and GRO γ activate human neutrophil and basophil leukocytes, *J. Biol. Chem.*, 268, 15419, 1993.

156. Jinquan, T. et al., Recombinant human growth-regulated oncogene-α induces T lymphocyte chemotaxis. A process regulated via IL-8 receptors by IFN-γ, TNF-α, IL-4, IL-10, and IL-13, *J. Immunol.*, 155, 5359, 1995.

157. Li, J., and Thornhill, M.H., Growth-regulated peptide-α (GRO-α) production by oral keratinocytes: a comparison with skin keratinocytes, *Cytokine*, 12, 1409, 2000.

158. Walz, A., Generation and properties of neutrophil-activating peptide 2, *Cytokines*, 4, 77, 1992.

159. Walz, A., Strieter, R.M., and Schnyder, S., Neutrophil-activating peptide ENA-78, *Adv. Exp. Med. Biol.*, 351, 129, 1993.

160. Schnyder-Candrian, S. and Walz, A., Neutrophil-activating protein ENA-78 and IL-8 exhibit different patterns of expression in lipopolysaccharide- and cytokine-stimulated human monocytes, *J. Immunol.*, 158, 3888, 1997.

161. Gerszten, R.E. et al., MCP-1 and IL-8 trigger firm adhesion of monocytes to vascular endothelium under flow conditions, *Nature*, 398, 718, 1999.

162. Loetscher, P. and Clark-Lewis, I., Agonistic and antagonistic activities of chemokines, *J. Leukoc. Biol.*, 69, 881, 2001.

163. Olson, T.S. and Ley, K., Chemokines and chemokine receptors in leukocyte trafficking, *Am. J. Physiol. Regul. Integr. Comp. Physiol.*, 283, R7, 2002.

164. Ogilvie, P. et al., Eotaxin is a natural antagonist for CCR2 and an agonist for CCR5, *Blood*, 97, 1920, 2001.

165. de Boer, W.I. et al., Monocyte chemoattractant protein 1, interleukin 8, and chronic airways inflammation in COPD, *J. Pathol.*, 190, 619, 2000.

166. Cambien, B. et al., Signal transduction involved in MCP-1-mediated monocytic transendothelial migration, *Blood*, 97, 359, 2001.

167. Zhang, Y., Ernst, C.A., and Rollins, B.J., MCP-1: structure/activity analysis. *Methods*, 10, 93, 1996.

168. Aaron, S.D. et al., Granulocyte inflammatory markers and airway infection during acute exacerbation of chronic obstructive pulmonary disease, *Am. J. Respir. Crit. Care Med.*, 163, 349, 2001.

169. Lydyard, P. and Grossi, C., Cells Involved in the Immune Response, in *Immunology*, Roitt, I., Brostoff, J., and Male, D., Eds., 5th ed, Dianne Zack, London, 1998, chapter 2.

170. Blease, K. et al., Chemokines and their role in airway hyper-reactivity, *Respir. Res.*, 1, 54, 2000.

171. Lloyd, C., Chemokines in allergic lung inflammation, *Immunology*, 105, 144, 2002.

172. Gerard, C. and Rollins B.J., Chemokines and disease, *Nat. Immunol.*, 2, 108, 2001.

173. Horuk, R, Chemokine receptors, *Cytokine Growth Factor Rev.*, 12, 313, 2001.

174. Ludwig, A. et al., The CXC-chemokine neutrophil-activating peptide-2 induces two distinct optima of neutrophil chemotaxis by differential interaction with interleukin-8 receptors CXCR-1 and CXCR-2, *Blood*, 90, 4588, 1997.

175. McQuibban, G.A. et al., Matrix metalloproteinase processing of monocyte chemoattractant proteins generates CC chemokine receptor antagonists with anti-inflammatory properties in vivo, *Blood*, 100, 1160, 2002.

176. Baggiolini, M. and Moser, B., Blocking chemokine receptors, *J. Exp. Med.*, 186, 1189, 1997.

177. Moser, B. et al., Interleukin-8 antagonists generated by N-terminal modification, *J. Biol. Chem.*, 268, 7125, 1993.

178. Gong, J.H. and Clark-Lewis, I., Antagonists of monocyte chemoattractant protein 1 identified by modification of functionally critical NH2-terminal residues, *J. Exp. Med.*, 181, 631, 1995.

179. Opdenakker, G. et al., Gelatinase B functions as regulator and effector in leukocyte biology, *J. Leukoc. Biol.*, 69, 851, 2001.
180. Azuma, C. et al., Cloning of complementary DNA encoding T-cell replacing factor and identity with B-cell growth factor II, *Nature*, 324, 70, 1986.

Index

R

S

T

U